e-Healthcare
Harness the Power of Internet e-Commerce & e-Care

Douglas E. Goldstein

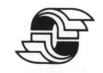

AN ASPEN PUBLICATION®
Aspen Publishers, Inc.
Gaithersburg, Maryland
2000

The authors and publisher have made every effort to provide current and accurate Web site addresses, but some may have changed after the book was printed.

Library of Congress Cataloging-in-Publication Data

Goldstein, Douglas E.
E-healthcare: harness the power of internet e-commerce & e-care/Douglas E. Goldstein.
p. cm.
Includes bibliographical references and index.
ISBN 0-8342-1365-6
1. Medical telematics. 2. Medicine—Computer network resources. 3. Internet (Computer network) I. Title.
R859.7.E43 G65 2000
362.1'0285—dc21
99-058554

Orders: (800) 638-8437
Customer Service: (800) 234-1660

About Aspen Publishers • For more than 40 years, Aspen has been a leading professional publisher in a variety of disciplines. Aspen's vast information resources are available in both print and electronic formats. We are committed to providing the highest quality information available in the most appropriate format for our customers. Visit Aspen's Internet site for more information resources, directories, articles, and a searchable version of Aspen's full catalog, including the most recent publications: **www.aspenpublishers.com**
Aspen Publishers, Inc. • The hallmark of quality in publishing
Member of the worldwide Wolters Kluwer group.

Editorial Services: Kathy Litzenberg
Library of Congress Catalog Card Number: 99-058554
ISBN: 0-8342-1365-6

Printed in the United States of America

1   2   3   4   5

To the e-leaders that are using the power of e-healthcare for optimum health and healing in the twenty-first century.

Table of Contents

**Chapter 7—Telemedicine Becomes a Reality with Web-Enabled
Applications and Net Devices 189**
Richard L. Nevins and Ronald J. Pion

**Chapter 8—Real-Time Customer Information and Health
Management Centers 211**
Loree Jurgens and Douglas E. Goldstein

Contributors

Mark L. Braunstein, MD
Chairman and Chief Executive Officer
Patient Care Technologies, Inc.
Atlanta, Georgia

Matthew B. Calish
Managing Director, Custom Solutions
Health Online, Inc.
Columbia, Maryland

Joan DeClaire, BA
Principal
DeClaire & Turrill Creative
    Services for Healthcare
Seattle, Washington

Randy Dulin, BS
Senior Vice President
Sales and Marketing
Health Online, Inc.
Columbia, Maryland

Sandra J. Feaster, RN, MS, MBA
Regional Vice President
Business Development and
    Government Affairs
LifeMasters Supported Selfcare, Inc.
Newport Beach, California

Margaret Fisher, MA
Vice President, Operations
BCS webservices.net
Vienna, Virginia

Mark Garvey
Freelance Writer and Editor
Catholic Healthcare Partners
Cincinnati, Ohio

David J. Howell, PhD, RRT
Manager of Marketing
    Communications
LifeMasters Supported Selfcare, Inc.
Newport Beach, California

LuAnn Joy, RN, BA
Director of Field Operations
LifeMasters Supported Selfcare, Inc.
Newport Beach, California

Loree Jurgens, RN, MHA
Director
Health Online, Inc.
Columbia, Maryland

Kathi Marshall
President, Chief Executive Officer
Marshall Educational Health
   Solutions, Inc.
Scottsdale, Arizona

Richard L. Nevins, MD
Vice President, Medical Affairs
McKesson HBOC
Phoenix, Arizona

Daniel Newton, PhD
President
The NewSof Group, Inc.
Redmond, Washington

Laura J. Oberbroeckling, JD
Mintz Levin Cohn Ferris
   Glovsky & Popeo, PC
Washington, DC

Ronald J. Pion, MD
Chairman and Chief Executive Officer
Medical Telecommunications
   Associates, Inc.
Los Angeles, California

Carroll Quinn, DNS
Director of Research
Mercy Caring of Catholic
   Healthcare Partners
Interim Director
The Health Connection
Cincinnati, Ohio

Francis H. Rhie, MD, MBA
Chief Medical Officer
Alteer Corporation
Irvine, California

S. Michael Ross, MD, MHA
Chief Medical Officer
Health Online, Inc.
Columbia, Maryland

Neal Sofian, MPH
Chief Executive Officer
The NewSof Group, Inc.
Redmond, Washington

Michael Stull, MBA
President
Technology Transformation
   Group
Bethesda, Maryland

Steven Sutor
Director
Content Development
Health Online, Inc.
Columbia, Maryland

Pamela Tanton
Health Online, Inc.
Columbia, Maryland

Cheryl L. Toth, MBA
Principal
Tothie, Inc.
Phoenix, Arizona

Karen A. Zupko, BS
President
KarenZupko & Associates, Inc.
Chicago, Illinois

Foreword

As THE NEW millennium approaches, it is popular to look back in history to discern the fundamental advances that have shaped the world we know today. The discovery of fire may have been the first, enabling control over our environment. The development of machine tools that enabled the industrial revolution made possible productivity advances over the past century. More recent discoveries—computers, high speed communication networks, and interactive technologies—are converging to enable the e-revolution that now dawns. These fundamental advances, like their predecessors, will enable profound changes in all aspects of our lives.

E-*healthcare* focuses on the impact of the e-revolution in one important arena—health care. The convergence of computing, carriage, and content that support the e-revolution will profoundly change how we experience health care. The changes that will occur are inevitable. E-revolution changes, in how we experience health care, will occur because they enable the only viable long-term strategies that improve the quality of health care delivered while also reducing the costs of providing that care.

Today health care is characterized by extraordinary advances in new technologies and therapies that are increasingly unaffordable. Every day, announcements of new diagnostic and therapeutic procedures occur. Pharmaceutical companies have new drug pipelines unmatched at any time in their history. Virtually every newspaper and newsmagazine have a regular column devoted to new advances. At the same time, health care costs continue to rapidly rise with no apparent end in sight.

Controlling health care costs in the future will not occur by focusing on the problems in one of the principal health care system segments. Health plans and managed care organizations face uncontrolled rising health costs that are occurring at a faster rate than the increases in premiums they can secure from employers. Hospitals each year face increased fixed expenses and costs due to regulatory changes that outstrip the increases they can negotiate from health plans for services provided. Physicians and other caregivers have reached their limit; they are being paid less to do more, as reimbursements each year are ratcheted down. Strategies these organizations pursue, which seek advantages for one component of the system at the expense of another, can at best provide only temporary relief since all of the components are under siege.

Where then will the changes occur that control health care costs and make possible the quality improvements in health care delivery to consumers and patients? Changes will occur principally in two areas. The first is in the management of how care is delivered. The "right" care is the "right" test, therapy, or procedure, provided at the "right" time, in the "right" setting, in the "right" way, by the "right" health care provider. Currently, there is great variability present in health care provided that does not appear to be related to changes in outcomes experienced in different patient populations. A substantial body of evidence has accumulated that suggests significant improvements in health care delivery can occur at considerably reduced costs with improvements in each of these "rights." Consumers will become much more involved in their health care as their role is transformed from recipient to partner. The consumer connection facilitated by the e-revolution will change how consumers and patients interact with all components of the health care system. The information base created from the new connections will provide the underlying empirical base of information that supports our understanding of what care is needed and the best way to provide it.

The second area of transformation is in the financial infrastructure that supports the health care delivery system. Significant overhead costs are present in each of the health care system components. These costs will be substantially reduced as new end-to-end solutions are provided in the e-healthcare revolution.

The senior management and boards of many health care organizations currently debate their role in the e-healthcare revolution. Where and when should investments be made by the organization at a time when too little capital is available? What should be the organization's role in e-commerce? Answering these questions requires that each organization develops its strategy and participation in the e-healthcare revolution. The strategy can only be developed after assimilating an understanding of the opportunities provided in the e-healthcare revolution. This book by Douglas Goldstein and the contributors will improve that understanding. The issue is not whether the organizations will need to participate, but when and how. Organizations that fail to develop a successful strategy will not be competitive. Participation in the e-healthcare revolution will be a requirement for survival, just as fire became essential for man's survival at home or the assembly line became essential for cost-efficient manufacturing.

David B. Pryor, MD
Senior Vice President, System Health Services
Chief Information Officer
Allina Health System

Acknowledgments

Cheryl Toth, quality editor, contributing author, and project manager for *e-Healthcare* delivered critical expertise, insight, and effort that made this book possible. Cheryl's in-depth understanding of health care and the Internet provided invaluable assistance in helping me organize and edit my research, insights, and more than twenty-three Medical Internet columns from *Managed Care Interface* magazine into this unique book. Her work in coordinating the contributing authors' chapters was even more important in achieving the depth and breadth of the overall book and CD-ROM.

E-xcellence in the "bits and bytes" world of cyberspace is only possible through e-team work. This book is no exception. Special thanks to all the contributing authors who took time out of their busy schedules to share their knowledge and experience in on-line health information and e-service markets. Their energy and time led to a series of invaluable perceptions and e-action steps for health care executives, physicians, and other providers to reduce costs, enhance marketing, and improve patient care in the next century.

Special thanks go to my wonderful wife, Lorraine, and enthusiastic young son, Jared, who supported me during an exciting year. Their love and support encouraged me to share my perspective and insights on the Internet revolution with the health care community.

Introduction

WELCOME to the e-healthcare revolution! Moving at the speed of "Internet time," the health and medical industry is experiencing an explosion of cyberchange, the likes of which have never been seen. From health care e-communications and e-communities to e-commerce and e-care, new developments and e-services roll out by the day, by the hour, and by the minute!

By scanning, absorbing, and applying the strategies in this book, you will embark on an exciting, challenging, and stimulating journey. Each chapter challenges the traditional "bricks and mortar" paradigm of the health care industry, and delivers knowledge and know-how for the new business paradigm of e-commerce and e-care in the twenty-first century. The chapters also provide insights about how the health care industry is undergoing a fundamental shift that will forever change consumer, patient, and health care professional behavior and interaction. This information has been uniquely packaged with tables, Web site examples, diagrams, and tips for success, so that you can take it to your board, your associates, your allied doctors, and your stakeholders and say, "I have seen the future, and the future is 'e.'"

SOURCE OF "E" INSIGHTS AND INSPIRATION

For the past several years, I have been covering the Internet revolution through a "Medical Internet" column published monthly in *Managed Care Interface Magazine* (www.MedicomInt.com). Some of these columns—such as "Surf, Shop, Ship = Spend"—chronicled the rapid increase in on-line expenditures evident during the Christmas of 1998, dubbed "e-Christmas." Others—such as "Consumers Are Using the Internet for Better Health"—described how many consumers are using the Net to manage their chronic diseases.

The collective wisdom and insight from my cyberspace adventures have led to the development of this book and CD-ROM version. Many of the Managed Care Interface columns have served as primary research for key chapters of the book, written by me and by several contributing authors. The knowledge gained from the monthly column was instrumental in developing the predictions, insights, and e-Trends in the book.

AN INTERACTIVE BOOK

You may wonder why anyone would write a traditionally published book about this fast-moving Internet target. There are several reasons. First, I am dedicated to educating and empowering doctors and health care executives about cutting-edge trends that affect their businesses and their livelihoods. Second, this is no ordinary book—because it is also available in a CD-ROM format. You can read the print version or spin the CD and click through the numerous Web site examples covered in the book.

THE BIG E-BANG

Power to the patient! The passive role of the patient is changing as consumers educate themselves with information they find—any time of the day or night—on the Web. "Health" is partnering with "medicine," which too often in the past focused only on treating patients when they were sick. Tens of millions of Americans are on line, and they have become accustomed to making purchases and executing daily activities such as banking, stock trading, grocery shopping, and e-communicating with friends and relatives. Guess what? They want to educate themselves about health and execute health care transactions, too. Medical services are periodic, unwanted purchases that most reasonable people try to avoid. The health and wellness approach of the twenty-first century is to empower and energize human beings to be healthier and to take responsibility for their own well-being—and the Net is one of the most cost-effective distribution channels for accomplishing this.

The thought leaders who have contributed to e-Healthcare share trends, statistics, and know-how that can be summed up in one sentence: The health care industry is on the verge of making a gigantic business model and care delivery shift, from "care delivery" to "e-care." This shift is not simply about accessing health and medical information on a national Web portal. We believe that health care is about service, not just information, and that most health and medical purchases are *local*. Patients want their own doctors—and they can't generally

---

The Shift to e-Healthcare

Manage	▶	Energize
For and To	▶	With
Discipline	▶	Pleasure
Risk Assessment	▶	Healthstyle
Provider Managed	▶	Consumer Centered
Bricks and Mortar	▶	Clicks and Mortar

Source: Copyright © 1999, Douglas Goldstein.

---

access them on a national, commercial Web site. Health care organizations and providers must take the lead in delivering e-communications, e-communities, and e-care directly to local and regional consumers and patients to improve outcomes. This is your challenge and also your e-opportunity.

We are not talking about adding additional layers to your organization or to the industry, as the cost-cutting strategies of managed care and physician practice management companies did. We are talking about completely revolutionizing the way care is delivered in the first place, using Web technologies that make sense. For instance, the number of face-to-face doctor visits will decrease, as will the number of phone calls to the doctor's office, because patients will be able to find basic information and eventually e-service through the doctor's interactive text, graphics, audio, and video Web service.

The home is rapidly becoming the new site of health and medical services for many health care interactions through Internet technology. People with chronic diseases or conditions are participating in e-care on a daily basis by entering health data, joining on-line support groups, downloading information related to their conditions from secure Web services (sanctioned by *their* doctors), and much, much more. Patients are becoming more involved and spending more time on their health care decisions. They are building long-term relationships with organizations that support cost-effective, efficient access to health and medical products and services through the Internet.

IT IS ABOUT "E," NOT JUST "I"

This book is about how "e" is creating a new health care world. Throughout the book, we refer to this as the world of *e-healthcare*, as opposed to *i-healthcare*. The "e" stands for electronic communications. "i"—which stands for the Internet—is a data, voice, and video delivery pipeline. Internet technology is a tool, not a strategy. The tool is allowing the rapid shift of transactions, services, and activities from phone-space to cyberspace. Your organization cannot be "e" without the Internet, but becoming "e" takes a lot more effort than installing a corporate Intranet and getting employees and doctors on line. Becoming "e" means that the digital mindset becomes part of the fabric of your organization. It means thinking about electronic "bits and bytes" rather than physical "bricks and mortar," or print and other traditional media. It means delivering true e-services for customers that save time and money!

As you "download" the bytes of knowledge contained in each chapter, challenge yourself to be realistic about how well your organization has harnessed e-communications, e-commerce, and e-care in your past efforts. Think about how fast your organization is moving compared with the market and other industries. Consider your strategy and time to market. Is the impact of the Net considered at every one of your strategy and business plan sessions? Are you employing strategies and tactics for becoming "e?" How fast are high-speed broadband connections expanding into your market? (These connections make delivering audio and video as easy as delivering text and graphics over 28.8 dial-up modem connections.) Think hard about whether your organization is taking aggressive action to be ready.

It is not *whether* health and medical care delivery services will be Web-enabled, but which ones will appear first, and when, and who will be leading the way.

TAKE THE "E" TRAIN

History tells us that Wall Street analysts and investment bankers both analyze and make markets, and in 1999 they were hard at work making markets in the Health.net industry. ("Health.net" is a term coined by Hambrecht & Quist to describe the merger of health and medical care with the Internet.) Wall Street is working to support, nurture, and grow the health.net industry revolution, just as it did for outpatient services, for-profit hospitals, prescription benefit management, and physician practice management (PPM) segments of the health care industry.

The PPM industry rose fast and fell, but this is not likely to be the case with the health.net industry, mainly because of the Internet's ability to lower per-unit costs of delivering information and service. In fact, the economic models of business across industries are being turned upside down because the costs of disseminating information have been so drastically reduced. Just think about the economics of mailing 20,000 printed flyers versus sending 2 million electronic Webcast flyers. A fundamental factor such as that one is very different from trying to "manage doctors" by integrating financially driven companies into a patient service business. Certainly, health and medical care are more complex than selling books on line. But that complexity will affect the timing and rate of deployment of e-technology in the health care services and products industries, not the ultimate outcome of the Health.net revolution in revolutionizing the entire industry.

Throughout this book, the terms *e-healthcare* and *care support* or *e-care* refer to a new generation of health improvement and disease management products and services that use the Web and other interactive communications e-tools. Care support refers to the next generation of managed care, which has as its core a *customer focus* or *patient-centered care model*. This is not the managed care of the 1980s and 1990s, which sought to restrict access, deny care, and micromanage doctors in an effort to get costs out of the systems. E-healthcare is truly aimed at empowering customers and patients, improving outcomes, and providing hospitals, insurance plans, and practices with e-commerce tools that will improve operational efficiencies and e-care technologies that will connect doctors and their patients.

E-healthcare is moving from risk assessments and provider management to a healthstyle (choosing our lifestyle from a health perspective) and a consumer-centered model. Electronic digital communication across cable, telephone lines, satellites, and wireless technology is delivering health and medical information, products, and services. The world is moving from bricks and mortar to "clicks and mortar." Clicks and mortar focuses on blending the best of the physical and digital world to streamline processes.

BEYOND WEB SITE BUILDING

If you bought this book to learn how to build a Web site or what to post on it, you may be disappointed. This book does not talk about how to build a Web site—it goes light-years beyond Web sites to the strategies and services of e-transactions, e-healthcare destinations, and e-care delivery. We do not talk about how to publish content on the Web. There is already enough of that, and besides, health care organizations are not publishers—they are service organizations. This book is about how to create e-communications and e-communities within your own health care community, with allied doctors and partners. It is about how to create e-service opportunities that combine cyberspace transactions with air-space services, such as a face-to-face doctor appointment or a first aid class at the hospital. It is about health care e-commerce and e-care.

This book is also not about how to Web-enable every last byte of health care. Instead of attempting to make everything high tech and put it all in cyberspace, we believe that some transactions are best done in phone space (on the telephone) or in air space (face-to-face, high touch contact). The contributors to this book are leaders in the e-healthcare industry and deliver insight, strategy, and imperatives as only health care experts who know technology, media, and patients can. But the authors are doctors, nurses, management consultants, disease management experts, and former hospital executives—not Silicon Valley technicians. Thus, they do not recommend throwing it on the Web if the Web way is not a lot better than a telephone call. They recommend nothing that will erode the consumer or patient relationship, because that relationship is vital in health care, if we are to improve outcomes.

For example, is text-based chat nurse triage more effective than calling a nurse at the hospital call center? Probably not. However, there are opportunities to reduce costs by moving some call center functions to the Web. Serving up Web-based audio and video streams about breast self-examinations, for example, saves on videotape duplication and mailing costs. A Web-based self-triage module that allows consumers to educate themselves about certain key conditions can reduce the number of phone calls into the center or a doctor's office.

The delivery of on-line triage self-care services under the supervision of a doctor is very different than the delivery of self-care services with the "entertainment" or media focus of the numerous general health Web portals populating the Net. A truly valuable on-line triage service provides nurses in a medically oriented call center to monitor the on-line activity, in case the consumer's or patient's responses indicate that he or she may have a more severe problem. The intervention may be a pop-up video window or an immediate telephone call, but it is not a flat text query.

The information in this book is focused on the prudent use of technology—not the use of technology for its own sake. The contributing e-thought leaders aim to preserve the doctor–patient relationship, support more efficient e-care, and improve the health care system through appropriate use of e-commerce and e-care in the twenty-first century.

NAVIGATING YOUR E-WAY

This book contains a lot of information and knowledge. Some chapters describe the fast-moving trends in both e-commerce and e-healthcare—others serve up leading-edge strategies and insight about what the future holds for e-care and on-line disease management.

The book is divided into four sections. The first section focuses on the e-trends that are revolutionizing health care and the entire world. The second section describes how the old models of care delivery, disease management, and demand management are evolving into care support and e-care models that allow consumers and patients to guide their own care. The third section suggests ways to put the Web to work in health care organizations, hospitals, and doctors' offices; and the fourth section provides a management roadmap for implementing "e" into your organization—and avoiding legal pitfalls along the way.

Identify the chapters that are of most use to you and your organization, and scan through them first. Check out the Web sites and services that are featured in each chapter—visit them on line to get a feel for them. If some of our cyberdialogue—such as phone space, air space, etc.—needs further definition, use the Glossary at the end of the book. It will help you add "e" to your organization's jargon.

PART I. E-TRENDS THAT WILL FOREVER CHANGE THE HEALTH CARE LANDSCAPE

Chapter 1. *The e-Healthcare Revolution*

A fast and furious introduction to the e-world, this chapter will challenge the way you think about the health care delivery system. Key e-trends, with built-in statistics and metrics, support the case that "e" is changing life, clinical care, and business as we know it. Numerous e-predictions, e-trends, and recommended e-actions about how to implement "e" into your organization are offered for you and your e-team.

Chapter 2. *e-Commerce: The New Business Model*

Challenge the thinking, change the attitude, and take e-action! The economics of the Internet are changing the very foundation of how business operates across every industry. Take key e-business lessons from market and thought leaders in other industries and apply them to your health care organization to achieve your critical clinical and business goals through new e-technologies.

Chapter 3. *The New Health Care e-Consumer and e-Patient*

Meet the new, empowered health care e-consumer and e-patient, who find reams of information on the Web, then take it to their doctors for validation. The e-consumer or e-patient is a new breed: folks who are perfectly comfortable assessing their own health on line and participating in their doctors' plan of treatment. The providers and executives who understand how to deal with these people and deliver consumer-centered care will be winners in the e-healthcare revolution.

Chapter 4. The Explosion of Alternative Medicine Information and Products on the Web

Kava Kava, St. John's Wort, acupuncture, Chinese medicine-complementary and alternative medicine (CAM) has become a multibillion-dollar business. On the Web, consumers and patients have access to vast numbers of alternative sites. This chapter guides readers though a list of popular CAM sites and what is available there. The authors deliver practical suggestions to clinicians about how to successfully handle patients who bring in data from these Web sites.

PART II. FROM TRADITIONAL CARE DELIVERY TO E-CARE

Chapter 5. Yesterday's Medical Model Versus Today's Customer-Focused e-Care

In the old disease management model, physicians worked one-on-one with patients who had chronic conditions, and there was little systematic control of quality or accountability. Web-enabled and other technologies give physicians real-time data and communication opportunities that base clinical decision making on best practice approaches. Combine this with the Web's ability to personalize data, and your organization can move past treating all people with the same disease the same way. It can truly provide customer-focused e-care.

Chapter 6. e-Communications and Interactive e-Care: The Next Generation of Disease Management

In the e-future of disease management, patients with chronic conditions perform self-care and monitoring on line to improve their own health. Citing a number of Web-based technologies, the authors (who created the very successful online and telephonic CancerSurvivorsNetwork.org for the American Cancer Society) offer significant knowledge about the applications that are helping disease management evolve into interactive e-care and the consumer behaviors that coincide with this shift.

Chapter 7. Telemedicine Becomes a Reality with Web-Enabled Applications and Net Devices

In the e-age, telemedicine includes much more than just academic or rural physicians communicating using expensive video-conferencing equipment. Two leading-edge physicians—one, who initiated a telemedicine program in rural South America, and the other, a leader in the field of home health telemedicine—use their combined knowledge to predict how the site of care will shift from the doctor's office to the home.

Chapter 8. Real-Time Customer Information and Health Management Centers

The former director of the Sutter Health System medical call center and the leading "e" expert describes the myriad applications that Web-enabled technologies have in the customer service center environment. In addition to a roadmap for implementing these strategies, the authors offer strategies and tactics on the implementation of real-time medical e-service centers that requires a significant shift in patient behavior and investments in enhanced infrastructure related to Web telephony.

Chapter 9. Technology and On-Line Care Management

The three case studies in this chapter show how the integration of Web-based and telephonic self-care can help patients with chronic disease. Key executives from Lifemasters (www.lifemasters.net)—a leading multimedia disease management, self-care, and health coaching company—share their experience about how to make these applications successful in your organization.

PART III. PUTTING THE WEB TO WORK IN HEALTH SYSTEMS AND PRACTICES

Chapter 10. Beyond Web Portals to On-Line Health and Medical Channels

The first generation of hospital "Web pages" were primarily on-line brochures that provided information and little else. In an e-healthcare world, these "pages" evolve into e-services and eventually into digital channels that offer consumers and patients on-line access to their doctors and hospitals. Performing transactions and getting things done are the goals of the interactive health and medical channel, which is integrated with the actual delivery of health care services. This chapter tells the story of how Allina Health System has developed its e-commerce and e-care efforts over the past several years.

Chapter 11. Meet the Empowered, Interactive SuperNet Woman

The SuperNet Woman makes most of the family's health care decisions, and she constitutes nearly 50 percent of the on-line audience. This chapter offers statistics and case studies to help you understand what drives women to return to your organization's Web service, and how to create and maintain a relationship with this savvy health care consumer.

Chapter 12. Physicians Get On Line

Patients are bringing in printed Web pages and asking if they can e-mail their doctors—what is a practitioner to do? Doctors are experiencing a significant shift in their practices, a shift that is brimming with opportunity. The authors, leading practice management consultants, provide practical tips for how physicians can use the Web to save time and money, and to improve patient relationships.

Chapter 13. Medical Extranets

Medical Extranets promise to reduce or eliminate the paper and logistical nightmares that exist in the health care system. Extranets also offer an opportunity for physicians and other providers to take back control from managed care organizations by gaining access to data that can be used to prove cost-effectiveness and effective outcomes. This chapter describes what can happen when providers, payers, and suppliers link themselves, using secure connections through e-technology.

Chapter 14. Pharmaceutical Companies Ride the e-Power of the Net

Furthering their reputation as creative and successful marketers, pharmaceutical companies have devised many strategies to lure consumers and patients to their Web sites for education, information, and a better understanding of their drugs. Leaders in the data capture arena, the pharmaceutical companies are collecting a lot of information about people who visit their sites. Learn how to collect and use these data in your organization.

Chapter 15. Searching for the Holy Grail: Integrated Medical Records and Beyond

It has been a long time coming, but technology may finally have a reasonable solution to the problem of integrated medical records: hybrid applications that connect doctors to the Web and help doctors and other providers work smarter. The medical directors of two emerging e-record companies give their thoughts and caveats on implementing this Holy Grail in physician practice.

PART IV. IMPLEMENTING "E"

Chapter 16. e-Health and the Law

As your organization works through the process of becoming Web-enabled and e-focused, there are a variety of legal pitfalls to avoid. A leading e-healthcare attorney provides the checklists to keep your organization out of the cyber-courtroom.

Chapter 17. e-Services: Planning Process for e-Business Development

You are ready to become "e," but how do you start? Using the authors' strategy, planning, and development model, this chapter takes you through the step-by-step process of building an action-oriented e-commerce and e-care business plan. It also delivers tips and recommendations about how to structure the effort inside your organization to achieve the necessary speed to market that is essential in the Internet Age.

Chapter 18. Invent the e-Healthcare Future

The new Internet economy and a series of fundamental market forces have forever changed every business model on the planet. Get energized to gain an "e" advantage for the twenty-first century e-healthcare future through hard-hitting wrap-up observations and recommendations.

This book and its electronic companion are starting points for thinking about and doing e-healthcare. These resources go beyond the numbers and metrics, outlining and integrating the proven methodologies and approaches applied by well-known e-thought leaders. Buy extra copies of the book for your employees, your customers, and your clients. Distribute books, CD-ROM versions, and bookmarks to your e-teams to strengthen the e-knowledge base in your organization. Surf the Net and share what you have learned and how you have used the knowledge to further your own e-strategy by e-mailing me at DigitalDoug@aol.com.

Now go forth, learn about "e," and do "e" better than the competition. Your future depends on it!

CHAPTER 1

The e-Healthcare Revolution

Douglas E. Goldstein

IN 1875, Alexander Graham Bell took a new communications device to William Orton, the chief executive officer (CEO) of Western Union and Telegraph. At that time, Western Union dominated the communications market in the United States. Bell showed Orton this new communications device—the telephone, he called it—and offered to sell the rights to the device to Western Union for $100,000. Bell thought this a pretty fair offer.

But Orton did not. He asked Bell what Western Union "could possibly do with an electronic toy." By responding this way, Orton sealed the fate of Western Union. The company missed the telecommunications revolution, which changed the way Americans communicated about everything.

Until now.

Fast forward to the present. A new communications revolution is under way. Only this time it is not telecommunication—it is *e-communication*. Every business, every individual, and every industry will be tremendously and irrevocably affected—and that includes health and medical care. E-communication will dramatically change how the American health care system operates and how its participants communicate. On the horizon is a connected world, linked by fast, cheap e-communication, where speed and e-service are vital. In the new e-healthcare galaxy, e-communities, e-communications, e-commerce, and e-care delivery are revolutionizing the way people market and deliver all health-related products and services.

Welcome to the e-healthcare revolution.

The last several years of the twentieth century will go down in history as the period when Internet technology and Web-enabled applications began to shift the power structure in health care. Empowered "e-patients" now seek health care information on line. Traditional referral patterns are undergoing a fundamental shift. Physicians are being threatened by cyberdocs whom e-consumers and e-patients can conveniently reach on line—from their own home via their personal computer (PC) or Net TV. The days when patients remained mute and simply followed "doctor's orders" are over. So are the days of "hospital-centric" care delivery. By the year 2001, the number of e-consumers who surf for medical information is expected to increase to 30 million, up from 17 million in 1998.[1] And health information and content are only the beginning. In the next wave will come e-products, e-services, and then the e-tsunami—e-care delivery.

The pipeline will not stop with the PCs connected to the Net. PCs and televisions are converging, and video cameras are being added for two-way connectivity. There is a rapidly proliferating number of information appliances, such as WebTV and iPhones, that will bring the power of Internet technology into American homes through cheap, easy to access broadband e-pipelines through the next generation of telephones, televisions, and wireless hand-held devices powered by Palm or CE Windows technology. Empowered e-patients are doing on-line self-care, completing health assessments and surveys, as well as accessing information about local health workshops, buying products, and finding e-healthcare services in their communities. Cybervisits are increasing, as are the number of on-line patient management applications for those with chronic disease; these applications allow better service and lower per unit costs than nurses connected by telephone in centralized medical call centers. Accountability, personal responsibility, and a take-action "just do it" attitude are being broadcast across the Internet from health care companies committed to supporting patients' demands for health care services. These health care companies are managing chronic disease with smart on-line applications. Also emerging are an increased respect for the mind-body connection, the legitimate role of prayer and meditation in healing, and alternative medicine practices.

Just take a look at what the Wall Street analysts are saying and doing. ING Barings uses the term *e-Health* and Hambrecht & Quist uses the term *Health.net* to refer to the new industry of health care and the Internet. According to Hambrecht & Quist, the Health.net market represents a series of multibillion-dollar opportunities that are categorized into three major segments: e-commerce, connectivity/communications, and content/community/services (see Exhibit 1–1).[2]

The e-commerce segment refers to the selling of health-related products, ranging from pharmaceuticals to personal care items, over the Internet. The connectivity/communications segment refers to such applications as data exchange and transaction processing. This market, estimated to represent a multibillion-dollar opportunity, is just emerging due to the complexity and fragmentation of the health care delivery system. Billions of dollars will continue to be invested

Exhibit 1-1 Health.net Industry Opportunities

Hambrecht and Quist's Health.net Market

1. *e-Commerce*—selling health-related products over the Internet—from pharmaceuticals to personal care items.
2. *Connectivity/Communications*—using Web applications for data exchange and transaction processing.
3. *Content/Community/Services*—providing health information, two-way communication between e-patients and providers, and on-line services.

Source: Data from www.hambrecht.com, © 1999, Hambrecht & Quist.

throughout the next decade by health care, technology, communications, and other e-business companies that aim to revolutionize the health and medical industry. Internet technology and interactive communications are revolutionizing all aspects of health and medical communications, communities, commerce, and care delivery. The last wave of on-line e-care challenges every provider and health care organization to get on board.

As the number of Net-connected Americans moves from 100 million to 200 million, and with billions more internationally surfing the Web for daily health and medical needs, the distribution of health and medical care delivery is fundamentally shifting. In the health care market for e-information, e-communities, e-commerce, and e-care delivery, the "branding" and "e-services" battles are just beginning. Many competing entities are vying for leadership spots in this new cyber health marketplace. Where is *your* organization today? How fast is it moving? Does it have the Net know-how to compete? What do you have to do to light the fires of change to prosper in the e-healthcare revolution?

E-HEALTHCARE IS ALSO AN E-BOOK

This is health care's first interactive e-book. There is a CD-ROM version that delivers the same valuable knowledge on e-commerce and e-care, but in an electronic form. The CD delivers the added benefits of live links to the hundreds of Web sites cited in the book.

The e-healthcare book and CD-ROM are dedicated to delivering practical, appropriate knowledge quickly.

E-healthcare is a short- and long-term market opportunity. The Wall Street analysts and investment bankers both "analyze" and "make markets." Just as Wall Street worked to support the growth of the physician practice management (PPM) industry, it is supporting the e-healthcare industry revolution. The PPM industry rose fast and fell hard, but this is not likely to be the case with the e-healthcare industry because the Internet offers lower per unit costs of delivering information and service. In fact, the economic models of businesses across industries are being turned upside down because the costs of disseminating information have been drastically reduced.

Health and medical care is more complex than selling vitamins or books on line, but that affects only the timing or the rate of deployment of e-technology. It is not *whether* care delivery services will be Web enabled, but which ones *first,* and *when.* This e-healthcare book, CD-ROM, and future e-newsletters and Web sites are your knowledge partners as you navigate the cyberfuture.

"DO IT BETTER ON LINE TODAY!"

The Internet offers health care companies unparalleled opportunities for reducing health care costs and improving service and outcomes. So why have health care organizations lagged behind other industries in embracing e-business? Cries of "health care is different," "patients won't want their records on the Net," and "technology will destroy the physician–patient relationship" have reverberated throughout the industry—but they have begun to fall on deaf ears. If the leaders of your health care company still have their heads in the sand about e-healthcare, your company's long-term outlook is about as good as that of the two-pack-a-day smoker who refuses to quit.

"Do it better—on line!" Use e-communications, e-communities, e-commerce, and e-care to support better health, reduce costs, and seek new business. The e-healthcare revolution is rapidly changing the health care landscape. Do not get Amazoned—be the first and the best in your market segment or region to roll out e-services, e-products, and e-care delivery. In less than three years Amazon.com became one of the best known names in book selling through the on-line media with only "bits and bytes" and no "bricks and mortar" bookstores. In 1999, Amazon.com went on line to gain prominence as the leading on-line retailer for videos, music, auctions, toys and games, electronics, and e-cards. Invest now in high-quality e-business action plans and the technology and people necessary to make your vision a success.

Understanding the evolution of health and medical Web sites is essential to effective Web service development. Exhibit 1–2 outlines the five major stages of

Exhibit 1–2 From Web Page to Channel

1. Web page—marketing presence
2. Web site—health library
3. Web service—customer service and transactions
4. Web health portal—information, products, and advertising
5. Interactive health and medical channel—information, products, and e-services

Source: Copyright © 1999, Douglas Goldstein.

Web services development in health care. A Web page often represents an initial marketing presence for an organization, much like an on-line brochure. A Web site adds co-branded or private label information to provide a richer experience for the visitor. A Web service moves beyond information to various service transactions such as physician selection or product sales. A Web portal is a gateway to an array of licensed information modules, product sales opportunities, and links to other Web sites. An interactive health and medical channel is a destination that supports repeat visits and enables an improved medical relationship between physician and patient by connecting them to information, products, and the actual site of care. If an organization is to leapfrog into the twenty-first century, its leaders must expand their thinking beyond just Web pages and e-commerce so that they fully understand e-care.

E-TRENDSCAPE = PREDICTIONS + TRENDS + ACTIONS FOR HEALTH CARE

This chapter delivers four e-predictions about the e-healthcare revolution, then describes key, observed e-trends supporting the e-prediction of the ongoing .com revolution. Within each e-trend there is a straightforward e-action on how to leapfrog the competition. Examine the prediction, read the trend, absorb the e-action, and then, most important, think about how to achieve e-success in your target markets. Use the five tips at the end of the chapter as you plan the future of your company's e-strategy. E-success depends on thinking differently, acting quickly, investing wisely, and empowering your team members to excel.

e-PREDICTION #1: "e" WILL FOREVER CHANGE THE PHYSICIAN–PATIENT RELATIONSHIP

e-Trend #1: More and More e-Consumers, Doing More On Line

Most people are into "e," and if they are not, they plan to be. Figure 1–1 illustrates the tremendous surge in consumers jumping on line. By 2000, 100 million Americans are expected to be on line, according to IntelliQuest.[3] And not everyone is connecting with a PC. Approximately 3.7 million Internet users use a hand-held computer, and television set-top boxes such as WebTV are used by 3.1 million.[4]

Rethink old data—e-consumers are not just "early adapters" or the techno-savvy or even the "young." These two groups of early Netizens were typically profiled as highly educated, highly paid, white, and male. As Exhibit 1–3 shows, 1999 trends made the Internet much more mainstream. Many of the 40 million who planned to go on line in 1999 are over the age of 35, have a high school education or less, and make less than $50,000 a year.[5]

Women are one of the fastest-growing groups on the Internet. CyberDialogue reports that in 1998, 42 percent of Internet users were women—up from 20 percent in 1995. AOL claims that 51 percent of its 13 million members are women—up from only 16 percent four years ago.[6] And according to the survey "NetSmart III—What Makes Women Click," the average SuperNet Woman is 41 years old and has a household income of $63,000.[7] The Internet has empowered interactive women who are taking care of many of their daily living activities on line. Forty-seven percent of Internet users were female—up from 20 percent in 1995—and these SuperNet Women are managing their family's health, trading stocks, purchasing vitamins, and much more. See Chapter 11 for more in-depth information.

The Internet has become the place where middle Americans search for information and shop for products and services. Executives from every industry are figur-

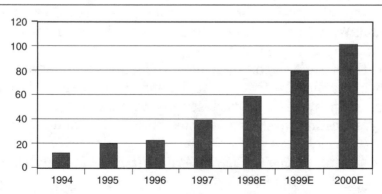

Figure 1–1 U.S. Internet Use Explodes. *Note:* E = estimated. *Source:* Data from Healthcare Information Services, © 1998, ING Baring Furman Selz LLC.

Exhibit 1-3 The Spread of Internet Use, 1999

> - 51% of the 40 million who planned to go on line in 1999 were over the age of 35
> - 49% of them had a high school education or less
> - 58% made less than $50,000 a year
>
> *Source:* Data from Cyberatlas.com, © 1999, Internet.com.

ing out ways to reach these savvy consumers and launching new .com, .net, .org, .edu, .biz, .sex, and .arts sites, and numerous other extensions are being created. Company uniform resource locators (URLs) have become as ubiquitous as telephone numbers on everything from letterhead to billboards to television commercials. IBM is investing hundreds of millions of dollars to educate consumers, business owners, and executives about the benefits of e-business (www.ibm.com/e-business/). Visitors to the IBM Web site learn specifics about e-business and how to formulate a strategy for their own company. In health care, the revolution has begun and will continue well into the twenty-first century.

Beyond the e-consumer to the e-patient! From downloading health tips off global health Web portals, to joining on-line support groups, to questioning their physician's course of treatment because of something they found on line, e-consumers are the driving force behind the prolific on-line access to medical information and care delivery. The e-healthcare revolution is about the empowerment of the American consumer and patient. It is about the evolution from self-serve health information and products, to medical services any hour of the day, in the patient's home via Internet technology. It is about giving all people—not just members of the medical community—access to information on line. And it is about *customer service*—formerly a lower priority than technical expertise or quality care.

Today's American e-consumers (and, more important, today's e-patients) want more than information. They want knowledge of and access to health services that can help and heal. E-patients want the power to participate in and lead their own medical care. For example, research companies such as cyberdialogue// :findsvp have identified a highly active segment known as HealthMed Retrievers (HMR). Using the Internet on an almost daily basis, these e-healthcare sleuths use the Net as an electronic support group as they struggle to overcome the paucity of health care information about topics such as injuries, prescription drugs, health insurance, and child development.

Baby Boomers, especially, are seeking their own answers. A 1998 Press-Ganey study showed that Baby Boomers are much less satisfied with the quality of health care services than are older generations.[8] A highly consumer-driven generation, Boomers have grown accustomed to convenience and choice—and they are a force to be reckoned with. For Boomers, self-service and customer service rule. And not only are they the largest generation ever to push through the American health care system, they are the first generation to make decisions for themselves *and* their ailing parents or relatives. The decision-making power of the Baby Boomers is significant—and many of them are fueling these decisions with information from the Web.

HealthMed Retrievers are a large, unsegmented group of on-line consumers. What health care needs is a truly effective segmentation system for chronic health seekers. If you work in a managed care organization or an at-risk health system, it is important to know whether diabetics use the Internet more or less than other people. In managing their disease, would they be more likely to use an on-line application or service or to place a call to a nurse in a call center? Information on specific patient populations' use of the Internet is only now becoming available. It is imperative to design on-line health and medical services based on target customer preferences. Harris Interactive has identified and profiled a group of cyber patients with chronic diseases that spend a lot of time on line getting information and managing their chronic conditions.

- *e-Action #1: Go Beyond the Numbers by Identifying What e-Patients Are Doing On Line!* To design any on-line service or to justify an investment in licensing an on-line application or service developed by a third party, obtain the necessary knowledge on use patterns. It is amazing how many health and medical Web sites were launched without any customer input. Ask customers what they want to do on line, design your services, and then ask customers for advice and involve them in periodic review. Be the leader in "e" innovation and service, or risk losing the market to competitors. Be smart. Be first. Be better.

e-Trend #2: From On-Line Information Today to Medical Decision Support Tomorrow

E-patients are connecting with global health information services, and increasingly with their providers, on line for a host of reasons—information, knowledge, self-care tips, access to lab results, Webcast daily health tip e-zines, appointment scheduling, registration, disease management, nurse triage, and, in the future, actual e-care delivery. On-line care delivery? Many executives do not think consumers and patients will want to replace air-space physician visits with on-line cybervisits because technology is impersonal. Think back a few years to when banking executives said the same thing about automatic teller machines (ATMs). "Customers won't want to use them," they said, "because people want to interact with a live person." Today customers *pay* to use ATMs. Very soon, operating a health and medical care system without a robust, integrated multimedia Web service and call center "care support" services will be like running a bank without an ATM network. With a video camera in every television sold and high-speed access to millions of homes...here come e-house calls!

Today, e-patients collect credentialing information about their physicians on line and can go to www.healthcarereportcards.com to see how their local hospital fares against others in the region, based on the number of procedures performed. Armed with health information from the Web, e-patients bombard their physicians with questions about treatments, drugs, and procedures from Health-Online.com (Figure 1–2), AHN.com, Thriveonline.com, and Ask Dr. Weil. (Health-Online.com, for instance, integrates health systems, physicians, and patients to enable true e-care delivery. Patients can register for local health and wellness classes, receive lab results, refill prescriptions, and manage disease. Physicians benefit from Web-enabled applications that make managing their practice more efficient.) How physicians respond to these exam room inquiries will depend on their own knowledge base and level of comfort with e-communications. But you had better believe that the e-patients of physicians who are unwilling to acknowledge the e-information will find a physician who is on line and connected; these patients are busy and looking for better service and more efficiency.

A good example of on-line decision support is the Medformation.com channel, shown in Figure 1–3, which is a robust Web addition of the call center of Allina Health System in Minneapolis. The call center handles over 500,000 calls a year. The Web service goes *beyond* supplying just information and products; it supports community and care delivery through the seamless extension of Allina's continuum of care into cyberspace. Care delivery is achieved by integrating the Medformation Online Health and Medical Channel with a 50-seat medical call center—consumers and patients always have access to a human, whether nurse or referral specialist, through the telephone or through Web telephony. More important, the Medformation Web channel is closely connected to the entire continuum of health and medical services of Allina Hospitals and Clinics throughout Minnesota and the surrounding states.

Health issues are different from medical needs. Many consumers need and want information on line, but medical care is really about who can treat it, heal

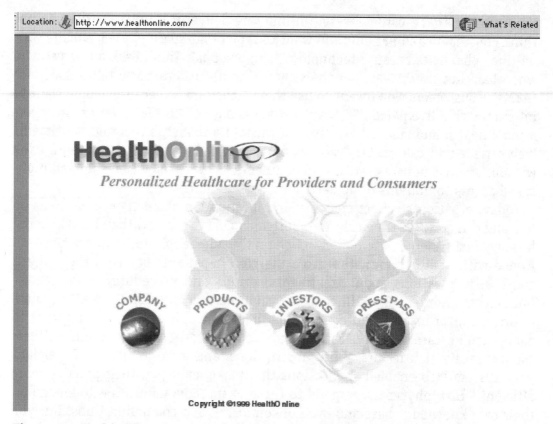

Figure 1–2 Health Online.com. *Source:* Reprinted with permission from www.HealthOnline.com, © 1999, HealthOnline.com.

it, and care for it. There are tens of thousands of health and medical Web sites, but most are based on a modified publishing/e-commerce business model. Medformation and other affiliates within the HealthOnline.com network of digital channels go beyond this, providing information that supports rapid access to health and medical providers and services in a specific community or region of the country.

As Allina's leaders sought to go beyond the two existing Web sites Allina.com and Medica.com, the strategic matrix in Figure 1–4 guided them in assessing what kind of additional Web services to design, implement, and operate. On the left side of the figure are education, triage, diagnosis, and treatment. Along the bottom are information, self-care, supported self-care, and professional care—things that consumers seek through phone calls to doctors, 800 helplines or on the Web. The Medformation.com on-line channel is being integrated with the site of prevention and care. It goes beyond information and products to include access to care through Web-enabled applications and integration with a medical call center and eventually actual doctors' offices. KPonline.com for Kaiser Permanente members is another example of an on-line channel for actual appointments and on-line dialogue with physicians and nurses.

Medformation.com and KPonline.com are examples of a new generation of interactive services that are focused on supporting consumers and patients with a robust, regional Web channel that can connect people in need with local commu-

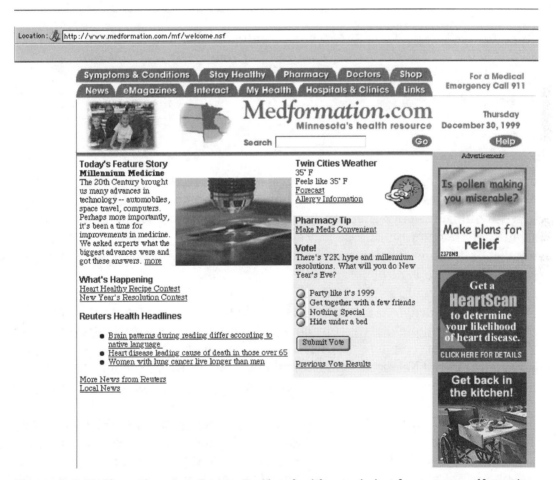

Figure 1–3 Medformation.com. *Source:* Reprinted with permission from www.medformation. com, © 1999, Medformation.com. Medformation is a registered trademark of Allina Health System.

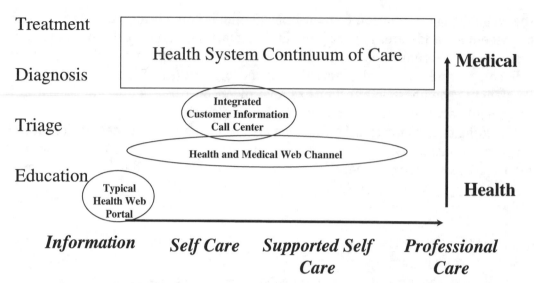

Figure 1–4 e-Care Delivery Business Model versus Health Information. *Source:* Copyright © 1999, Douglas Goldstein.

nity knowledge and actual medical services. It is true that cyberspace visits will not replace all visits to physicians or home visits by home health care agencies, but early in the twenty-first century people will monitor "MedNet" metrics (the science of tracking on-line health and medical use of the Net) that show the number of cybervisits being conducted by low- and high-speed connection to the home. The future is now.

- *e-Action #2: Leapfrog the Competition by Doing It Fast and Right!* It is now the time to develop effective consumer and patient Web outreach strategies and systems that compete against known and unknown competitors. Three months in the Net world is like a year anywhere else. On-line branding battles are just beginning in health care. How many of us recognize the names "Amazon.com" or "Yahoo.com" today? Many of these brands did not even exist in the mid-1990s. Mediconsult.com, OnHealth.com, Medscape.com, Healtheon.com, Achoo.com, drkoop.com, iVillage's All Health, and many others are trying to be the Yahoo! of health care. If your health care organization is not the leading on-line service in your market, the competition will take the lead and embed its name forever in the minds of customers. Amazon.com evolved rapidly, going beyond books to music, gifts, e-cards, videos, auctions, and so on. Perhaps when you read this book, Amazon will have added tabs for "physicians" and "drugs," thus bypassing the traditional health care business of the twentieth century!

e-Trend #3: Everything Is Connected to the Net

In the past, PCs were the primary information device that delivered Internet connectivity to individuals. But like the hula hoop and New Coke, the PC was not meant to last. E-consumers want access to a burgeoning array of Net services— but they do not want to be stuck at their bulky, complex PC every time they need to get on line to buy stocks or order a refill on a prescription. E-consumers are mobile, they are busy, they want convenience, and, most of all, they want it now. Given this profile of today's e-consumers, consumer products and medical device manufacturers are working hard to develop various wireless information devices that will both augment and supersede the PC—which in the year 2010 will conjure up analogies to those "big, expensive calculators" of the 1960s.

Devices for tapping into the Net's endless stream of information now include interactive telephones, television with video cameras, wireless personal data/ information assistants (PDAs), and integrated devices such as combined PDA/cell phones. E-consumers will be Net enabled in their living rooms, in their kitchens, in their cars, and in their pockets. Round-the-clock access to information—and, more important, to various knowledge databases that help people do their jobs and keep on top of the e-service tidal wave—are becoming increasingly commonplace.

On-line service providers such as AT&T, cable companies, utilities, and www.home.com—as well as Microsoft—are all clamoring to get a foothold in this new interactive marketplace. When Microsoft bought WebTV, an on-line service that then had only 60,000 subscribers, many laughed. But Bill Gates is no dummy; he knew that gaining control over the technology interface of the television and cable lines would bring his company greater influence. Now, the convergence of Internet and information devices such as Internet-connected iPhones® (www.MDtel.com) is dramatically increasing access to the Net. InfoGear's iPhone® enables consumers to surf the Web and talk on the telephone simultaneously. Since nearly every American already knows how to use a telephone, the iPhone® makes using new technology less scary. Microsoft's current challenge is to gain influence over television, PDA, and other interfaces that most consumers will use to research, buy, and obtain health services over the Net.

When elderly and chronically ill persons can easily access the Net on television or on their Netphone, the range of e-healthcare service delivery uses will be limitless. An America Online (AOL) initiative titled "AOL Anywhere" is gaining steam as there are more sales of new wireless connect devices that let AOL be the gateway to everything electronic. "E" as fashion is just emerging. Electronics are being wired into clothing. The Army is testing a T-shirt that monitors the site of injuries so that information can be transferred to MedVac units prior to arrival for a downed soldier, or, how about a cyber-connected toilet seat that could record a patient's vital signs several times a day. E-books that allow people for a small fee to download the latest Tom Clancy bestseller, and more and more innovations, are increasingly becoming part of every minute of our lives.

- *e-Action #3: Track the Rate of e-Change in Other Industries To Gain Insights into Opportunities in Health Care.* Health care often lags behind other industries in innovation. A few years ago, while other industries invested heavily in information services, for instance, the health care industry did not. Tracking other industries such as retail and financial services will help members of the health care industry see opportunities for e-change. Staying current with fast-breaking developments and alliances requires getting connected to great on-line and print resources such as www.thestandard.com, www.interactive-week.com, and wired.com. These are three of the best information sources on the e-revolution. They deliver weekly knowledge, ideas, metrics, and much more via e-mail, Web service, or print publications. The time is now to be informed and allocate investment wisely to ride the e-surf throughout the twenty-first century.

e-PREDICTION #2: PASSIVE WEB SITES WILL PERISH, TRUE DIGITAL e-SERVICES WILL PROSPER

e-Trend #4: Beyond Web Portals to Health and Medical Web Destinations and Channels

Internet rules e-volve fast. If yours was a health care company that felt content to establish a marketing-oriented, no-service Web site last year, be careful not to rest on those laurels. E-commerce and e-services are fast moving away from "information" and moving toward "transaction." From information and transaction, e-commerce will then move to "community" and "care delivery." Like Phoenix rising from the ashes, your company must e-position itself to make this shift too. Push your organization's e-strategy from Web site to interactive digital channel. Exhibit 1–4 explains the evolution of health and medical Web sites from passive brochureware Web sites to interactive relationship-developing destinations called digital channels.

Exhibit 1-4 From Brochureware to Interactive Digital Channel

Phase I: Web page—Generally called "brochureware," a Web page is a strategy whereby an organization takes print brochures and shovels them onto the Net to establish a presence.

Phase II: Web site—A Web site is often referred to as an effort to share "value-added information" on health and medical issues. This could mean providing information on how to have a healthy pregnancy or how to cope with or cure various symptoms or conditions. The goal of most Web sites is to build relationships by giving away health education information. Implementation is generally directed by the marketing department.

Phase III: Web service—A Web service delivers a customer- or patient-focused service that saves time or money for both the consumer and the health care organization. It is a more advanced application of Internet service. For instance, a health plan that helps consumers find a doctor and answers members' service questions is delivering a better and faster solution for the customer, while also reducing health system operating costs by moving phone volume over to an automated Web solution. The goal of this phase is to build market share and manage health.

Phase IV: Commercial Web service—A commercial Web service focuses on Web solutions that service health care transactions. This could include everything from the purchase of a diet book to the delivery of actual e-care to a consumer's home to use with advanced health monitoring systems. The goal of Phase IV is services and applications that build e-patient relationships, decrease overall costs, and deliver e-care.

Phase V: Web portal—High-traffic, multiservice Web services that are an entry point to the larger Internet, Web portals offer extensive search capabilities, on-line shopping, and other transactions. A Web portal combines phases I–IV of Web development and services into a multifeature and multifunctional content gateway to the Internet. Examples of multipurpose portals include: Yahoo!, Netscape's NetCenter, Excite, AOL.com, and others. There is an emerging generation of regionally focused gateway portals that include Digital City, City Search, MediaOne On-screen Gateways, and Internet provider/cable company home pages.

Phase VI: Interactive digital channel—The PC disappears as interactive television and telephones take over as the information appliances of choice for most Americans. Health information streams through to e-consumers and e-patients via digital audio and video—right into the American family room and kitchen.

Source: Copyright © 1999, Douglas Goldstein.

Your organization's goal should be to create an interactive experience that brings e-patients and e-consumers back time and again for more e-products and e-services. Take a look at Web sites and search engines in both general and financial service sectors and you will find that they have moved from being simply Web sites or search engines to being gateways or "portals" to multiple services, transactions, and products. Charles Schwab, for example, has partnered with Excite to create www.myschwab.com. At My Schwab, e-consumers customize everything, from their stock watch list and daily news, to their horoscope and appointment calendar. A log-in button is easily accessible for Schwab customers to review the status of their brokerage account. Schwab is moving its Web site from a transaction site to a financial portal in an attempt to compete against Yahoo! Finance and Quicken.

Why are smart e-finance companies moving in this direction? In 1999, it was estimated that 2.4 million American households participated in on-line trading, and 1.9 million more were expected to start investing on line by 2000.[9] About 7 million households accessed their financial accounts via the Web.[10] These facts helped financial companies easily conclude why upstart cyberspace brands such as Quicken.com, Yahoo! Finance, and AOL Finance are beating out traditional brands such as Merrill Lynch for trading transactions. E*Trade figures, for example, that if the company builds a Web portal with great services that help people do more and save money faster, *they will come and stay awhile.* Similar viability and low-cost advantages are also evident in Amazon.com's ability to beat out Barnes & Noble, doing *10 times* the monthly sales of on-line books and records of its competitor. The other obvious advantage Amazon has is that it was first. In his 1992 political campaign, Clinton won with a motto, "It's the economy, stupid!" For the Internet, the slogan goes "It's the relationship, stupid!"

This is an important trend for e-healthcare because no one yet holds a primary position as the e-care delivery community or gateway. While an expanding number of health and medical Web sites are on the Web, only a few players, drkoop.com or WebMD.com, have begun to emerge as dominant e-healthcare Web portals—and there certainly is no one clear provider of e-care delivery on the Web. The question is not whether many care delivery functions will be Web enabled but when and how fast. With the stakes so high, it is never too late to vamp up your "e" efforts.

Furthermore, what the nationally focused portals and information aggregators do not generally provide is the ability for the consumer and patient to *complete* many types of health care service transactions. They cannot lead the charge of integrating cyberspace with air-space service transactions at the local level—for instance, face-to-face encounters, health monitoring, health assessments, workshops, and seminars. Liability is a factor, and in cyberspace there is no way for an e-physician to perform a hands-on examination. Remote telemetry of patient vital signs, however, is developing quickly, and certain visits can be replaced through a cyberphysician or e-nurse using fast connections and a video camera.

Allina Health System, Catholic Healthcare Partners, and dozens of other leading health systems realized this fact early on and have developed a digital interactive health and medical channel that delivers health knowledge, product sales (transactions), and nearly seamless integration with their own network of providers and services. For instance, Allina has over 14 million annual contacts—in person, on line, on the telephone, and via fax—with the local population. Its Medformation.com e-community serves up health information, products, local news, workshops, and events, as well as medical breakthroughs and local customized information based on a consumer's health interests and needs. E-consumers can find a physician on line, identify products that treat specific conditions, order from local merchants, schedule an appointment, complete the new patient registration, get support from a nurse in a Web-enabled call center, and much, much more through the HealthOnline.com network of affiliated on-line channels.

This network of health systems smartly transitioned its Web site from a cost center to a profitable e-care delivery business model. At one time, a Web site was seen as a necessary marketing expense—one whose return was in "intangibles" such as information, image, and "feel good" communications. No more. Investments in e-products and e-services can and should yield a return on investment. E-communities that offer e-services and transactions have business models that are based on cost reduction or new business revenue—such as product sales or advertiser support.

There is significant growth in the advertising and sponsorship dollars available for health care sites on the Web. Forrester Research and Jupiter Communications (www.jup.com) both report projections for on-line advertising to exceed $4 billion by the end of 2000 (unpublished data from ING Baring Furman Selz). Growth in pharmaceutical direct-to-consumer (DTC) advertising topped $1 billion in 1998—up 38 percent from a year earlier. Estimates are for DTC pharmaceutical advertising to exceed $5 billion by 2005, with a significant portion going to the Web due to the Web's ability to target consumers with specific conditions.[11] According to Jupiter Communications, on-line health and medical advertising will grow from $12.3 million in 1997 to $265 million by 2002, with on-line DTC advertising representing 50 percent of the total.[12] Jupiter also concludes that health Web portals will be uniquely positioned to capture a lion's share of the revenue.

If your organization is a provider-based network, do not lose your e-patient relationships for health care information to global cyberphysician services—develop, license, and private label your own solution so your patients stop at your Web service before going on to other sources. As your health care organization prepares to upgrade and enhance its e-consumer health and medicine Web applications, services, and e-care delivery, look at other industries for guidance. Lessons learned in financial services, retail, and business-to-business can create a framework for your e-healthcare initiatives. You do not necessarily have to invent and innovate; you can license and private label. The key is to make your Web services a destination where people can do things more quickly, more cheaply, and better.

- *e-Action #4*: *Position Your e-Healthcare and Medical e-Care Delivery Strategy on the Web—Be the Leading On-Line Service in Your Markets*. Integrate cyberspace health information with air-space medical e-care delivery transactions and services. Go beyond Web portals to interactive e-community channels where e-patients, e-consumers, and providers gather and manage care delivery in your air-space community.

As you move your health care organization from Web site to e-community, think e-service, e-transactions, and e-care delivery. Shift into high gear and bypass passive phases of the e-healthcare revolution—serve e-patients better and get a return on investment with e-communities and interactive on-line channels that enhance medical relationships between people and their physicians and community hospitals.

The key for health care organizations is to determine how much to invest and whether the investment is guided by experienced Internet advisors and executives who understand the health care industry and the new, interactive Internet medium. Automating certain health care transactions and medical services on the Net can reduce operating costs, but these processes are frequently much more complex than just buying a book or PC on line. Be sure you hire seasoned advisors who understand health care, the Internet, new media, and do the necessary "think through."

e-Trend #5: *e-Care Support—Next-Generation Disease and Demand Management*

Challenge the paradigm and change the attitude. Managed care is out and consumer "e-care support" is in! E-care support puts consumers and patients at the center of the equation to reduce unnecessary health care expenditures. This approach empowers appropriate supported self-care though information and knowledge and rapid access to health care services through multimedia Internet and real-time customer management call centers. In efforts to achieve total health management and prevention, health care organizations are increasingly tapping the power of the Net and other media to communicate with and serve the needs of vendors, physicians, diverse groups of members, prospective employees, and other constituencies. Optum's® Health Forums is one example (Figure 1–5). It provides information, education, and support services that contribute to a better quality of life and overall health and well-being. On-line discussions with nurses and counselors through live events, frequently asked questions about health and well-being, interactive health quizzes, searchable databases, and e-newsletters. In addition to exploiting the Net as a tool for marketing, education, research, and customer service, health care organizations are using it to virtually connect and improve relationships with physicians, other providers, and community groups as well as fulfill social responsibility goals, promote and manage special events, and raise funds from sponsors and individual contributors.

The Web can deliver better service at lower costs for either business-to-business transactions or consumer-to-business transactions. From a human perspective, however, the applications that a customer or target market is ready to use vary. While everybody hooked up to the Internet uses e-mail, not everyone trades stocks on line. Therefore, you must ask, "What is an appropriate use of Internet technology and services relative to the current and future needs of my customers in our local and regional health care market?" And "How can we Web

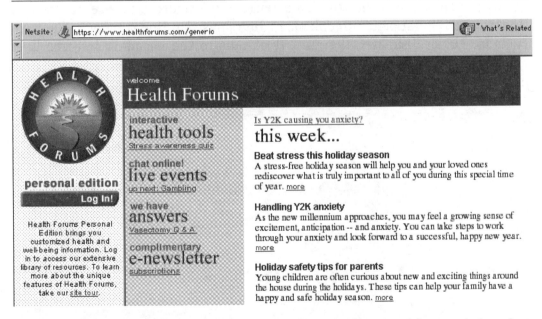

Figure 1–5 Optum's® Healthforums.com. *Source:* Reprinted with permission from www.healthforums.com, © 1999, Optum.®

enable a high-touch call center service like nurse triage and ensure it still allows consumers to get a high-touch human interaction when needed?"

E-care support involves a suite of services—a series of demand/disease management services that complement and augment the medical management efforts of foundations, independent practice associations, management service organizations, and physician organizations to foster appropriate patient utilization of health care services. This suite of services is not a replacement for case management because it targets at-risk or inappropriate utilizers prior to a referral by a physician or system resource. The e-care support system uses a variety of interventions based around the telephone and Internet as primary telecare tools to target and support high-risk populations, chronic care populations, or populations that consume a high level of inappropriate resources, as identified from claims analysis and health/cost risk assessments. Figure 1–6 illustrates the use of a Web-enabled medical call center to achieve key corporate objectives related to achieving better marketing and new business to enhance cost reduction and disease management within at-risk populations.

- *e-Action #5: Do Better Customer Service through Integration of Phone Space and Cyberspace.* Swedish Medical Center in Seattle, Washington (www.swedish.org), is another health system that saw the opportunity to expand from a Web site to Web service. The Swedish e-service generates a return on investment through an on-line physician finder service. The Web-based finder decreased the number of calls to the hospital's toll-free lines

Integrated Customer Information Centers

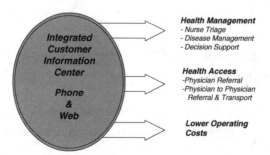

Figure 1–6 Integrated Customer Information Centers with Web Services. *Source:* Copyright © 1999, Douglas Goldstein.

from prospective patients seeking physician referrals. Since October 1997, the usage of the site's physician referral system has climbed steadily, and telephone calls have decreased from 800 to 400 per month.[13] With a savings of $6 to $8 on each call, that's an annual cost reduction of more than $33,000. Swedish's plans include progressively Web-enabling additional call center and related transactions to achieve lower per unit costs, while maintaining service levels and supporting consumer efforts to connect with physicians and caregivers.

Delivering a robust e-care support service means developing an enabled e-community that allows e-patients and e-consumers to select a physician and schedule appointments at the same time, purchase self-care products and have their use encouraged by cybercoaches, request free videos, or use special on-line applications to help manage diseases and conditions. It is time that your health care organization reassess all of its on-line strategies and potential applications and be sure that they support better consumer health and reduce health care costs. To achieve this goal, the Web front end must not be simply "rip and read" e-mail (this refers to first generation Web sites where e-mail to the site was printed out and circulated for response). The Web customer interface must be integrated to the legacy systems of call centers to support better customer service access to health and medical products and services. Improved service through on-line technology means better, cheaper, faster!

e-PREDICTION #3: e-COMMERCE IS THE DRIVING FORCE OF CHANGE FOR HEALTH CARE BUSINESS PROCESSES

e-Trend #6: Biz-to-Biz—Better, Cheaper, Faster On Line

The e-healthcare revolution is about more than just e-communications, e-communities, and e-care delivery. E-commerce is a driving force. Business-to-business e-transactions are fast replacing purchase orders and ordering lag times. In virtually every industry—from steel to electronic parts, computer networks to employee uniforms—e-customers can access on-line catalogs and place orders directly with manufacturers. As Table 1–1 shows, the savings are dramatic. Companies such as Cisco Systems see a significant portion of their sales from direct on-line orders. About 57 percent of Cisco's revenue comes from its Cisco Connection Online (www.cisco.com). That is $11 million a day, $1.3 billion each quarter. Cisco Connection Online also provides 70 percent of the company's customer ser-

Table 1–1 e-Commerce Savings by Category

	Traditional System	Internet	Percent Savings
Airline Tickets	$8	$1	87%
Banking	$1.08	$0.13	88%
Bill Payment	$2.22 to $3.32	$0.65 to $1.10	67%–71%
Term Life Insurance Policy	$400 to $700	$200 to $350	50%
Software	$15	$0.20 to $0.50	97%–99%

Source: Data from *The Industry Standard*, p. 86, May 3, 1999, Reprint Management Services.

vice—which saves Cisco Systems $70 million per year in customer service staffing costs.[14]

Total business-to-business transactions are expected to reach $1.3 trillion by 2003,[15] and health care companies stand to receive a tremendous boost in efficiency, cost savings, and revenues from e-commerce solutions. The result of e-commerce in health care will be lower labor costs, decreased claims payment and purchasing lag times, and increased operational efficiencies.

Let us start simply—buying material and supplies for the hospital. Age-old systems have been paper intensive and include purchase orders, verification processes, and a dedicated department. Connecting directly to suppliers such as Cintas, however, would reduce these components significantly (www.cintas-corp.com/online_shopping/). With e-commerce connectivity, paper trails are digitized, and fewer people are needed to stock the supply rooms.

Medical offices and front-line operations at the hospital will see surges in productivity as automated management tools emerge on the Web. A significant portion of administrative and clinical staff time is spent running after authorizations, eligibility, and other "mother, may I?" processes for managed care plans. When offices, hospitals, and plans are connected via e-commerce solutions, these processes can be digitized, eliminating burdensome paperwork and time-consuming protocols. On-line eligibility verification, referral authorization, claims submission, payment and explanation of benefits payment posting are all good examples of how e-commerce will make operations run more smoothly. Health care companies can also take advantage of e-commerce options that other industries enjoy: on-line banking and purchasing computers and office supplies.

- *e-Action #6: Automate the Top Priorities for Reduced Operating Costs through e-Commerce—and Save Money!* E-commerce is different from e-care. Although your e-strategy will include both, most likely different teams will be involved in creating each one. Their efforts will be coordinated through several key executives—often the senior operations and information systems executives.

Many, many health care services and transactions can be Web enabled. There are several important questions here: If we Web enable, is it better than the way we have traditionally done it? Are our customers ready to use the technology? Will it cost less? Consider, as an example, employing on-line nurse triage (Exhibit 1–5) as opposed to nurses in a call center environment. Is a Web-enabled triage application where consumers and patients communicate through e-mail or text-based chat better than a traditional telephone call? Because of the time delays involved and lack of audio feedback to correctly assess a patient's condition, the answer may not always be "yes." Those providing general service nurse or physician-on-the-Web services have to be trained to be perceived as giving advice but not actually give advice because of the legal exposure and the fact that there is no physician–patient relationship. Also, a nurse or physician responding by text-based chat or e-mail rather than a simple telephone call has a higher cost of delivery profile and lower effectiveness. On-line nurse triage is best when it is integrated with a call center supported by a health plan, physician, or health system.

E-care delivery and e-care support focus on using Internet technology to do cyberservice visits and support patients in the home. This includes replacing a certain number of home visits through the use of broadband connections to the

---

Exhibit 1–5 On-Line Nurse Triage

Opportunity: Reduce costs by moving calls to the Web.
Options:
   — e-mail to a physician or nurse
   — text-based chat with physician or nurse
   — on-line self-care triage module (unsupported)
   — on-line triage with Web telephony support to a health care call center with nurses and referral specialists
   — on-line triage with Web video connection to a health care call center

Source: Copyright © 1999, Douglas Goldstein.

home and various clinical Web applications that allow nurses to see, hear, and support patients in the comfort of their own homes.

E-commerce focuses on reducing transaction costs and simplifying supply chain purchasing in a way that reduces operating and staffing costs. E-commerce also focuses on re-engineering a variety of administrative processes involved with managed care and hospital operations. One imperative is certain: Explore e-commerce opportunities for your organization now and prepare for e-care delivery when high-speed bandwidth connections are in more homes and actual care support is possible. The only thing you have to lose is excess labor costs and inefficiencies.

e-Trend #7: Surf + Shop + Ship = Rapidly Accelerating On-Line Spending

The Christmas season of 1998 is viewed as the first e-Christmas. On-line consumer sales were estimated at $13 billion in 1998, and projections go as high as $40 billion for the whole year 2000.[16] The Gap stores' Christmas windows in 1998 held a 12-foot vertical banner in every window that said "SURF, SHOP, SHIP" and delivered the message, "If you are going to spend money in cyberspace, spend it with us." The Gap knows that if cyberspace is going to deliver e-tailing, it had better encourage consumers to shop with Gap, not the other guy. Even if e-consumers do not buy on line, Web research influences their buying decisions for even more billions of dollars of traditional purchases. The fear of supplying credit card numbers on line has subsided precipitously—now, e-consumers are wondering "why don't they offer it to me on line in a way that is better and faster than other methods of transaction?"

E-consumers already buy books, flowers, computers, cars, and more on the Web—why not carefully selected products and services from your health care organization? Not only is this a customer service/self-service advantage, it creates new revenue streams for your organization. It can convert what has traditionally been a cost center (like marketing and information systems) into e-revenue centers. And guess what? The international health Web portals are already doing it. E*TRADE's transition from a stock-trading single application to a financial services supermarket in three short years illustrates the speed that "e" is taking over e-commerce throughout the world (see Exhibit 1–6).

AllHealth, at iVillage, peddles GreenTree's multivitamin made just for women. America's Health Network's Health Mall channel offers MEDIC ID bracelets, ear thermometers, and portable whirlpools for tired feet. Ask Dr. Weil sells complementary and integrative medicine books in its bookstore. MotherNature.com (Figure 1–7) offers "motherly" health advice as well as herbs and other health-

Exhibit 1–6 E*TRADE.com—Transaction to Portal

- Customizable market data and news
- Mortgage loan information from E-loan
- Real-time research from BancAmerica Robertson Stephens
- Subscription fee for some services
- Financial profile
  —$70,000 per quarter from advertising
  —Sells all ad space
  —72 percent of revenue from transactions

Source: Data from an assessment of E*TRADE.com, 1999, E*TRADE Securities, Inc.

related products. If you are wondering what your patients would think about your prestigious nonprofit or academic institution selling products, here is the answer: they will love it, and they will keep coming back for more. Regional physicians and health systems risk losing their patient relationships because they have fallen far short of venture-backed Web portals and e-commerce players such as www.drugstore.com and CVS.com, which acquired on-line pharmacy Soma.com in 1999 for $30 million (Figure 1–8). At the time, Soma.com was only a six-month-old on-line initiative. CVS, one of the largest retail pharmacy chains, and its CVS.com partner illustrate the key principle of blending "clicks and mortar."

E-consumers—and your institution's e-patients—are already surfing, shopping, and shipping a whole variety of health-related products from the national health care Web e-commerce sites. Why let them make their purchases at these Web sites when your organization can sell books written by your renowned physicians, supplements, and other health-related products locally and regionally?

- *e-Action #7*: *Diversify Health and Medical Web Sites from Information to Products and Services.* The fact is, managed care has reduced reimbursement revenues. Outpatient procedures are becoming the norm for many surgeries. Federal funding is not what it used to be. E-tailing is popular with e-consumers and e-patients, and it can deliver new revenue. Low-cost e-transactions via a Web-enabled storefront should be considered in your e-healthcare services strategy and part of the evolution of your Web site to a true service center. Consider e-tailing the following items:
  - vitamins and supplements
  - allergy-free products—pillowcases, aerators

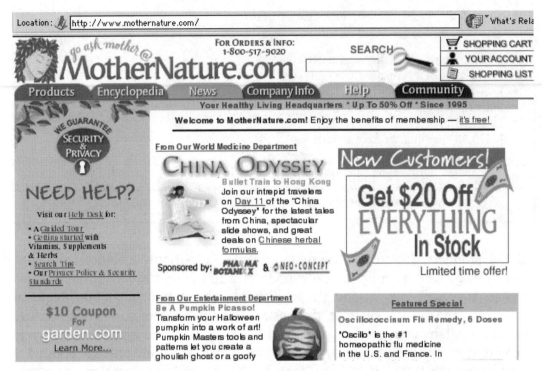

Figure 1–7 MotherNature.com. *Source:* Reprinted with permission from www.mothernature.com, © 1999, MotherNature.com.

- skin care products
- kids' games such as Bronchiasaurus, a CD-ROM game to keep asthmatic kids healthy
- local health and medical products and service companies that deliver everything from massage therapy to flowers

For some health care leaders, e-tailing may seem a bit too progressive. But remember that your e-consumers and e-patients are already shopping e-health e-tail at the global health Web portal sites and e-commerce services. If the money is going to be spent, why not have it spent through a Web service offered by your organization?

e-Trend #8: e-Medical Category Killers

If your organization is a health system or hospital that has a pharmacy or durable medical equipment company, it is probably under attack by on-line cat-

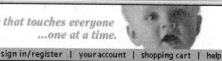
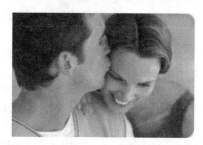

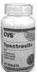

Figure 1–8 CVS.com. *Source:* Reprinted with permission from www.CVS.com, © 1999, CVS and Soma.com.

egory killers. On-line category killers are Web services such as www.drug-store.com or www.eToys.com that focus on delivering products or services on line in one particular market niche. These companies do business with the high over-head of fixed cost bricks and mortar facilities. Etoys.com only exists in cyberspace, whereas Toys R Us must support the high staff and facilities costs of operating toy stores throughout the world. This means on-line category killers can sell to everyone on line cheaper than their bricks and mortar competitors.

Local vendors no longer have the stronghold on consumers and patients when it comes to health and medical product purchases. Take the pharmacy industry, for example. For years, small pharmacies have been squeezed out by giants such as Walgreens and CVS. Now these behemoths have a new competitive threat from a new breed of pharmacy—the e-drugstore. Drugstore.com and PlanetRX.com are examples of how historic product lines can be disintermediated by new players in the market. Disintermediated refers to the use of on-line services to eliminate entire layers of distribution between a seller and a customer. BeDirect Dell (www.dell.com) is a great example. At mid-year 1999, Dell was selling $36 million in computers direct to consumers without the use of a computer superstore or other retailer. The traditional bricks and mortar retailer has been cut out of the transaction and the consumer gets a lower price and potentially better service. Surf on over to Drugstore.com to get a prescription refill, and you will probably find yourself sidetracked by all the other products—and the sales. There might be on-line-only prices for Advil. Click on the "hair care" page and select from hundreds of hair care product brands. Before your script is cyberfilled, you might find that your shopping basket is filled with toothpaste, soap, and vitamins.

Thousands of e-consumers and e-patients are taking advantage of the conve-nience and low prices available at on-line drugstores. And Drugstore.com is not the only category killer here: Cyberdrug.com, PlanetRX.com, and others are hit-ting the Net—along with traditional players Walgreens and Rite Aid. All of the major bricks-and-mortar pharmacies are taking different actions. As previously mentioned, CVS bought Soma.com and used Soma.com's e-commerce abilities to enhance www.cvs.com. Rite Aid made the strategic decision to buy into Drug-store.com and be a retail outlet for Drugstore.com's services. Not only do on-line pharmacies offer direct-to-your-door next-day delivery; they offer confidential-ity that eliminates embarrassing price checks on Ex-Lax and Preparation H.

- *e-Action #8: Automate the Top Priorities for Reduced Operating Costs through e-Commerce—and Save Money!* E-consumers love the convenience of buying on line—at home, on their own schedule. Do not let category killers such as on-line pharmacies or medical device manufacturers kill your product lines. Set up e-shop against these competitors. Web-enable your durable medical equipment service or in-house pharmacy and establish regional alliances that will drive a high volume of consumers to your Web services. One significant advantage of a regional Web service is that it can focus its advertising efforts on a regional market and leverage existing brands that have name awareness in a particular community. And in the case of on-line pharmacies, your organization can do better than the Web portals, since you are connected to the physicians who write the prescriptions. Two-way communication between e-patients and e-providers can execute on-line scripts and refills—and still push the product to the e-patient's door the next day.

The only way for regional pharmacies to fight back is to deliver great on-line and air-space service. It may take Drugstore.com one night to deliver a request, and consumers want many items immediately. A regional pharmacy chain can deliver something in a hour, or a consumer can pick it up the same day. If regional chains do not fight back, they will find their business declining while they are forced to fulfill same-day requests for global on-line pharmacy services. Success in the twenty-first century will truly depend on being "clicks and mortar!"

e-PREDICTION #4: e-CARE DELIVERY WILL BE THE DOMINANT FORM OF MEDICAL DELIVERY IN THE YEAR 2010

e-Trend #9: e-Healthcare @ Home

Accessing the Internet using "information appliances"—from Internet-enabled telephones to WebTV to the PC-in-the-door Frigidaire—is changing how physicians and health systems offer and provide medical care. Allowing patients to be cared for in their own home, via a device such as an iPhone or two-way video connection, is the way of the future. "Cybervisits" will become as commonplace as the annual physical—which will most likely evolve into a cyberphysical. Elderly patients can be treated in the security and comfort of their own homes, and those with chronic disease can perform their own daily e-checkup—such as testing their blood sugar level or performing a pulmonary function test—and log it so physicians, nurses, and other providers can monitor care on line.

Companies such as Patient Infosystems are making this type of at-home care possible, using Internet applications, PCs, and the telephone. Diabetic patients, for example, enter their glucose levels into a Web-enabled application, and the data are monitored by qualified clinicians. Unless there is a problem, the e-patient does not have to see a physician. A recent program for asthmatics cost $1 per patient and returned $8 per patient.[17] Patient Infosystems (www.health-desk.com/web/products/internetapps.html) has programs for hypertension and on-line nutrition counseling and evaluation. All the programs are designed to keep people at home for their care.

During the twenty-first century, the primary site of care delivery will be the home. Telemedicine in the home is rapidly becoming a reality. Significant portions of outpatient care will take place in the home—via both personal visits by caregivers and cybervisits through interactive, broadband connections. With the increasingly widespread implementation of cable modems, high-speed digital access through digital subscriber lines, and fast wireless satellite connections, technology and bandwidth are no longer limiting factors. The factors slowing the dissemination of telemedicine in the home are reimbursement, medical and legal factors, and the ability of patients to learn to use the interactive programs to support better health. Time and pressure from consumers who want convenience and want it from their home, along with the fact that operating costs for delivering care in the home will be significantly reduced, will force payers to figure out the reimbursement methodologies sooner rather than later.

- *e-Action #9: Start Paving the Way for Health Care at Home Now.* New e-communications technology will improve the cost, quality, and convenience of care delivery. Empower your e-patients to manage much of their own care. If you are part of a health plan, consider implementing in-home monitoring for two common disease states—diabetes and asthma. Give away Net devices such as iPhones (www.MDtel.com); the return on that investment will far outweigh their cost! If you are a hospital or health system, sponsor a program for patients to get connected with on-line support groups. Share the cost with a pharmaceutical company that makes a drug that supports a certain condition—for example, your hospital and Marion Merrill Dow, maker of Cardizem, could pay for WebTV for seniors with cardiovascular disease so they can connect with others on line about their condition. The bottom line is, do not view the distribution of "free" Net devices as an expense. It is an investment that will reduce costs and lower medical loss ratios in the long term; plus, it will enable your organization to control the consumer health interface to the Net.

The bandwidth available drives the nature and type of e-services that are possible. As the world moves from 28.8 and 56K modems to high-speed connections, the amount of information and e-services that can be cost-effectively sent directly to the consumer home changes radically (Figure 1–9). In the low-

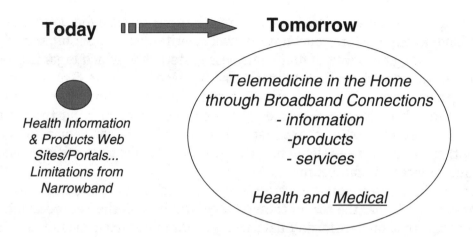

Figure 1–9 From Information to Relationships. *Source:* Copyright © 1999, Douglas Goldstein.

bandwidth world, text and pictures push the limits unless various approaches to data compression are used. In the high-bandwidth future of tomorrow, all applications need to be interactive and look and feel like television programming in order to meet consumer expectations. With high-bandwidth Net services reaching more and more homes each year, the reality of telemedicine in the home is here!

Physicians must be an integral part of marrying high tech with high touch. Medicine at home represents a significant change in the way they currently practice; obtaining input and buy-in from them and their managers is critical to success. And speaking of behavior change, those plan executives or government officials reading this chapter must begin to re-assess the old reimbursement model—which rewards taking care of sick people—and re-invent, *e-invent,* new methodologies that address e-communication and e-care in a digital world.

e-Trend #10: Being Med Digital

The Internet and "e" technology can no longer be viewed as simply aspects of temporary business strategies. Being med digital has to become part of the fabric of a health care organization. If "e" is not one of the CEO and management team's top three initiatives, then your organization is likely to be "Amazoned," perhaps by a competitor you did not even recognize in last year's strengths, weaknesses, opportunities, and threats analysis. (Because they were late to the on-line game, Borders Books was Amazoned, and the CEO lost his job.)

If you are part of a national chain of regional pharmacies, did your organization have www.drugstore.com on its 1998 competitor list? If your organization is not reinventing your way of doing business better, then which organization is? Why has the growth of on-line stock trading been so rapid? E-consumers can make trades more quickly, at lower cost, and with more information than when going through a broker! When the speed of the connectivity and the software application allow people to experience better on-line services or transactions than they could on the telephone or in person, organizations without leading on-line services will fall behind.

One of the basic economic forces driving the current and future transformation of health care is that the cost of transferring data through the Net is dramatically lower than that of transferring data using electronic mechanisms of the 1980s and 1990s. Today and in the future, the lower cost of moving data through the Net through "packet" rather than dedicated "circuit" technology means that organizational processes and structures will be altered forever (see Exhibit 1–7). Success today depends on speed to market within an environment of coached chaos, common goals, connection, and creativity.

As the cost of moving data is reduced exponentially, the organization of companies changes. The top-down hierarchical structure of the industrial age is all but dead. New "e" models of structure are evolving where customers are in the center, supported by a nexus of e-service and staffing (Figure 1–10). The "e" organization is linked through virtual connections, relationships, and a flexible team structure that can evolve as the challenges of the marketplace are addressed.

Take the short quiz in Exhibit 1–8 to determine whether your organization has gone fully digital. If you cannot answer "yes" to all these questions, you are not

---

Exhibit 1–7 Costs of Data Transfer Drives Processes

Industrial/Info Age	Internet (Web) Age
• Consistency	• Creativity
• Control	• Coached chaos
• Continuity	• Connection
• Channels	• Common goals
• High cost of transmitting data	• Very low cost of transmitting data

Source: Copyright © 1999, Douglas Goldstein.

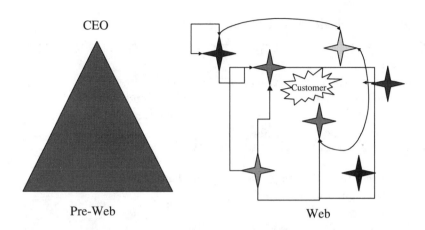

Figure 1–10 Pre-Web and Web Management Structures. *Source:* Copyright © 1999, Douglas Goldstein.

yet med digital! It takes a forward-thinking leader to usher an organization into the new millennium of e-healthcare. If you answered "no" to any of these questions, you have to do much better.

- *e-Action #10: Imagination Is More Important Than Information or Knowledge.* Your organization will have truly embraced the e-healthcare revolution only when "e" penetrates every area of the organization. When that is the case, the entire health care process will look very different. Consider the example that follows.

Sally, her husband, and her two children have just moved to town, and they are looking for physicians and other health care providers. Sally logs on to the regional health system's Web channel from her interactive television one evening to select a physician, order disposable diapers, obtain reviews on local physicians, and send flowers to her mother, who just went home from the hospital. After Sally enters the women's health area of the channel, an article about a medical breakthrough catches her eye—apparently, a particular brand of birth control pill reduces the risk of ovarian cancer. The pharmaceutical manufacturer of this brand has an ovarian cancer risk assessment next to the article. Sally decides to participate interactively on line and then downloads a fact sheet about discount coupons for the brand.

"I want a woman physician," Sally thinks as she completes a series of questions through a Web-based voice recognition questionnaire about her prefer-

Exhibit 1–8 Is Your Health Care Company Med Digital?

	Yes	No
Our CEO and senior management team are "e" literate.	___	___
We do not print out e-mails and then have someone respond.	___	___
Our Web services offer interactive e-products and e-services, and we're planning our strategy for e-care delivery.	___	___
Our Web front-end interface is tied into our legacy systems for customer service.	___	___
We have less paper to sort through every day; our corporate Internet helped save the rain forest.	___	___

Source: Copyright © 1999, Douglas Goldstein.

ences regarding obstetrics/gynecology (OB/GYN) physicians and pediatricians. When she is presented with the top three matches based on her criteria, she begins to review an audio-video stream profile on each one. She stops on Dr. Mary Winkle because she likes the soft tone of her voice and the fact that Dr. Winkle has a daughter about the age of Kristin, Sally's oldest child.

Sally then connects directly to Dr. Winkle's physician–patient Web service, completes her on-line registration, and schedules an appointment for two days later. Then she moves on to completing a health risk profile, new patient history, and background, and she is able to attach medical records stored in the family WebMedVault. During the new patient history on-line process, Sally was webcast three different education videos concerning prevention and early diagnosis of the conditions that Sally indicated existed in her family history. Sally then clicks over to her previous OB/GYN's site, logs on to her personal chart, copies the records, and attaches them to an e-mail for Dr. Winkle's staff.

Sally performs a similar process to find a pediatrician and schedules a checkup for her children. Before logging off for the night, she realizes that she needs vitamin supplements and an antibiotic ointment, so she orders them through this regional health and medical channel's e-commerce service.

As the children are getting ready for school the next day, a pop-up screen appears while Sally watches the *Today* show. It is a reminder about her appointment with Dr. Winkle, along with a list of what additional information to bring with her, how long the appointment will take, and how to get there. Later that morning, Sally receives the same information for the kids' new pediatrician, along with two recommended local channels that focus on attention-deficit hyperactivity disorder—which Kristin has—and offer psychologist-monitored on-line support groups for moms.

The day of Sally's appointment with Dr. Winkle arrives. Registration is simple. Sally provides a few signatures; her copayment is automatically deducted from her cyberwallet, which she set up with a credit card when she registered. The staff have previously done a Web-based eligibility check, so there are no delays as she registers, but they tell her that her health plan requires her to pay out of pocket for any lab tests.

Dr. Winkle is as nice as she seemed on her video. She discusses Sally's endometriosis and notes that she should e-mail Sally a list of on-line community resources, including on-line and off-line support groups, useful regional Web sites, and several educational video streams. She also suggests that Sally join a live cyberforum being held on endometriosis next week. After Dr. Winkle performs her examination, she dictates into a Web-based transcription service. Embedded in the Web dictation service is an artificial intelligence function that automatically codes relevant Current Procedural Terminology codes and International Classification of Diseases, Ninth Edition, Clinical Modification codes, based on Dr. Winkle's dictation.

It is time for Sally to check out. No encounter form is completed, and no money changes hands. The staff tell Sally that her lab results will be e-mailed to her in about three days and suggest that she check the practice's frequently asked questions or on-line triage service monitored and supported by the office nurses and the health system call center after hours if she has further questions. Sally's claim is automatically transmitted over the Net to her insurance company by the end of the day.

This example shows the many opportunities to streamline the patient experience in the twenty-first century. Web applications and e-processes to support all of the above transactions exist today! Technology and the Internet will certainly be used in the medical service process to achieve significant cost reductions and improve customer service for the patient. The challenge is to create a consumer-friendly and well-organized Web interface integrated with the operating systems of the physician, health system, and other health care organizations sooner rather than later. Remember, every great idea was first a dream or thought before becoming reality.

RAPIDLY E-VOLVING FUTURE OF E-HEALTHCARE

Billions of dollars are being invested in developing regional, national, and international e-healthcare services. There is a whole generation of evolving health and medical Web services seeking to attract consumers and develop relationships with them, deliver business-to-business e-services, and much, much more. Many of the consumer health Web sites are focused on selling advertising and generating on-line sales revenue from selling vitamins or self-care products.

There are numerous e-companies seeking to improve the connectivity between the different trading partners in health care through Web-based solutions. Nearly every health and medical manufacturer is seeking to automate on the Web a number of transactions and customer service activities that have traditionally involved electronic data interchange or traditional call centers.

Intel thinks health care is one of the next big growth areas of the Net and sponsors an annual Internet e-Health Day (www.intel.com/ehealth). Intel has invested in some health-related Internet companies, including LifeMasters (www.lifemasters.net), an on-line care support company that monitors e-patients with chronic illness via various "e" technologies such as smart on-line disease support, telephones, pagers, the Web, and so on. See Chapters 6 and 9 for more information on on-line disease management.

Your organization must take e-action to apply Internet technology in all its forms, including Intranets, Extranets, public Internet @ HomeNet, and tobe-created.net. There are some key questions to address.

- How are you going to jump ahead of known and unknown competitors?
- How is your organization going to harness "e" technology to energize, empower, enhance, and expand your services throughout the twenty-first century?

If your health care organization wants to win in the e-healthcare revolution, it must continuously be aware of the health care e-trendscape. Track both business and health care e-trends and their implications for your business and markets. Ask, "What is the e-trend, and how will it affect how we deliver products and services? What actions do we take in the next three months or year to move proactively to be a leader in e-healthcare?" Lead your organization to e-healthcare understanding and action!

HEALTHCARE E-TIPS FOR SUCCESS

Race, do not walk, to executive management to discuss the key threats, opportunities, and solutions associated with your e-services efforts. Lead your organization into the e-healthcare revolution with the e-tips listed below.

Be a Leader and Deliver the "e" Message. Health care organizations have rarely jumped on a new business trend or been the first to use new technology. But if your organization does not shift into high e-healthcare gear fast, it stands to lose revenue, brand relationships, and market share! Take a risk and deliver the message: the Web is here to stay, and interactive televisions and iPhones are rapidly being deployed. If your organization does not do something "e" fast, it will get Amazoned—or worse yet, get steamrollered by demanding e-consumers and e-patients. Yes, it has taken longer for the efficiencies of the Web to affect health care than to affect books, real estate, and stock buying. Health care transactions are notably complex. But now, with Web acceptance widening every day, enhanced communications and links, and better security features, e-healthcare is going full force into the e-future.

Use Jujitsu on the Resistance. Scout out the William Orton(s) in your organization. The principle in jujitsu is to channel opponents' energy against themselves. When opponents advocate sticking with the "tried and true" ways of delivering care, then share knowledge on how the Internet revolution compares to other great communication revolutions of the past 90 years—radio and television, for instance. Use e-mail, Web sites, Web tour buses, and interactive approaches to illustrate how to do things better and faster with Net technology. Resistant health care leaders must ultimately realize that e-business Darwinism will prevail. Slow-moving Compaq CEO Eckhard Pfieiffer was ousted by his own board because of his inability to embrace the new world of e-commerce. Your board may do the same if your organization gets Amazoned like Borders (whose CEO was also ousted) did!

Change the "Thinking" and "Business Model." Say aloud the new e-mantra: "Traditional business models do not work on the Net." Repeat. The saying "you can't teach an old dog new tricks" comes to mind. Old habits are hard to break, but the new generation of e-consumers and e-patients will change that. Just watch.

Famous for committees, task forces, and meetings, health care organizations love to test, research, and ponder new ideas before putting a plan into action. Cancel the meetings and shorten the discussion. *Do something fast.* If your biggest e-proclamation is "we use e-mail!" you are missing the bigger picture. E-business is about e-communication, e-commerce, and e-care delivery with everyone—that means with e-patients and all e-consumers.

Do e-Healthcare. Thinking and building support are good, but to be success-ful you have "to do" something. There will be a number of imperatives for physi-cians, health systems, and health care organizations in the twenty-first century.

- Build your brand—across all media, including cyberspace.
- Enhance your medical relationships.
- Reduce Web service costs through alliances and group purchasing.
- Build health and medical Web e-services that deliver information, products, and services.
- Support behavior change based on the pleasure principles, meaning that people respond much better to incentives and positive reinforcement than they do to harsh discipline.

To achieve these goals, an interactive Web service that is customized to your medical e-community is essential. This means Web-enabling health and medical e-communities, e-commerce, and e-care delivery. It means integrating cyber-space with real-time interactions between caregivers and patients in the home and your organization's facilities and providers. Use your e-service to facilitate mission-critical health care transactions.

- Develop customized interactive Web services such as on-line health risk ap-praisals for submission and feedback, medical records, downloadable diaries, logs, and journals to support healthier behaviors.
- Support your brands and those of allied physicians by creating Web services for communication from provider to provider and provider to patient. The next generation of Web application must be designed to evolve rapidly with new features and plug-in applications.
- Provide patients with opportunities for interaction in the form of on-line resource and database searches, as well as high-involvement, fun-focused activities such as clubs, games, contests, bulletin boards and forums, and on-line and air-space chat rooms and support groups.
- Look for resources that address the mind-body connection and alternative or holistic approaches to medicine; and provide guidance on health care fraud, quackery, and misinformation within the Web, mailing lists, and newsgroups.

Remember to make it personal and make it fun! When consumers hit a medical Web service, it must address whether they are first-time visitors or regular e-patients. It must deliver information, products, and services based on the plea-sure principle. Consumers do not want to be managed. They do not want to be disciplined. They do not want to "have to do" something. Creating behavior change in health and medical care depends on personalizing and using the pleasure principle. The pleasure principle is focused on encouraging behavior change based on incentives and positive reinforcement rather than discipline and negative feedback. This means promoting wellness on your Web service by offering resources on fitness, nutrition, health conditions and problems, and stress and psychological issues—personalized to the e-patient's lifestyle and health needs. You will not be able to discipline behavior change, but consumers certainly do respond to the incentives.

Build e-Databases with Customer Approval and Involvement. You cannot get to e-care tomorrow without e-databases today. The first and often missed step is to start building an e-database now. For instance, why are the majority of health systems and physicians not collecting e-mail addresses at the site of the care transaction? Because they never have in the past, no one thought about it, a form has to be changed, or no one has instructed front-line staff to do so. The Web is about "unique visitors on a monthly basis," which is how Web services measure their success in marketing. Health care companies that are digital tout their number of registered users: "Here are the physicians and health systems with tens of thousands of customers who interact with our Web channel on a daily basis."

To begin with, modify these out-of-date forms and gather e-data. Just like the telephone, the Internet will change communications forever. Would you do business today without a telephone number? Of course not. But ask your Web task force or technology department, "How many consumer or patient names do we have in our e-mail databases?" "Do we have e-mail addresses for at least 5 percent to 60 percent of our customers?" In most cases, the answer will be "no."

In the next year, you will not be able to do business without one or more Web services that deliver information and services to key audiences—via e-mail, live chat and other on-line services. Amend registration and intake forms to include e-mail addresses, survey e-patients about their on-line needs and wants, and start building an e-database today.

The message to health care organizations is clear. Consumers and patients want on-line services now. Do not allow other Web players to steal your thunder. Mobilize the marketing, education, and customer service power of the Web in your organization. Do something smart. Do something fast. Start your strategic Internet and Intranet planning and development initiative *now*.

Take control of Web-enabled applications and e-care delivery in your market and win the e-healthcare revolution.

REFERENCES

1. S. Fitzgibbons and R. Lee, *The health.net Industry* (New York: Hambrecht & Quist, 1999), 8.

2. Fitzgibbons and Lee, *The health.net Industry,* 8–10.

3. Fitzgibbons and Lee, *The health.net Industry,* 10.

4. "More People Online without PCs," http://cyberatlas.internet.com/big_picture/demographics/quest.html (20 April 1999), accessed 17 June 1999.

5. "38 Million Americans Getting Wired," http://cyberatlas.internet.com/big_picture/demographics/mainstream.html (14 January 1999), accessed 17 June 1999.

6. J. Ledbetter, "Men Are from Mars, Women Are from AOL," http://www.thestandard.com/articles/display/0,1449,1750,00.html (18 September 1998), accessed 9 March 1999.

7. B. Tracy, "Survey Says Women Want Web Sites That Build Relationships," http://adage.com/interactive/articles/19970922/article1.html (September 1997), accessed 17 March 1999.

8. D. Bellandi, "Consumers First," *Modern Healthcare,* 26 January 1998, 30.

9. "Online Investing Goes Mainstream," http://www.cyberatlas.com/market/finance/forr.html (11 March 1999), accessed 18 June 1999.

10. J. Cohen, "Everybody's a Banker," *The Industry Standard,* 15 March, 1999, 36–40.

11. eHealth, inc., *Business Plan,* 22 March 1999, 24.

12. eHealth, inc., *Business Plan,* 24.

13. D. Goldstein, "Do It Better...Online! Energizing Improved Customer Relations through Internet Technology," *Managed Care Interface,* January 1999, 46–47.

14. D. Goldstein, "Do It Better...Online!," 11.

15. M. Leibovich et al., "Internet's E-Conomy Gets Read," *Washington Post,* 20 June 1999, A1.

16. "Online Holiday Shopping Triples," *Catalog Age Weekly,* 31 December 1998.

17. http://www.healthdesk.com, accessed 24 August 1999.

e-Commerce:
The New Business Model

Douglas E. Goldstein

EVERY COUPLE OF DECADES, business in the United States undergoes a fundamental shift. The 1950s had Main Street. The 1970s saw Americans get hooked on shopping malls. In the 1980s Americans fell for franchises, and giants such as Wal-Mart led the superstore craze of the 1990s. As each new retailing paradigm toppled its predecessor, a new group of company leaders emerged. For example, Sears never made it out of the mall. Home Depot squashed the mom-and-pop hardware store. And who was really paying attention when Ray Crock bought a hamburger joint from the McDonald brothers in 1955?

Time and again, company leaders missed early warning signs. Had they attended to these signs, the leaders could have prevented their company's demise. Their failure to recognize that a new business model was about to be built often resulted in historic disasters. Can you say Wal-Mart? Microsoft? E*TRADE.com? Dell? Amazon.com? If you can, now is the time for health care chief executive officers (CEOs), board members, and physician leaders to stand up and take notice of the new business models that are being built. These models center on e-technology.

Forget the hype, forget the sales numbers, and forget the fact that in mid-1999, 92 million people were surfing the Web in North America.[1] This paradigm shift is not about numbers. And frankly, it is not just about "I" for Internet. *It is about "e" for electronic multimedia.* It is about the emergence of e-commerce, which is proving to be the foundation of an entirely new industrial order. E-commerce will change the relationship between companies and customers in ways no one has yet predicted. Try to build a new business model on that! The reality is that the only way to try is to get in the game with a series of well-funded initiatives that can rapidly e-volve over time. Learning by doing is the only way in the e-world of today. Frankly, your e-commerce effort is equal if not more important than the Y2K effort of the late 1990s.

Simply put, e-commerce is revolutionizing the entire business world—the way people compare prices, buy groceries, find information, advertise products, facilitate transactions, see physicians, and so on. If the exponential rise of on-line retail revenues from 1997 to 1998 is any indication of things to come, 1999 will likely go down in history as the year when e-retailing—or e-tailing—and e-commerce really began to take off. On-line holiday shopping alone more than tripled in 1998—$13 billion, up from $2.6 billion in 1997. Boston Consulting Group predicted that on-line sales in 1999 would reach $30 billion to $40 billion.[2,3] Exhibit 2–1 offers more information about today's e-growth, which is reshaping American business.

During 1999, mainstream Americans took to the Internet. According to IntelliQuest, 51 percent of those who planned to get wired in 1999 were over the age of 35, 49 percent had a high school education or less, and 58 percent made less than $50,000 a year.[4] When the "average" American began to surf in cyberspace, the Internet ceased being a novelty and became a source of e-information and a site of e-commerce and e-communication. As a result, holiday on-line shopping figures were predicted to triple from 1998 expenditures, which were just over $3 billion, according to Jupiter Communications.[5] Yes, these projections could be wrong, but when it comes to the Internet, they probably are too low.

The speed of change and transition is awesome. Just think, in four years, Yahoo.com has become one of the world's most recognized brands. The speed of Net communications and the ability to disseminate information, knowledge, and deliver e-service are unparalleled in history. Just as dogs live seven years for every human year, one calendar year in the non-Net world equals three or four

---

Exhibit 2–1 E-Growth

1. More Americans doing "e-verything" on line. By 2002, International Data Corporation predicts that 136 million Americans will be on line—about 50 percent of the U.S. population.
2. Consumer buying on line "e-xplodes." On-line consumer sales have been estimated at $40 billion by the year 2000. In addition, on-line research influences billions of dollars of traditional purchases.
3. Rapid acceleration in on-line advertising and sponsorship. Forrester Research projects that on-line advertising will grow from $1.9 billion in 1998 to $7.7 billion by 2002.

Source: Copyright © 1999, Douglas Goldstein.

Net years. Just think about it as if your quarterly plan was your annual plan. If your organization does not act, a known or unknown competitor will be planning your Net demise!

Powered by the Internet pipeline, the e-consumer of the new millennium has access to voluminous amounts of information on which he or she can base purchase decisions. The e-consumer has easy one-touch access to new levels of service and transactions. On the World Wide Web, health care organizations compete for market share and the attention of their region's consumers. Health care organizations have only just begun to recognize the Web's unique ability to cost-effectively build long-lasting customer relationships through improved e-service delivery.

As more and more Americans are wired and can easily access the Net from interactive televisions, computers, and Internet-enabled telephones or iPhones, the following trends will continue:

- E-consumers will have access to everything very quickly across information appliances (telephones, computers, televisions, cell phones, PalmPilots, etc.).
- Transactions will move from lag time to real time, anytime, anywhere—24 hours a day, seven days a week.
- One-to-one marketing and relationship development with e-consumers and e-patients will really be possible and affordable.
- Telephone-based customer service and medical call centers will become one with the Net or Web telephony or voice over Internet protocol.

Health care executives who maintain that the Net is a fleeting fantasy should call the former CEOs of Compaq and Borders for some advice. Both CEOs were ousted in 1999 for failure to successfully lead their companies into the age of e-commerce.

From a consumer's perspective, health care is not an information business. It is a service business where information is part of the process, not the destination. Consequently, for the health care industry, the current wave is e-commerce and the next cyber tsunami is e-care delivery. The time lag between waves is minimal.

If e-commerce in other industries is an adolescent, then e-commerce in health care—and most especially, e-care delivery—is still a newborn. Nearly all other industries have outpaced the health care industry in on-line growth, but the genie is now out of the bottle. It is time that health care executives and physicians learn from other industries and begin to apply these e-principles to America's health care system.

Does this mean your health care system, medical practice, health plan, or health organization is going to become a full-fledged e-retailer? Not necessarily. The delivery of health care is far more complex than selling a product on line and collecting credit card payments. But count on the shift beyond e-commerce to *e-care delivery*—to bust existing health care delivery paradigms wide open.

E-care delivery is the right way to meet e-consumer and e-patient needs on line—and at the same time recognize that, unlike retail, health care is personal, confidential, and private. E-care delivery strategies recognize the fact that not all aspects of health care fit neatly into a simple cyberspace transaction. Integration of cyberspace, phone-space, and air-space visits is important to an e-care delivery strategy, as Exhibit 2–2 shows. And yes, e-retailing is part of e-care delivery too. If your organization does not rapidly evolve and shift its business model to one that contains e-commerce and e-care strategies, one of your known or unknown competitors will.

If you do not want your health care organization to go the way of the dinosaurs, it is critical to understand the e-trends that are shaping e-commerce in other industries. These trends illustrate the ways retailers, manufacturers, and service providers are re-creating their business models to "clicks and mortar"—just as your organization should clearly understand how the Internet is revolutionizing health care e-communication, e-commerce, e-communities, and e-care.

This chapter highlights ways that the Net and "e" services are revolutionizing our lives and offers key e-actions for health care that accelerate your Net learn-

---

Exhibit 2–2 E-Care Delivery

1. E-communication between e-patients and their physicians
2. E-services such as real-time call centers—Web-enabled call centers where e-patients can receive triaged medical e-advice from qualified professionals via cyberspace, telephone space, video streaming, audio streaming, or e-mail
3. E-communities where e-consumers and e-patients share information and support about particular health concerns and disease states
4. E-care delivery—on-line monitoring for chronic conditions via personal computers, interactive televisions, and iPhones
5. E-commerce such as offering health-related products and services on line and interfacing with related business partners such as insurance companies and suppliers

Source: Copyright © 1999, Douglas Goldstein.

ing so your organization can leapfrog known and unknown competitors that seek to erode your market share.

CHANGING THE WAY AMERICANS DO "E-VERYTHING"

E-commerce lesson number one comes from bookstore retailers. Several years ago, a little Web site called Amazon.com offered consumers the option to search for and purchase books on the Internet. Before companies such as Barnes & Noble could say "business books are in aisle 4," Amazon's initial public offering had become legendary. "Bricks and mortar" booksellers were left holding their book bags and wondering what hit them. Look at Table 2–1, which lists the number of monthly visitors to each of the three major Web booksellers. Even though these retailers' e-commerce responses to Amazon have been admirable, their on-line sales still lack luster. At the end of 1998, Amazon had grown to amass 6.5 million visitors a month—versus Borders' 256,000 and Barnes & Noble's 2.9 million—and Amazon's market capitalization of $18 billion at the end of 1998 was more than four times that of Borders and Barnes & Noble combined. This market cap is even more amazing given that Amazon.com has less than half the revenue of the other two organizations (around $600 million and lost nearly $160 million on the year) while the other air-space booksellers had in excess of $2 billion in revenue each and both made profits.

What is so fascinating about Amazon.com? Part of the lure when it launched in the mid-1990s was the fact that consumers could get more than just a book. Amazon.com felt like a coffeehouse; visitors could post their own opinion of a book they had read and read others' opinions. Not just professional reviewers, not just publishers, but other real people. They could "talk back," demanding

Table 2–1 Traditional Booksellers Get "Amazoned"

Bookseller	12/98 Online Visitors per Month	1998 Revenue	1998 Profits (Losses)	1998 Market Capitalization
Amazon.com	6.5 million	$610 million	$(160 million)	18 billion
Barnes and Noble, Inc.	2.9 million	$3 billion		2.2 billion
Borders, Inc.	256,000	$2.27 billion	$79 million	1.8 billion

Source: Data from Charles Schwab Online Research Library, 1999, Direct S&P Stock Reports, and Barnes and Noble 1998 Annual Report.

unique products and customized services. Further, the click of a mouse would bring up even the most obscure titles on just about any subject. If the book was out of print, Amazon.com would find it. Amazon's focus has first and foremost always been customer service. That focus has resulted in book sales of $610 million in 1998—313 percent higher than 1997 sales.

After adding music, videos, and gifts and forging a 46 percent stake in Drugstore.com, Amazon (www.amazon.com) continues to be a driving force in Internet commerce—regardless of the fact that the e-bookseller has yet to make a profit. "Helping people find and discover the things they want, and helping folks make better purchase decisions" is what CEO Jeff Bezos says it is all about. Amazon's OneClick service "remembers" consumers when they return to the site, and Gift Click offers a unique way to send presents.

- *e-Action for Health Care: Do Not Get "Amazoned."* The biggest lesson for health care companies is not to get "Amazoned"—the term used to describe what happened to companies who were flattened in their industry when the first competitor with hundreds of millions in venture capital set up shop on the Internet. The historically slow-to-change culture of health care organizations and providers can be deadly in the age of e-commerce; resist the temptation to be reactive, and be proactive instead.

Rapid consolidation in the hospital industry in the 1980s and 1990s left most regions with two to four health systems that compete with each other as well as scattered independent hospitals. Amalgamation of the insurance industry has resulted in similar oligopolies. If your health care company is not the first, with enough capital, e-thought leaders, and an e-business model that works, your competitor will be. And you will be Amazoned before you know it. Step up to the plate by offering e-commerce, e-communication solutions, and e-care to consumers that save them time and money now.

SAVING TIME AND MONEY BY ELIMINATING THE STOCKBROKER

You heard all about it on CNN, CNBC, and the Today Show. Maybe you were even part of the boom. As the volatile and tumultuous stock market made millionaires out of many Americans in 1998 and 1999, on-line trading exploded. The on-line brokerage industry accumulated 3.6 million accounts in 1998, according to Piper Jaffray, Inc., representing a whopping $420 billion in assets. Of the approximately 336,000 trades each day during the fourth quarter of 1998, 27 percent were placed by individual investors, on line; that is more than 90,000 trades per day.[6] By mid-1999, E*TRADE (Figure 2–1) had over a million customer accounts and composed 7 percent of New York Stock Exchange volume and 18 percent of Nasdaq volume.[7] The company asserts that "someday, we'll *all* invest this way," and it is probably right. Individual investors can access free real-time quotes and gather their own information about stocks they plan to purchase. The best news: commission charges are as low as $14.95 per trade. A 1998 study by Cyber Dialogue and Booz-Allen & Hamilton estimated that 10 million brokerage account holders would be trading on line.[8]

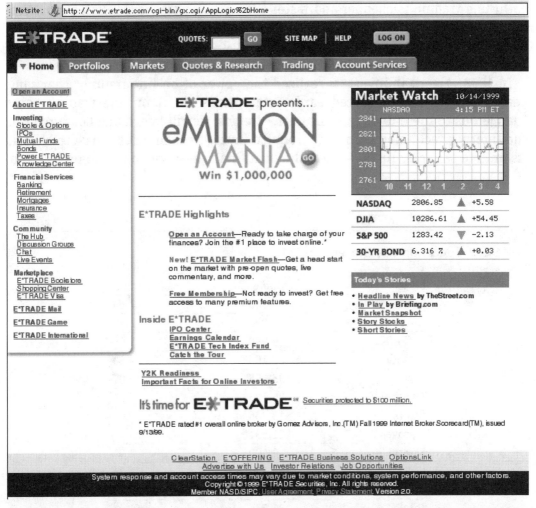

Figure 2–1 E*TRADE. *Source:* Reprinted with permission from www.etrade.com, © 1999, E*TRADE Securities, Inc. E*TRADE is a registered trademark of E*TRADE Securities, Inc.

Table 2–2 describes the trading volumes of the top 10 on-line brokers. E-consumers like the convenience of on-line brokers, and brokerage firms like the low cost of doing business this way. Charles Schwab (www.schwab.com) is the industry leader, Charles Schwab. The father of discount brokerages, Schwab was the first to realize the potential of on-line trading. The Internet broker logs, on average, more than twice the trades per day as the number two player. The comprehensive Schwab site allows investors to access reams of company, trend, and research data, and channels such as Schwab's OneSource mutual fund analyzer empower visitors to make informed choices. The newer www.myschwab.com can be tailored to suit a customer's preferences.

On-line trading is cheaper and faster than placing trades through a stockbroker. E-consumers have great access to information, knowledge, and research. Market mavens like Cheryl Peterson think on-line trading is better than talking to a person! See Exhibit 2–3.

In 1998, American investors realized the power of on-line trading. That same year, Merrill Lynch retracted earlier statements about on-line trading being "dangerous to the individual consumer." In fact, Merrill Lynch and Co. purchased the Internet technology group of troubled investment firm D.E. Shaw to beef up its on-line services. In 1999, Merrill Lynch finally responded to the on-line bro-

Table 2–2 Top 10 On-line Brokers

Broker	Trades/Day	Share
Charles Schwab	93,000	27.6%
Waterhouse	42,003	12.5%
E*TRADE	39,990	11.9%
Fidelity	33,100	9.8%
Datek	33,695	10.0%
Ameritrade	25,725	7.6%
DLJ Direct	13,366	4.0%
Discover	11,531	3.4%
Suretrade	9,600	2.9%
NDB	4,420	1.3%
Others	30,306	9.0%
Total	336,736	

Source: Reprinted with permission U.S. Bancorp/Piper Jaffray, © 1998.

Exhibit 2–3 A Market Maven Speaks Out

"I don't want to have to wait on hold to talk to a broker; I just go to my Schwab account, place my bid, and I get an e-mail when the order is filled." An individual Phoenix investor echoes the sentiments of thousands of savvy stock buyers across the country. On-line brokerages such as Charles Schwab, E*Trade, and Ameritrade empower do-it-yourself investors with the research data, news, and company statistics needed to make investment decisions without the help of a broker or financial advisor. Says the investor, "I'm no dummy—I can read the *Wall Street Journal* and the information at the Schwab site and know what I want without 'expert' advice. I also like being able to spend time in the evenings and on weekends doing research about potential stock buys—and traditional brokerage firms aren't open during those hours."

Source: Copyright © 1999, Douglas Goldstein.

kers with its own robust on-line alternative blended with real-time linkage with their extensive broker network.

The big market buzz for on-line brokerages is about electronic communications networks, or ECNs, that directly link buy and sell orders. These systems bypass traditional stock specialists and market makers and deprive them of the profit they squeeze out of the difference between the buy and sell orders they process. ECNs are growing at a fast clip and now routinely account for more than a fifth of Nasdaq's daily volume. In fact, investors now funnel one in seven trades through any of more than 100 Internet brokers—significantly cutting into Wall Street firms' commission business. The phenomenal growth of the networks has left the New York Stock Exchange, more than 200 years old, with little choice but to consider partnering with one of the nine established ECNs. But the Big Board better watch its backside; ECNs are seeking recognition as full-fledged exchanges—a move that would change the Wall Street landscape significantly.

- *e-Action for Health Care: Is a Service Business—Make Your Web Service Better Than a Telephone Call!* Just as the traditional stockbroker was the "expert advice giver" in pre-Internet days, so was the physician the first and last word on what was best for the patient. The evolution of stockbrokers from expert to information facilitator (individual investors still may consult with their broker—but they do it armed with research and statistics collected on their own) is an indication of what is to come for physicians and health care providers.

Already physicians are confronted in the exam room by patients with pages printed from the Web. This trend will continue as more and more Americans seek information about their own care, *prior to* scheduling a visit with the physician. The physician's role could evolve from "medical expert" to "facilitator of health information decision making" to help these e-patients decipher what they found on the Web.

To deliver better customer e-service, physicians must respond with their own robust "e" services, such as on-line patient registration, appointment scheduling, and on-line triage for typical medical problems. Integrating all of these functions into their customer service telephone systems will allow them to provide better service than cyberphysicians because local physicians hold a competitive advantage: A typical physician can link cyberspace to a nurse in the office to a patient's medical record to an actual visit, where a physician or other provider can heal and help.

Health care providers must also realize that consumers are not as security phobic as was once imagined. Tens of thousands of investors maintain on-line accounts and trust the accuracy of on-line transactions with what is often their life savings. About 60 percent to 75 percent of today's consumers have e-mail addresses. How many providers are capturing that information to lower practice expenses? Very few.

Patients are wired, your future competitor is wired. Why not you? If physicians build their e-mail databases just as they have collected telephone numbers, then this information can be used to lower practice operations cost and improve the physician–patient relationship. As the saying goes, "use it or lose it." E-communications with e-patients can solidify the physician–patient relationship; continuing to buck the trend will further erode this relationship. In the past, you could not do business without a telephone number. Today you cannot do business without knowing your customers' e-mail address and Net preferences!

FROM INFORMATION TO SHOPPING TO HEALTH E-CARE SUPPORT

It is no revelation that there are oodles of retail items to purchase on line these days. Consumers have access to a plethora of products from on-line vendors whose brand names range from the familiar Land's End and Williams Sonoma to newcomers such as iVillage's Shopping channel. One thing is certain: the convenience and choice on line are sure to impress even the most seasoned shopper.

Traffic to on-line shopping channels indicates that e-consumers are sticking, for the most part, to brand-name merchants and well-known product categories such as books, music, flowers, software, and toys. Case in point: home shopping network QVC's iQVC is a trusted brand in empowered home shopping. Consumers flock to the site to buy their favorite brand, learn more about QVC hosts, and access program guides. Other retailers such as Toys-R-Us and The Disney Store also enjoy significant on-line revenues due to their existing air-space brand-name recognition. Multilevel marketing companies such as the Amway Corporation (see Exhibit 2–4) have gotten on line too, revolutionizing their business

---

Exhibit 2–4 Amway Founders Go High Tech But Stay High Touch with Quixtar

The founders of Amway Corp., the undisputed king of multilevel marketing, created a sister company with a new business model in the fall of 1999—on the Web. The international, multibillion dollar company is already known for its sticky customers. Quixtar, its new cyberspace sister, offers a new way to purchase goods and services—and share with others how they can profit from doing the same.

Amway's founders have a tradition of reinventing their business model, while maintaining a strong relationship with the Independent Business Owners [IBOs] they support. It is due to the energy and creativity of more than three million of these IBOs worldwide that Amway has become the giant it is. These same IBOs are the driving force behind Quixtar.

On September 1, 1999, www.Quixtar.com opened for business, Quixtar, Inc. (pronounced Quick-Star), features a unique convergence of personalized shopping, member benefits, and business ownership. Anyone in North America can take advantage of the Quixtar opportunity and start their own Internet business—without the need to make huge investments in programming, warehousing, distribution, or product development. All volume and revenue generated through purchases made on the Quixtar^{SM} site is credited to IBOs affiliated with Quixtar.

How does this new business model relate to e-healthcare? Like the health care industry, it is a "high-touch" business—with IBOs meeting face-to-face for mentoring, meetings, and motivation. The Quixtar business model is a good example of how empowering the consumer does not have to sacrifice all real space relationships. Many IBOs affiliated with Quixtar still meet for specific training and informational sessions. Simplifying the distribution model on the Internet allows them to make better use of time when they are together. Less paperwork and automated tracking of billing information will create time in each business owner's schedule to pursue more business and massage existing business relationships.

The lesson here is that automating redundancies and paperwork, and empowering the e-consumer by offering access to significant amounts of information does not necessarily sacrifice relationships. In fact, it can help improve those that exist, and even create new ones.

Source: Reprinted with permission from Quixtar, Inc., © 1999.

plans in the process. The Amway Corporation has adjusted its business model many times since the 1950s, from door-to-door sales, to interactive distribution, to e-commerce.

On-line music seller CDNow.com, for example, launched its "My CDNow" in September 1998. My CDNow lets customers get a page designed just for them with music suggestions based on their stated preferences, past purchases, and ratings of artists and other CDs. The result: the number of pages viewed on My CDNow's "Wish List," which lets visitors name the CDs they may buy later, jumped almost 200 percent immediately.[9]

Smart e-tailers serve up more than just an on-line catalog for visitors. Disney (www.disney.go.com) offers consumers a family channel that includes tips on parenting, meal planning, at-home activities for kids, and a resource guide to Disney-like fun in every hometown, giving visitors a reason to come back. Avon (www.avon.com) offers a virtual beauty advisor as well as tips and ideas about makeup and beauty. Both of these sites are attempting not just to sell more products but to educate consumers to be informed buyers in the future.

iVillage.com (Figure 2–2) is a women's channel that specializes in health care and offers a comprehensive shopping experience with many brand-name retailers, the latest news, and information about women's issues. Visitors can take a health assessment quiz, join an on-line diet and nutrition support group, participate in weekly health polls, and store their medical records.

BabyCenter.com (Figure 2–3) is a leading source of information and products for parents. In addition to offering visitors shopping, child information resources, and bulletin board support groups, BabyCenter features a personalized guide for moms. Information is pushed to a personal page, based on the woman's stage of pregnancy or the age of her baby. Growth updates, checklists, and answers to common questions appear on the personal page.

What these Web sites have in common is more than simply pushing products. Each attempts to personalize a visitor's shopping experience in one or more ways. By doing this, these e-tailers encourage visitors to come back time and again to the site—and buy more. They focus on membership and relationships.

- *e-Action for Health Care: Health Care Is a Service Business—Combine High-Tech with High-Touch.* Many health care providers find analogies between retail and health care distasteful, but the reality is that health care companies can learn a great deal from the techniques e-tailers use to attract consumers and keep them coming back. The first lesson from e-tailers is the concept of Net personalization. On-line shopping sites encourage browsers to register, which creates a database of consumer names and preferences. Software "cookies"

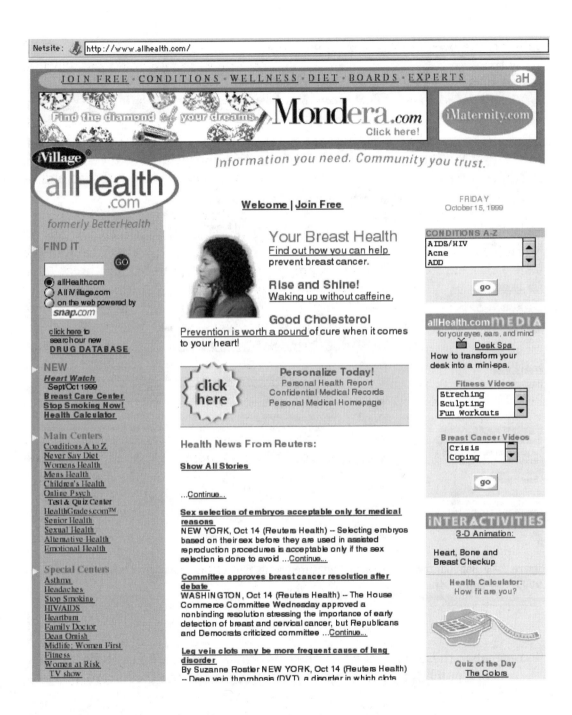

Figure 2–2 iVillage's allHealth.com. *Source:* Reprinted with permission from www.allhealth.com, © 1999, iVillage.com.

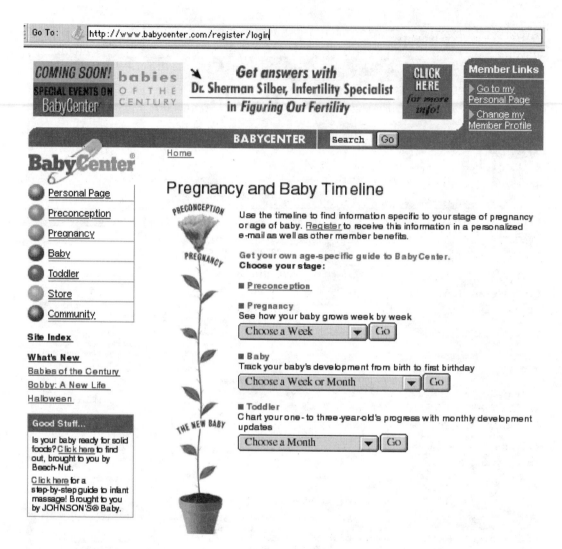

Figure 2–3 BabyCenter.com. *Source:* Reprinted with permission from www.babycenter.com, ©
1999, Baby Center, Inc./eToys.

remember these visitors when they return, which consumers tend to like.
One click purchasing cuts down on frustrating, repetitive credit card information entering.

How can new technology—which some health care providers consider one of
the primary reasons for the dehumanization of health care—be personal? Simply

put, storing a variety of information about consumer preferences can help push customized content their way, and *that* is what customer service is all about. After all, the single, 30-year-old vegetarian with a penchant for gardening, Hinduism, and adventure travel is a different consumer than the 38-year-old mother of two who likes to do home projects and is active at her conservative Christian church. Mass marketing this is not—it is "me" marketing.

Health care companies can make Net personalization work for them by collecting information specifically geared toward what they deliver. For example, a 50-year-old diabetic with a husband taking Viagra has different needs than a 25-year-old male with seasonal allergies. Whether you push custom health information or a personal medical record, Net personalization can recreate the "personal touch" that many feel health care has long since lost.

Lesson number two from e-tailers is about aesthetic appeal. Health care information on the Web is more about interactivity and media than it is about health care, and your Web service must be aesthetically appealing and interactive. Face the fact that you are dealing with the television and MTV generation, and they already have high expectations about how a Web service should "move."

The developers of first-generation health system Web sites unfortunately did not do enough surfing prior to putting up the first Web calling card, and the results were often clunky sites that contained a great deal of lengthy narrative in an unattractive format. Peruse 8 or 10 e-tailer Web services such as www.dell.com and www.amazon.com and you will quickly get some ideas about how to present information in an appealing way to consumers and deliver e-services that encourage repeat use. In addition to a robust on-line store, Dell has a state-of-the-Net real-time call center staffed by humans ready to talk to you over the Web or over the telephone to facilitate your order and cross-sell other products.

Many e-tailers are also good at keeping things interactive and interesting. Notice the way most copy is written at an e-tail Web service. It is typically hip and conversational. In other words, it is written so the average visitor can read and easily understand it. Think soundbites. Lose the passive or academic tone; be sure your health care company has good content editors who tighten and liven up the content of your Web service. When was the last time you saw a health and medical service that used humor?

Surf major e-tailers, visit your competitors—look, learn, and improve. This is not about just content, it is about community—no, e-community. Move beyond content to deliver e-services and e-care delivery. This means moving from a passive Web site to a true Web service environment that helps e-consumers and e-patients select and schedule an appointment. Remember that it is possible to Web enable almost any service or transaction function. The real trick for health and medical services is to make the Web version of the service better than the service normally used for the transaction (telephone, in-person exchange, etc.).

To succeed on the Net, health systems and networks of providers that deliver medical service must ensure that Web applications and services are truly integrated with various health care legacy systems. Real-time customer call centers with live representatives and nurses, core admission and discharge processes, and the practice management systems of medical groups are some examples. If integration is achieved, a Web click to select a physician can lead to an appointment and perhaps an on-line conference with a nurse to assess whether a person really needs to see the physician or can manage the symptom or condition with supported self-care solutions.

Some leading health systems across the country have formed an alliance (www.healthonline.com) to support consumers and patients connecting on line with their physicians and health systems. These on-line efforts go beyond using the Web for marketing but truly are focused on delivering better e-service.

NET TOOLING THE TRAVEL INDUSTRY

Travel agencies across the country are feeling the pinch of on-line competition. Airlines, car rental companies, and hotels have realized the power of the Internet, and three-quarters of the top 75 are reaching out to customers directly and inexpensively on the Internet.[10] With a simple mouse click, consumers can find bargain airfares to Ft. Lauderdale, detailed reports about Mediterranean cruises, and rental car rates for their visit to Aunt May's—anytime they want, 24 hours a day. No longer is using a travel agent the most efficient means of obtaining travel information. Agents have lost their exclusive access to airline, hotel, and rental car prices and information. The empowered consumer now has access too.

For instance, consumers can research prices and buy tickets directly on airlines' Web services. In just two years, airlines went from providing airline schedules on first-generation Web sites to building e-commerce Web services that sell tickets and support transactions faster and better than travel agents. Northwest Airlines (www.nwa.com/travel/cyber), Southwest Airlines, and others now offer last-minute deals for those who visit them on line. Even the best travel agents cannot look out for all of their clients up until the last minute of travel.

So e-consumers have begun to do it themselves, and they pocket handsome e-savings. Priceline.com[SM] (www.priceline.com) revolutionized the travel industry when it offered consumers the opportunity to "name their own price" on airfares, hotel rooms, and rental cars. The company buys large blocks of tickets from airlines, then resells them to the public, often for less than what it paid for them, which is one of the flaws of the company's business model. Few things appeal more to the American consumer than to be able to haggle over the price of a high-priced item—and get what they ask for.

Direct-to-consumer selling by airlines and hotels has meant significant decreases in commissions for travel agents. Although these have been steadily decreasing over the past several years, the Internet gives consumers the opportunity to bypass travel agents altogether. Agents now get paid less for performing the same service. Some agencies have begun to offer new services such as travel management and events management just to stay afloat, and many are closing. In fact, at the end of 1998, five firms in the Washington, DC, area had filed for bankruptcy. In the end, some experts say, travel agents will become obsolete.

- *e-Action for Health Care: Prepare for On-Line Price Comparisons for Medical Products and Services.* In some ways, the decline of the travel agent is similar to the decline of the expert stockbroker. By extension, some fear that health experts (i.e., health care providers) could likely become "health managers" rather than advice givers. Certainly it is within the power of physicians and providers to fight back with their own robust Web services that can be used to support the physician–patient relationship. If providers do not establish Web-based services that deliver information, products, and services, then the physician–patient relationship could be further eroded by the cyberdoctor experts delivering diagnoses and management on line through high-speed connections into the home.

As they did with airfares and hotel rooms, consumers will begin to shop for the best medical care "deal." Companies such as CompareNet (www.comparenet.com) allow e-consumers to compare prices on consumer products and household items. Next up: annual physicals, coronary bypass surgery, and breast augmentation?

If made easily available to consumers, information about National Committee for Quality Assurance and Health Plan Employer Data and Information Set indicators, as well as charges for hospitals and physician professional fees, could significantly affect the hospitals and physician groups consumers elect to go to. Healthcare Report Cards, shown in Figure 2–4, already lists comparative outcomes information on many procedures. Will the cost of these procedures be compared next?

The "e" revolution is upon us. The time to act is now. Because the Internet world moves at the speed of light, companies and individuals have little time to respond to cybercompetitors—much less time than they had to respond to competition in the pre-Internet era.

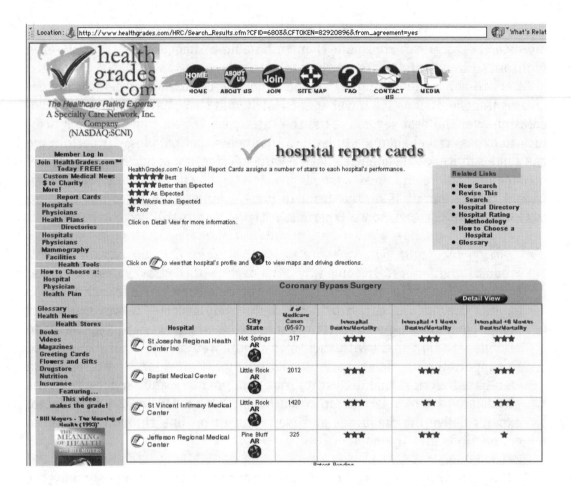

Figure 2–4 Healthcare Report Cards. *Source:* Reprinted with permission from www.healthgrades.com, © 1999, Healthgrades.com.

E-BANKING: BEYOND AUTOMATIC TELLER MACHINES (ATMs)

In 1999, 7,200 on-line banking application vendors and providers built transactional sites, according to the International Data Corporation. By the end of 1999, Internet banking applications accounted for nearly one-third of the U.S. banking applications market.[11] Powerhouses Citibank (www.citibank.com) and Wells Fargo (www.wellsfargo.com) offer a variety of on-line services to customers.

The lure of being able to check account balances on line, transfer funds, and pay bills electronically has consumers signing up for on-line banking services at a record pace. The number of people banking on line—through sites run by their financial institution or retailers—is expected to hit 15 million by 2001.[12] Why? As discussed above, consumers like to be empowered. In this case, they like having access to, and control over, their money while they are at home. Plus, on-line banking saves time and money. Table 2–3 shows just how much e-consumers love on-line banking.

And consumers are not the only ones who benefit from on-line banking. Companies seeking alternative sources of equity funding can find money on the Internet via on-line connections. One such company, Web Securities LLC, has built a full-service securities house dedicated to helping early-stage enterprises access the capital markets via the Web. Creating this virtual Wall Street—which Web Securities dubbed "Web Street"—fulfills Bill Gates' vision of "friction-free capitalism." Up-and-comers unable to find venture capital may just be able to obtain it through an e-commerce firm such as Web Securities.

E-banking also greatly reduces a bank's overhead. Fewer tellers and access to less expensive money are just two of the draws. Overhead reduction is a good thing, since the real-time application of e-banking minimizes the float that banks have historically made their primary revenue stream.

- *e-Action for Health Care: Consider This Question: Do We Need Health Insurance Intermediaries?* Are health insurance intermediaries necessary? The answer could be no.

About 25 percent of consumers' health care dollars go to administration, and profits go to the health insurance middleperson. How does this benefit consumers? In the Net world, allocation of 5 percent of the premium dollar for administration would likely be very generous! If the consumer is getting access to valuable services such as round-the-clock access to advice nurses by telephone and

---

Table 2–3 The Growth of On-Line Banking

Year	Number of Households Banking On Line
1999	4.8 million
2001	10 million

Source: Data from INTECO, The Industry Standard, © 1999, Reprint Management Services.

Web and other valuable disease and demand support services, perhaps it would justify a greater percentage of the premium dollar being spent.

Currently, the health insurance industry, with its high transaction volume, requires that people interact with customers to complete transactions, and using customer service agents is costly. But this will change in the e-age, when many transactions can be automated and computers talk to other computers to resolve issues. This saves money by replacing high-cost customer service agents spending valuable time handling an administrative transaction. A customer service agent's time is much better spent on high-touch service issues affecting care outcomes. ChannelPoint (Figure 2–5) is one company that understands this as it seeks to replace paper-based insurance processes with e-commerce transactions.

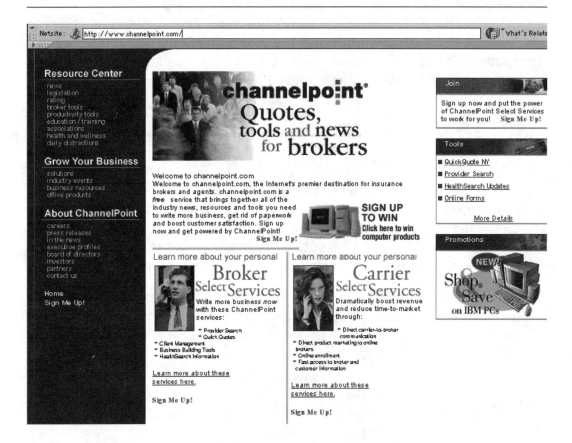

Figure 2–5 ChannelPoint. *Source:* Reprinted with permission from www.channelpoint.com, © 1999, ChannelPoint.

For example, ChannelPoint's Commerce Broker automates an insurance broker's everyday rating, quoting, request for proposal, and enrollment tasks—all within a standard Web browser. It also lets brokers give accurate product recommendations without the hassle of manually comparing and evaluating prices, benefits, and networks. The broker's time can then be more focused on the high-touch, more complex service issues with potential customers. ChannelPoint's services improve processes. The health care industry still needs various intermediaries, but there will be increased efforts to do administrative activities much more efficiently on line.

Internet banking reduces costs by eliminating positions at the front lines and branch level. After all, if consumers' paychecks are deposited electronically, they can move funds between accounts and pay bills on line, and they can withdraw cash from an automatic teller machine, there is little need for branch tellers. Insurance claim submission will experience a similar shift. With eligibility ensured via on-line verification and an electronically submitted claim on the Web, payment can be made and deposited directly into a health care company's account. With fewer people needed to process what historically have been labor-intensive transactions and processes, there will be significant cost savings.

The Internet and an ever-expanding array of great on-line services are forcing every element of the health and medical industry to reconsider the following questions: "What is our business?" "What value do we deliver to our customer?" "Does Internet technology offer a terrific chance to lower operating costs, build customer relationships, and create an e-business model blending Web clicks with existing bricks and mortar processes that will work throughout the next century?"

EVEN BIG ITEMS

Many people think of the Internet as the place to shop when you want books, CDs, and flowers. But what about big items—like automobiles? New battle lines have been drawn on line as automakers race to compete with on-line car buying services in order to obtain loyalty—and cash—from America's drivers. Several years ago, car buying services on the Net were merely matchmakers, allowing would-be car buyers to find information—prices and dealership locations, for instance. But these services have since evolved to offer much more than comparison and dealer locator guides. Some, such as CarPoint, now offer a full range of auto services to consumers—from financing and insurance, to ongoing maintenance reminders.

For example, only a few car owners can remember when they should have their next oil change. Not to worry—Microsoft's CarPoint (www.carpoint.com) allows owners to sign up and receive e-mail reminders about when to take their car in for an oil change, 30,000-mile checkup, and so on. Owners are also alerted to manufacturer recall notices. Autoweb (Figure 2–6) takes service one step farther by allowing consumers to schedule maintenance appointments on line, post questions to a mechanic, and browse a library of auto topics. According to MediaMetrix, Autoweb was the most heavily traveled auto site in December of 1998, and it boasts more than 400,000 registered users.

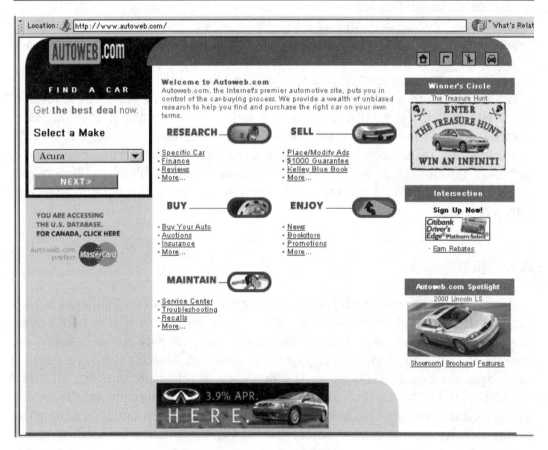

Figure 2–6 Autoweb. *Source:* Reprinted with permission from www.autoweb.com, © 1999, AutoWeb.

- *e-Action for Health Care*: *From On-Line Care Support to Medical e-Auctions.* Though it is not a pretty analogy, in some ways a visit to the physician is similar to a visit to the auto mechanic. Both the human body and your car require preventive maintenance and regular checkups, often not scheduled as frequently as they should be. Plus, there is always a wait, and you never know what the bill is going to come to until you check out.

Health care Web services can also automate maintenance checkups. Health care providers can send reminders for previously scheduled appointments, annual physicals, and well-woman visits. These reminders will lower overall treatment costs because they will encourage people to obtain the care they need. Consumers with chronic conditions such as diabetes and asthma will like the ease of scheduling an appointment on line and asking health care questions of the on-line expert, and managing their disease on line quicker and faster than other means.

"Going once, going twice"—could medical e-auctions be the next step? Organs, bypass surgery, plastic surgery—all to the right bidder, on line.

BUSINESS-TO-BUSINESS E-COMMERCE

Although revenue growth in the on-line consumer goods and services sector is and will likely remain very strong, the amount of money spent in business-to-business e-transactions is much greater. According to Forrester Research, business-to-business transactions were $43 billion in 1998 and are expected to reach $1.3 trillion in 2003.[13]

Take a lesson from the steel industry. Steel surely is not sexy, but MetalSite (www.metalsite.net) has at least made it more profitable. The service links mills around the world who have secondary and overrun inventory they need to dump. FastParts (www.fastparts.com) and Affiliated Networks (www.affiliatednetworks.com) do the same for computer parts and marine supplies, respectively.

E-business transactions include everything from one company buying another's products on line to linking businesses via Web applications that allow real-time auctions. In essence, e-business is any transaction that is done on line—and that reduces or eliminates the need for a telephone call or air-space transaction. Boeing has saved hundreds of millions of dollars by moving its monstrous system of spare parts sales and technical maintenance manuals on line. Airlines have reduced the cost of ticket processing from $8 to $1 per ticket.[14] In the computer networking industry, e-business makes it possible for Cisco Systems to sell its routers on line and handle customer service transactions. In the health care industry, e-business allows for on-line eligibility verification and claims submission, which can significantly reduce the number of rejected insurance claims.

Web services developer VerticalNet is one of many companies that is capitalizing on the business-to-business on-line craze. VerticalNet links multiple buyers with groups of sellers in vertical-industry network niches (Figure 2–7). The company offers content, industry news, product information, directories, classifieds, and job listings as well as a host of other services for the industries for which it develops services. VerticalNet also has created a community of professionals from across the globe that can exchange ideas, search for career opportunities, and monitor industry events. But the company's core business is to foster an environment in which buyers and sellers can do business. Take a quick look at www.verticalnet.com and explore their health care communities.

- *e-Action for Health Care: Reduce Operating Cost through e-Business Now.* Attention health care companies: business-to-business e-commerce is about more than group purchasing initiatives! E-business stands to finally end paperwork hassles and labor-intensive processes in health care. The industry has been so unconnected for so long that the same test is ordered multiple times within the same year—simply because no one can find the first test results. Patients complete a separate information sheet every time they see a health care provider. It is time to stop the madness.

The Net and the various e-service applications that are being developed, launched, and distributed to service tens of thousands of different health and medical information, product, and service transactions promise to significantly cut down on the amount of paper being moved. Net technology takes atoms of paper—costly to duplicate, handle, and distribute—and replaces them with electronic digital bits and bytes that, once produced, can be distributed at little cost once the customer's Web address has been captured and stored in a database.

In early 1999, American Airlines Webcast over 2 million e-mail messages to frequent flyers whose e-mail address is in an e-database. Based on the flyers' preferences, these customers were given special fares and deals that helped American Airlines sell unsold seats, move inventory, and increase profitability. All this *without* having to buy an ad or pay an ad agency to place the ad.

Hospitals always collect patients' telephone numbers. But patients' e-mail addresses are almost never collected. Just think, an e-mail database of patients' health interests would allow an organization to segment and target prevention or health services specials to improve utilization of beds, outpatient services, and thousands of other health care products and services.

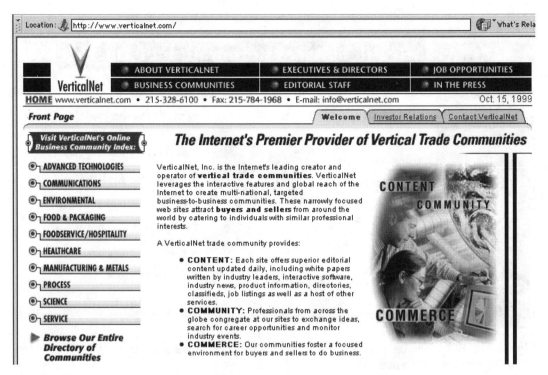

Figure 2–7 VerticalNet. *Source:* Reprinted with permission from www.verticalnet.com, © 1999, VerticalNet.

What is your health care company doing to connect itself to suppliers, physicians, consumers, and patients? Up until recently, electronic purchasing has been available for hospitals only via electronic data interchange and dial-up connections. One would think the reduction in paperwork and errors, as well as a quicker turnaround time, would have convinced health care providers to embrace this technology years ago—but that has not been the case.

Group purchasing cooperatives such as Health Services Corporation of America (HSCA; Figure 2–8) hope the Internet will change administrators' minds. HSCA's site offers an electronic catalog of 600,000 products. HSCA and information technology business leader McKesson HBOC are working together to link the purchasing software with existing materials management software in large health systems. Next steps including linking single hospitals, integrated delivery systems, and physician offices.

Many business processes need overhaul, and e-commerce offers a viable solution. On-line ordering of medical supplies is simple, but health care e-commerce

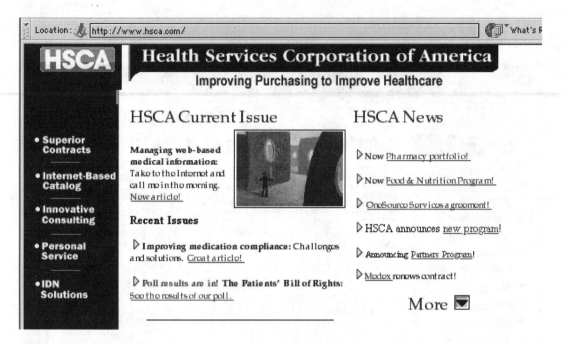

Figure 2–8 HSCA. *Source:* Reprinted with permission from www.hsca.com, © 1999, Health Services Corporation of America.

is about so much more. For instance, Extranets that make on-line eligibility verification a reality by partnering with e-commerce companies that deliver this service would save health care systems and providers millions in delayed and rejected insurance claims. Great cost savings would also come from serving up certified medical education for hospital staff, and management courses for administrators and physician office staff. And what about auctioning off magnetic resonance imaging, heart catheterization, or inventory overage to the highest local bidder? Now that is a smart way to use e-commerce.

E-HEALTHCARE—"DOING IT BETTER ON LINE"—THE COMPETITIVE ADVANTAGE

Applying Internet technology to the health care industry—whether it is by the Internet, Intranet, Extranet, or another Net yet to be invented—involves a complex set of value propositions that must be thought through carefully, but fast. The human body is a complex entity with an unlimited amount of variability that has to be understood. Health information and education is one business. Selling medical and health products by an 800 number or on the Web is another business.

Delivering health and medical services over the Internet is much more complex than product transactions such as selling books or trading stocks on line. Health and medical services are generally periodic, unwanted purchases. Very few people really want to go to the physician or hospital. These transactions have an entirely different set of factors that must be considered when developing Web services.

Ultimately, seeking to improve outcomes, reduce costs, and ensure appropriate application of professional services is about changing people's behavior. The complexity and fragmentation of the health and medical service transaction require appropriate research, feasibility, systems analysis, and application development. The cybercompetition is lurking, and the time to act is now. But there is time to develop on-line systems both quickly and well. Chapter 17 outlines a robust e-business planning process that can take your organization through the steps to creating a great Web service that achieves mission-critical goals.

There are many lessons to be learned from the e-commerce experts and e-tailers that already exist. Your role as a health care e-leader should be to understand these lessons, then integrate them into your health care company's e-solutions. One of the most important trends to watch is that of personalizing e-service. Mass marketing will not work in cyberspace. To get to know your e-customers. Key principles for success include brand building and delivery interactivity and services that keep people coming back. Just like physicians court their referral sources, so too must your health care organization court its e-customers. If it does not, someone else will—and that someone may be a seemingly unlikely player such as iVillage.com or eToys.com, which purchased BabyCenter.com in the late 1990s. Both of these e-companies have moved into the e-health space with information and e-products that meet consumer needs and build relationships.

Remember that the electronic landscape is evolving rapidly. Learn what to do and what not to do by evaluating non-health-care-industry success stories and failures. Surf over to industry rags such as *The Industry Standard* (www.thestandard.com), *Interactive Week* (www.Interactive-Week.com), *Cyberatlas* (www.cyberatlas.com), and *Internet.com* (www.internet.com) to stay abreast of the retail and other industry e-changes that can and will affect health care. Attend a conference like Internet World and have your eyes opened.

It is also essential to build internal talent that will lead your company's Internet effort. As you grow internal talent, it will be critical to partner with external organizations that support efforts to build your brand, your services, and your overall e-business. At the end of the day, Internet technology is designed to facilitate access to health care information, products, processes, and services. Every health care organization—from providers and health systems to medical products and pharmaceutical companies—has the responsibility to figure out how to apply technology to lower costs, improve service, and achieve better patient outcomes. The Internet and all Web applications are tools to achieve lower costs and better care.

Challenge yourself, your board, and your health care constituents to re-invent your health care organization's business plan and take e-action. Do not let the talk of e-revolution fall on deaf ears. Take advantage of the opportunity to become the Amazon.com in your target markets sooner rather than later. The health and medical delivery system is being reinvented at the speed of thought based on today's "e" strategies and e-services. Be an e-leader and be committed to developing great on-line systems quickly based on a strong understanding of the Net and customer needs and behaviors.

REFERENCES

1. "Females Lead Online Growth Spurt," http://www.cyberatlas.com/big_picture/demographics/nmr.html (17 June 1999), accessed 17 June 1999.
2. "Online Holiday Shopping Triples," *Catalog Age Weekly,* 31 December 1998.
3. "Online Holiday Sales Estimated at $1.14 Billion," *Catalog Age Weekly,* 31 December 1997.
4. "38 Million Americans Getting Wired," http://cyberatlas.internet.com/big_picture/demographics/mainstream.html (14 January 1999), accessed 9 March 1999.
5. "Holiday Shopping Will Soar in '99," http://www.cyberatlas.com/market/retailing/trak.html (22 February 1999), accessed 22 June 1999.
6. "Online Trading Erupts in 1998," http://cyberatlas.internet.com/market/finance/broker.html (5 February 1999), accessed 19 March 1999.
7. *Washington Post*, 2 June 1999.
8. "Offline Brokerages May Suffer," CyberAtlas, http://cyberatlas.internet.com/markets/finance/print/0,1323,5961 153001,00.html
9. R. Hof et al., "Now It's Your Web," *Business Week,* 5 October 1998.
10. J. Evans, "Travel Agents Feel the Squeeze," *Washington Post,* 27 December 1998, A16.
11. J. Borzo, "Net-Banking Market To Triple in '99," http://www.thestandard.net/articles/display/0,1449,3379,00.html (3 February 1999), accessed 22 March 1999.
12. J. Cohen, "Everybody's a Banker," *Industry Standard,* 15 March 1999, 36–40.
13. M. Leibovich et al., "Internet's e-Conomy Gets Read," *Washington Post,* 20 June 1999, A1.
14. Leibovich et al., "Internet's e-Conomy," A1.

CHAPTER 3

The New Health Care e-Consumer and e-Patient

Douglas E. Goldstein

I was diagnosed with breast cancer in 1996. I was only 34 at the time and felt isolated because I hadn't heard about any other women who were diagnosed at such a young age. After I started searching the Internet for support groups and information about breast cancer, I realized I wasn't alone.

My teenager had been plagued with acne for several years, and it was really starting to wear on his confidence and esteem. Our family physician tried different treatment regimes, which did help, but on the Internet I found a lot more information about how to help my son deal with the psychological effects of his diagnosis. The information helped him cope with his feelings.

I've had allergies and asthma since childhood and was tired of being on so many medications all the time to control them. I started searching on the Internet for treatment alternatives and found several Web services that explained herbal and holistic ways of treating my disease. The information enabled me to ask the right questions of my physician as well as a naturopathic physician I began seeing.

MEET THE NEW, empowered health care e-customer—both e-patient and e-consumer—who is fast becoming an expert at accessing reams of information, for free, on the wonderful World Wide Web. The three health care e-customers quoted above are by no means unique. They represent a tiny fraction of the growing number of Americans—dubbed "cyberchondriacs" by Harris Interactive (www.HarrisInteractive.com) Chairman Humphrey Taylor—who turn to the Internet for personal health information, advice, and support. Of the 60 million adults who searched the Web for health care information in 1998, 91 percent found what they needed.[1] Figure 3–1 shows which diseases interest these e-consumers the most.

Be healthy, be well. Millions of Americans are seeking better health, *without* the aid of a physician or care provider, by accessing information about vitamins, clinical trials, alternative medicine, fitness, and organic food. In fact, self-care is the largest form of health care in the country, bigger than hospital care, bigger than physician care, and bigger than home care. Approximately 80 percent of health care expenditures in the country are related to consumer self-care, and the Internet is fast becoming consumers' medium of choice when they are seeking health and wellness information.[2] Estimates vary, but at the time this book was printed, there were somewhere between 15,000 and 50,000 Web sites about health and more being created each day. Health-related sites such as the ones listed in Table 3–1 are visited by hundreds of thousands, or millions, of Americans every month. Like it or not, the power in health care is shifting from physi-

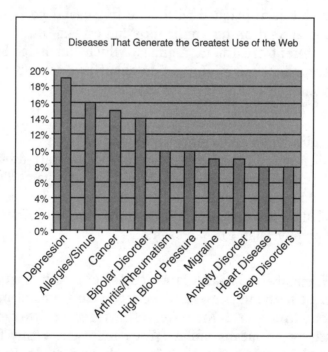

Figure 3–1 Different Diseases and the Percentage of Cyberchondriacs Who Search On Line for Information about Them. *Source:* Reprinted with permission from HarrisInteractive.com, © 1999, Louis Harris & Associates.

Table 3–1 Health-Related Sites Draw Significant Traffic

	Unique Visitors per Month
AOL Health Channel	2,142,000
Thrive Online	821,000
May Health Oasis	679,000
InteliHealth	666,000
Mediconsult.com sites*	545,000
America's Health Network*	325,000
OnHealth	316,000
Medscape.com	308,000
Health Answers	281,000
Empower Health/DrKoop.com	255,000
Phys	240,000

*An aggregation of commonly owned, branded domain names.

Source: Adapted with permission from Media Metrix, The Industry Standard, © 1999, Reprint Management Services.

cian to nonphysician and from physician's office or hospital to the new primary practitioner: the e-consumers and e-patients themselves.

Net researcher cyberdialogue://findsvp has a name for these empowered e-consumers—HealthMed Retrievers (HMRs). HMRs are a very upscale group and are sophisticated and proactive in their use of the Internet for a wide variety of applications. According to a 1998 study completed by Michael Brown and cyberdialogue://findsvp, evidence suggests that HMRs are more educated, earn higher incomes, and are more likely to use the Internet each day than non-HMRs (Exhibit 3–1).[3] This HMR demographic is nothing to sneeze at. By December of 1998, 22.3 million sought health information on line, and cyberdialogue://findsvp predicts that the number of these surfers will hit 30 million by 2001.[4] Regardless of whether 30 or 60 million Americans looked for health information on line in 1998, the fact is that the vast majority of Americans and others throughout the world will be doing health and medical e-actions on line in the twenty-first century.

What are e-consumers doing on line? Any number of things—all of which are empowering them to ask their physicians more questions and manage more of their own health care. At least for now, they primarily seek health information—

Exhibit 3–1 How HMRs Compare with General Internet Users

- Women are more prevalent in the HMR group: 53% vs. 46%
- HMRs' household income is higher: $61,700 vs. $56,800
- HMRs are more likely to be college graduates: 48% vs. 41%
- HMRs are more likely to use paid sites.
- HMRs are more likely to use e-mail discussion groups (listservs).
- HMRs are more likely to read advertisements to access premium information.

Source: Data from cyberdialogue://findsvp research, © 1998, Healthcare Information Services, ING Baring Furman Selz LLC.

answers to questions they have not been able to ask or not had answered by their personal physicians. Health topics such as cancer, heart disease, children's health, diet and nutrition, and women's health have all been investigated by curious e-consumers and e-patients who know how to scour the Web. Alternative medicine, fast becoming less "alternative" and more mainstream, is often investigated by e-consumers. Long a topic that traditional physicians refused to discuss, alternative medicine is of great interest to Americans, and Web companies such as Ask Dr. Weil (www.askdrweil.com) and drkoop.com know it. Sites that discuss alternative therapies, herbs, and supplements attract hundreds of thousands. Dr. Andrew Weil's Web site and others have become a common bookmark for many empowered e-consumers.

While understanding that HMRs exist is certainly helpful, it is important to note that HMRs are not a well-defined e-consumer market. Okay, so those who surf for health information are a desirable demographic. But this information is not useful for marketing or cost management in a health system or organization—it is too general. What about chronic disease-plagued e-patients? Are they on line? What are they looking for? What are they doing? Those with chronic disease stand to benefit most from interactive monitoring and on-line health management. The cost of managing these e-patients on line is significantly less than the cost of managing them over the telephone or in person. But unless you know what people with chronic illness are accessing on line, it is impossible to target chronically ill e-patients with a defined, transactional application. What is your health care organization doing to find out? And what are you planning to do to attract them and support them in improving outcomes? HarrisInteractive.com is actively identifying and surveying e-patients with chronic conditions. Tune in to their Web site for their latest findings.

E-CONSUMERS ARE *NOT* PASSIVE

As Figure 3–2 shows, interest in on-line health information is growing—and surfers are seeking answers to their own health issues. E-consumers take a much more active role in their health care than others have. They search the Web and print out articles and opinions and cart them along to visits with their physicians. The number of times patients ask about a specific procedure or drug therapy is increasing significantly. Consumers review the credentials of their health care providers—which are available on the Web—as they assess the quality of their current physician or consider local specialists.

E-consumers know how to locate information quickly—without having to interact with a physician, nurse, or other health care provider in person or on the telephone. They are used to real-time, on-line transactions and already buy airline tickets, books, and personal computers (PCs)—as well as trade stocks and access daily news—on the Internet. Of course, they also search for information about Viagra side effects, cancer prevention, and other health issues. Interactions with medical offices have never produced such voluminous amounts of information so quickly. E-consumers are busy and do not want to be put on hold, wait three weeks to schedule an appointment, or get the runaround from office staff. They want information, they want it now, and they can get it on line through the World Wide Web. The empowered e-consumer in Exhibit 3–2 is much different from the passive patient of old.

It is critical that health care organizations realize that e-consumers are no longer just "early adapters" or the techno savvy. These two groups of early Netizens were typically profiled as highly educated, highly paid, white, and male. But 1999 trends show that the Internet is becoming much more mainstream. About 51 percent of the 40 million who plan to go on line in 1999 are

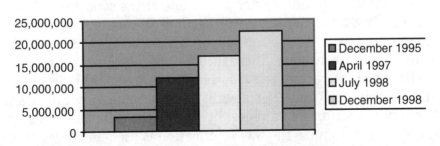

Figure 3–2 Number of U.S. Adults Retrieving Health or Medical Information On Line. *Source:* Data from cyberdialogue://findsvp, © 1998, and *The Industry Standard*, 1999.

Exhibit 3–2 Passive Patients versus Empowered e-Customers and e-Patients

Old Think—"Patient"	New Think—Empowered e-Customer and e-Patient
• Took a passive role in his or her care and typically followed "doctor's orders" • Sought medical advice from a local physician • Assumed that as long as a person had a medical degree, he or she was a good physician • Rarely questioned treatment plans or physician's opinion • Was hospital centric; knew what only local hospital had to offer • Relied mainly on physician for medical information—few alternative sources	• Takes an active role in his or her own care • Has access to treatment protocols, clinical trials, and discussion groups worldwide—will bring in printed Web pages with questions • Seeks doctor profiling, board certification information, and malpractice claim information for physicians • Uses information to have an interactive session with the physician; asks questions and does not just "do what the doctor ordered" • Often asks about alternative therapies and treatments, in addition to traditional Western medical protocols

Source: Copyright © 1999, Douglas Goldstein.

over the age of 35, 49 percent of them have a high school education or less, and 58 percent make less than $50,000 a year.[5] The Web is fast becoming the place where middle America searches for information and shops for products and services.

It is also essential for health care executives and providers to understand that although many in the existing patient base may not have a computer at home, that does not mean they can be ruled out as one of the soon-to-be Web enabled. In fact, the PC is a transitional device that now is part of a family of Internet appliances that are easier to use and support a more mobile—or computer-illiterate—e-patient and e-consumer. These include Internet-enabled telephones with color monitors and interactive television services wired to the Net.

"Internet appliances" and "Net devices" will become very important in the next millennium, according to a report by Hambrecht & Quist.[6] These appliances stand ready to revolutionize the way information is used and accessed by giving e-consumers the ability to obtain information from any device. Interactive telephones and televisions are the hottest tickets.

After years of moving at a snail's pace, the Internet television market is poised to take off. When Microsoft purchased WebTV for $300 million (with only 100,000 subscribers), many laughed. But Bill Gates saw the great future of this technology. After all, every American knows how to turn on the television. Even people who are elderly or uneducated do not fear the television. Now, Microsoft is perfectly positioned to control the access between the television interface and the broadband Net data pipeline into American homes.

When access to the Internet becomes this easy, even couch potato Americans will begin surfing and spending. The collision of the Internet and television means average Americans will use the Internet to access information, shop, and surf. Seeking e-care support for health and medical needs is becoming as much a part of everyday life as turning on Oprah or the evening news.

The interactive telephone is another device that is making Net access easier. InfoGear's® iPhone® is a nifty gadget that allows e-providers and e-patients to view each other during a cyberappointment. Equipped with a keyboard, the iPhone® also acts as a personal scheduler and allows e-consumers to surf the Web.

Re-focus your health organization to attract new, empowered e-consumers *before* they begin to purchase new information appliances. Armed with these easy-to-use devices, e-patients will find Web-enabled care delivery much more comfortable and will catch on quickly.

SUPERNET WOMAN LOGS ON

Faster than a speeding modem. Able to change Web sites with a single mouse click. Look, there at the PC, iPhone®, or WebTV—it's SuperNet Woman!

Look behind that Net screen and there is often a woman clicking the mouse. More and more, wired health and medical information seekers are women. Recent data definitively show that the number of women using the Internet has grown significantly over the past three years. The Internet has empowered these women to make a variety of important decisions for themselves and their families.

The Bureau of Labor Statistics says that women accounted for 46.2 percent of total labor force participants in 1997 and will compose 48 percent by the year 2005.[7] That means women have plenty of their own money to spend. Women have gained purchasing power and are using it freely, as *they* choose, and many of them are choosing to spend it on the Internet. SuperNet Woman is on line, and she's part of an important target market for your health care company's Web service strategy.

The bottom line? This is not your father's health care system. In mid-1999, 92 million Americans were on line through various information appliances,[8] and the number continues to grow. From Internet-enabled telephones and interactive television Net interfaces such as WebTV, to newer and faster computers, innovative ways of jumping on the Net will continue to attract e-consumers, HMRs, and "Chronic Care e-Seekers" (a term used by the author to describe patients with chronic conditions that are using the Net to improve their health and lower costs).

SEEKING A CURE FOR THE COMMON HEALTH SYSTEM

It comes as no surprise that e-consumers have become increasingly dissatisfied with the U.S. health care system. Overall, the public holds a fairly negative view, and most people believe the system has problems and needs more than minor change in order to work better. In addition, growing numbers of adults believe managed care does more harm than good to the quality of care.[9]

So it should not surprise health care executives or providers that e-consumers are logging on to the Internet to find medical information that is seemingly unattainable elsewhere. E-consumers are fed up with the bureaucracy and inefficiency of the health care system. In response to rising out-of-pocket costs, health maintenance organization (HMO) gatekeeper models were created. HMO health care did not sit well with many Americans, who want access to specialty care at their own discretion—they want choice! They also want convenience and are willing to work to get what they want.

An e-revolution is brewing. E-customers of health care demand more options and are determining the direction of their care. A recent *Modern Healthcare* survey showed that 59 percent of all Americans say the current U.S. health system needs "major change," and consumers are demanding it.[10] They arrive in their physician's office, printed Web pages in hand, and announce exactly which drug will treat what ails them. And they do their homework—no longer taking "doctor's orders" as their only choice.

If health care organizations do not wake up, smell the coffee, and get on line with real services, transactions, and something for these e-consumers and e-patients to *do*, the new empowered e-consumer will become even more disgruntled with the hornet's nest of paperwork that plagues the system. The trillion-dollar health care beast is wrought with frustrating inefficiencies—referral processes and inaccurate billing among them. If America's health care leaders do not embrace Web technology fast, the e-consumer will angrily wonder, "How come I can compare product prices using Inktomi or CompareNet, retrieve full-text articles from the early 1980s, watch a laparoscopic hysterectomy live—all on the Web—but you can't get me a referral and an appointment to an orthopaedist the same day via a Net interaction!"

Health care executives and providers beware. The balance of power is shifting, and access to e-communication and information on the Web will forever change passive patients into informed e-customers who manage their care as they see fit. A 1998 KPMG Peat Marwick study listed the following three primary reasons why Americans are taking control of their own care.

1. **Evolution of "consumerism."** Like it or not, health care providers must realize that they offer goods and services like any other business does. Consumers are used to choice, efficiency, and convenience in other areas of their lives, and they demand it in health care too.
2. **Cost shifting.** Consumers are shouldering more of their own health care costs as employers offer them more plan choices.
3. **The Web explosion.** The Internet makes it easier for consumers to access reliable medical information on line—and they are doing so in greater numbers than ever before.[11]

Not just health information but medical care knowledge, products, and services being delivered over the Internet. The evolution of consumerism is demanding it, and e-consumers and e-patients seek it. Health care organizations must be ready to offer over-the-Web and over-the-telephone healing—as well as face-to-face patient encounters—to the almighty e-consumer. A few important facts about the e-consumer are listed below.

- **E-consumers want knowledge.** E-consumers and e-patients want to connect to the right information or service easily and quickly on the Web. They like to feel connected to their and other *trusted* providers. They want their information intelligently routed so that all providers will have it and be able to act on it. This need can mean very different things for different populations, but it existed well before the wired world. More important, e-consumers and e-patients want decision support related to their symptoms and conditions. This is really about getting answers and solutions, not just information.
- **E-consumers are already connected in cyberspace.** On-line support groups, chat rooms, and voice-over Web bulletin board services all carry useful information to help e-consumers make decisions. In fact, a recent study showed that e-patients liked on-line support groups better than their physicians in 12 of 14 categories (Exhibit 3–3).
- **E-consumers want convenience.** Americans are becoming increasingly demanding about how they spend their time—they do not want it wasted. Anything that makes things easier and quicker with the same value will win

Exhibit 3–3 E-Consumers Assess Which Resource Is Best—On-line Groups, Specialists, or Primary Care Providers (PCPs)

	Online Grp	Specialist	PCP
Most cost-effective	82.68%	8.38%	8.94%
Best in-depth information	76.92%	20.88%	2.20%
Help with emotional issues	74.73%	9.89%	15.38%
Most convenient	72.68%	14.21%	13.11%
Best practical knowledge	68.48%	23.37%	8.15%
Help with death and dying	57.50%	15.00%	27.50%
Most compassion and empathy	52.46%	17.49%	30.05%
There for me in the long run	49.43%	21.02%	29.55%

Source: Adapted with permission from T. Ferguson and W.J. Kelley, "E-Patients Prefer e-Groups to Doctors for 10 of 12 Aspects of Health Care," *The Ferguson Report*, 1:1, pp. 1–3 © 1999 http://ferguson-report.sparklist.com.

out. That means people who have been used to completing a prescription refill transaction in 20 minutes want the Web to do it for them in 2. If they can avoid taking time off work (and waiting 25 minutes in the reception area before they are seen) for a physician's appointment, they will. You must do it fast, do it better, and make them happy in order to keep them coming back. Make your company's new e-goal the 60-second transaction that goes from information, to product, to service! Now that is e-service!

- **E-consumers want it to be all about them.** People want to feel that they are being paid attention to and that things are being done just for them. Some still have a vague memory of, or at least have been told about, a time when physicians made house calls. E-patients still want this, even though the medium may be completely different. The next major site of care in the twenty-first century is the home, where care will be delivered by cyberphysicians and cybernurses through broadband high-speed connections.
- **E-consumers and e-patients want control.** The more patients feel in control, the less stressed and the happier they are. The shared decision-making research that has been done around cancer surgeries has illustrated this fact very strongly. This is why people want some control and access to their own patient records and lab results, along with explanations of what it all means.

A very high number of consumers already use the Web to research items before they buy them. Ask most e-comparison shoppers and they would tell you that lower prices and convenience are the biggest reasons they shop on line. They are looking for the best deal, and they usually find it on the Net. Who is to say they are not comparing you and your competitor? The Internet busts secrets wide open: your secrets are revealed with the click of a mouse as Web sites offer information such as credit histories or the names of Web sites being registered through public sources.

Talk with and listen to the new, empowered e-consumers. Every health care organization will have patients who are e-consumers. The cure for the common health system is the virtual health system of tomorrow. Connected into customers' homes through broadband connections that have video cameras, vital sign monitoring, and so on, as well as allowing e-consumers and e-patients virtual access to a variety of health e-transactions, education, and cybermedical visits will replace many in-person medical visits—and increase e-patient satisfaction tenfold.

GIVING PHYSICIANS AND HOSPITALS A CHECKUP

Empowered health care e-consumers are testing their newfound access to reams of information about physicians and hospitals nationwide. Information once kept from patients—information on credentialing and licensing, outcomes, and malpractice suits—is now readily available on the Web. After the mainstream media provided consumers with a flood of information about these sites, empowered consumers visited them in droves. Where are these e-customers going for data? Companies such as CSS Credentialing (www.tese.com/cas/) will check on a physician's credentials, schooling, malpractice claims, and more for only $15, a small price to pay for an e-customer's peace of mind. Certified Doctor (www.certifieddoctor.com) allows consumers to verify the board certification status of any physician certified by one or more of the 24 member boards of the American Board of Medical Specialties. Do you know what the data at these Web services say about your organization's physicians—or *you?*

All the press about provider profiling and "report cards" has facilitated the launch of Healthcare Report Cards (www.healthcarereportcards.com)—a Web site for those who want to see how their local hospital or health system fares. Select your city and state, and clinical outcomes for cardiac care, orthopaedics, neurosciences, pulmonary care, and transplants are readily available. The National Committee for Quality Assurance (NCQA; www.ncqa.org) has also gotten into the e-information game. Consumers can search to determine if their health plan is on the NCQA's accreditation list.

Attention health systems and providers! E-customers and e-patients are much more aware of your outcomes than you might think. Their access to the National

Practitioner Databank could make them think twice about seeing a specialist in your network. And the fact that the local hospital has performed only 10 total hip replacements in the past year may compel a patient to go elsewhere for the procedure. Decisions about where e-consumers receive their care will be based on more than local marketing and public relations efforts.

If health care e-consumers have choice built into their health plan, of course they are likely to go to the facility that performs the procedure they are about to have most frequently, with the best results, for the lowest cost. Order a reality sandwich and punch up the data about your health system to see what e-consumers and e-patients are learning.

PHYSICIANS ARE NOT MEETING E-CUSTOMER AND E-PATIENT DEMANDS

Although the e-world is an active one these days, physicians and other health providers have been slow to get on line. As shown in Table 3–2, using the Internet for delivering health and medical information is low on their list. Why?

- Health care organizations have always lagged behind in technology expenditures. Typically, if providers cannot see an immediate impact on the bottom line, they are reticent to spend money on a technology solution. This is unfortunate, since automation and Web-enabled networks present the solution to most if not all of the hassles of health care's fragmented and paper-ridden systems.
- Health care organizations—from hospitals to medical practices to health care plans—are strapped with old legacy information systems that are expensive to upgrade or to link to the Web service front end.

Table 3–2 Physicians' Preferred Patient Education Methods

	% of All Physicians	% of Physicians Who Use the Internet
Print Materials	73%	80%
Charts and Models	60%	65%
Videocassettes	52%	57%
Audiocassettes	37%	41%
Internet	19%	25%

Source: Data from cyberdialogue://findsvp, © 1998, 1997 Interactive Healthcare Professionals Survey, *The HealthMed Retrievers*.

- Health care organizations have difficulty seeing how the ability to buy books and research purchases on line has anything to do with health and medical care.
- Technology is often seen as "impersonal" by physicians and other providers.
- The culture of health care organizations is change resistant. In fact, many health care providers and companies ride the tail end of many business trends—for instance, they were loathe to get a computer in the first place. As nonprofit, helping enterprises, many organizations find it hard to admit that, in the end, they are running a business.

It is clear that many providers are ambiguous at best about patients getting information on line. E-customers and e-patients want health information on line and would prefer to receive it from national experts or their own physicians—but most physicians do not deliver information on line! Physicians surveyed state a preference for providing information to patients and consumers through methods other than the Internet. A commonly cited worry is that consumers might get inaccurate information at some of the top health care information sites and might incorrectly self-diagnose. But a recent Harris Interactive (www.HarrisInteractive.com) study shows that 67 percent of consumers prefer to print out information they find on line and bring it to their physician for discussion. About 90 percent say they want their physician involved before deciding what action to take. So while people might access information on America Online's (AOL) Health Channel (Figure 3–3), they most likely will discuss what they find with their physician before making a final decision. This reinforces the need to go beyond information to knowledge and decision support. Success on the Net in health and medical care depends on integrating Web services into the customer service function and then into the product/service delivery within whatever health care transaction.

Another provider argument is that consumers will not understand the information they are exposed to on line. That one does not hold water either. Health information on Web sites such as drkoop (www.drkoop.com), medscape.com, www.intelihealth.com, and OnHealth (www.onhealth.com) is packaged in clear, easy-to-follow form. No academic studies or complex statistical analyses here—just the outcome of these scientific studies, and news consumers can actually use in everyday life.

Finally there is the theory that most patients are seniors and that older Americans do not like computers. Wrong again. About 36 percent of seniors between the ages of 50 and 64 owned a PC in 1998, up from 27 percent in 1996. People over age 50 use a PC 14 days per month for an average of 130 minutes per day.

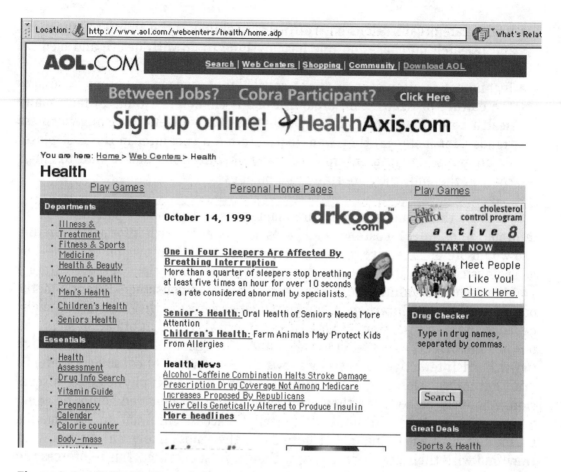

Figure 3–3 AOL Health Channel. *Source:* Reprinted with permission from www.aol.com, © 1999, America Online Health Channel.

Senior-focused Web site Third Age (www.thirdage.com) draws 250,000 senior cybervisitors a month by offering information on health, exercise, nutrition, and relationships. The fastest-growing group of Americans jumping on line are women over the age of 50.

The impetus is clear. Health care professionals and organizations must start playing catch-up. Whatever the reason for lagging behind e-consumer demands, it is time to get down to business. The Internet revolution rolls on—and the number of on-line Americans continues to increase—whether your health care institution likes it or not. E-customers and e-patients, not providers, are the ones leading the way.

GLOBAL WEB PORTALS ARE LEADING THE WAY, BUT WHERE ARE THEY HEADED?

National Web portals such as drkoop Online (Figure 3–4), medscape.com, OnHealth, Thrive Online (www.thriveonline.com), America's Health Network (www.TheHealthChannel.com), InteliHealth, and America's Doctor (www.americasdoctor.com) drive hundreds of thousands of unique visitors to their Web sites each month. drkoop Online and InteliHealth (sponsored by Aetna U.S. Healthcare and Johns Hopkins Medical Center) have brand names that consumers are coming to trust. drkoop Online offers comprehensive health content for women, seniors, men, and children. The Personal Drugstore, Personal Insur-

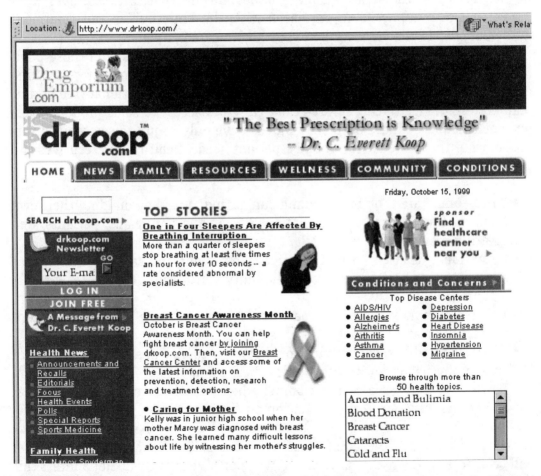

Figure 3–4 drkoop Online. *Source:* Reprinted with permission from www.drkoop.com™ (http://www.drkoop.com).

ance Center, and Personal Health Profile are just a few of the customized features offered to e-customers. drkoop Online boasts more than 90 support groups in its community.

Dr. Andrew Weil, a leader in the field of alternative health, has capitalized on his brand name as well; his Web site includes information about self-healing, supplements, and sexual health. At Thrive Online, launched in 1996, consumers can find information on medicine, fitness, sports, diet, and sexuality. In late 1998, Thrive Online began to focus primarily on women's health. America's Doctor (www.AmericasDoctor.com) serves up informative health quizzes and other health content and features television and movie stars talking about their health issues on video. Physicians are available round the clock to answer questions but not dispense medical advice—liability issues prevent that. Even so, does what America's Doctor's physicians say mesh with the philosophies and treatment methodologies of the physicians in your health care system?

The national health Web portals have received a lot of press, and those planning to go public stand to rake in big bucks as Wall Street clamors for anything combining the Internet and health care. But what are these national Web portals really offering? Health care information, tips, and access to some products, yes, but not much else. These on-line resources have only begun to scratch the surface of what the new e-customer and e-patient needs. Health care executives and providers need to ask the following questions of on-line resources:

- Whose brand are they building and supporting? Are they building their own brand at the expense of the relationships among physicians, patients, and health systems?
- Do national health Web portals offer transactions and services that reduce administrative health care costs (eligibility verification, call center e-transactions, etc.)?
- Are they integrated with "air-space" or "telephone-space" physician–patient relationships at a regional or local level?
- Do they facilitate communication between physicians and patients—or among physicians within the local medical community?
- Do they operate on a secure channel where e-patients can access personal and confidential medical information on line?

Today, the answer to each of these questions is "no." Tomorrow, the answer will be different. The reality is, national Web portals currently do not address this set of needs of the new e-customer or e-patient beyond providing health tips, support groups, and physician-finder services. And while these features are useful in their own right, when patients need care delivery, they want their physician or their hospital. Via the national Web portals, e-patients cannot communicate with their physician, receive e-care from local nurses or hospital staff, or enter an e-community that addresses their needs at the local level. The Web portals in 1999 tend to be text-based information warehouses that cannot even give medical advice or triage—it is too big a risk.

Given these facts, the opportunity for health care organizations is astounding. But if credible, trustworthy, and compassionate local or regional health systems and providers do not respond to e-consumers' desire for self-service, the national health Web portals stand ready to drive health care out of the local market through cyberdoctors.

No one knows who is the physician behind the keyboard at these various Web portals. He or she could have a medical philosophy that is very different from that of the physicians in your health system. Do e-patients really want medical care delivered by a faceless cyberphysician who is trained to be perceived as giving advice but cannot actually give advice because there is no physician–patient relationship? With high-speed connections, will cyberdoctors be able to diagnose and treat? The answer is yes, but the question remains whether it will be widespread in one year or five. Health care organizations need to aggressively seek ways to court e-consumers and e-patients. Let us not forget Chapter 2's tale of three bookstores—two bricks-and-mortar stores and one cyberspace store. Who continues to lead in on-line sales of books and music? Amazon.com, of course.

The fate could be the same for your bricks-and-mortar health organization! Be a maverick in your market—be the first to provide e-care on line and combine the benefits of "clicks-and-mortar" to better serve patients.

E-CUSTOMERS AND E-PATIENTS WANT SELF-SERVICE

In his book *NetFuture,* Chuck Martin describes seven cybertrends, one of which is the emergence of the "open-book corporation." Sure, health care organizations have given lip service to the idea of the customer being in charge. But in an open-book corporation, the customer is really in the driver's seat—if the producers of products and services are willing to sit in back. Let your e-customers and e-patients take the wheel by giving them access to literally everything about your business, make them do everything themselves—search for prices, schedule their visit, manage their account—and they will *love* you for it.[12]

The best consumer health and medical Web services offer great customer service through supported self-service through the Net. Take a look at Chapters 6 and 9 for some great examples of this, including Lifemasters.net. On-line media give you the opportunity to provide extraordinary customer service through supported self-service. E-customers can get handfuls of cash when banks are closed, and they can fill their tank at midnight without the assistance of a gas station attendant. E-patients do not want to be restricted to physicians' hours for answers to their health care questions—they want to find answers themselves, anytime. Supported Web self-service involves linking the Web service front end.

Look at the benefits of on-line trading of stocks. Gone are the days of calling a broker. E-customers place on-line trades by themselves at any time during the day. The individual investor has greater control, makes his or her own choices, and can access a broad range of research and analysis—at a time that is convenient. Web browsers and the Internet enable consumers to get better e-service, and the organization reduces its cost of supporting it. The e-customer is ecstatic that he or she pays less for the trade and gets to do it without making a call. The brokerage likes it because bypassing a broker reduces the overall cost of the trade.

What are the implications for Web-enabling health care transactions? A significant reduction in costs, for one. Empowering consumers by feeding them information that encourages better health care decisions and choices means fewer visits to the physician and fewer admissions. Monitor the blood sugar of diabetics, and there are fewer amputations and less retinopathy. Ensure asthmatics perform regular pulmonary function tests, and emergency department visits are reduced.

Re-engineer your call center to carry integrated real-time on-line Web telephony transactions as opposed to just phone-space transactions and services, and improve physician–patient communications. Obviously, some nurse triage issues do not lend themselves to e-mail or on-line text-based chat and must remain telephonic interactions until it is very easy to be surfing a Web site and open an audio/video window to a real-time medical call center when a live nurse is really needed. Today there are a whole bunch of health questions that can be answered simply by telling e-patients to log onto your Web service and access your frequently asked questions. Over the next decade, integrated Web real-time call centers will improve access to health and medical knowledge and decision support with lower operating costs.

Health insurance companies are turning on the Web services for e-consumers too. Prudential offers e-consumers health tips, extensive coverage information for each of its products, and a way to find a local physician. Blue Cross Blue Shield of California goes a step further and has Web-enabled its application and underwriting process. E-consumers can help themselves to any number of the insurer's plans and apply on line. Responses are quick, and Web-enabling the process has decreased the number of first applications that have to be sent back because information is missing; the on-line forms server does that in real time.

This is the time to form a task force that can rapidly plan strategies and actions. Health care systems and providers must be willing to provide this e-communication and supported self-service now. The lines of battle are already being drawn in cyberspace; if you want medical care delivered to patients in your community based on the philosophical norms of the physicians within it, do not wait to get on line. Be the first to structure e-care delivery that meets the needs of the eager e-patient. If your health care organization does not act now, the national Web portals will continue to "deliver" more and more care to your local patients. Total self-service in health and medical care can lead to disaster in many cases. The key is monitored on-line e-care support and integrated cyberspace and phone space real-time call centers. Check out Chapter 8 for indepth discussion of the next generation of medical call centers.

E-PATIENTS HAVE FILLED THEIR OWN E-VOIDS

While health care systems and providers were busy building physician–hospital organizations, e-patients were busy setting up their own support Web site and Net "portals." In fact, as noted above (Exhibit 3–3), consumers with chronic and serious illnesses find on-line support communities more helpful than either specialists or primary care physicians in 10 of 12 medical care areas. On-line groups ranked significantly higher than either generalists or specialists for convenience, emotional support, compassion/empathy, help in dealing with death and dying, and other indicators.[13]

Many physicians consider the Internet to be impersonal—to dehumanize the physician–patient relationship. E-patients disagree. They have gone ahead and empowered themselves and others who suffer from chronic illness or disease with access to information, on-line chats, and helpful bulletin board services. Somehow these e-patients figured the on-line experience—on their own time—was more effective and satisfying than the 9 to 12 minutes (on average) spent with their physicians face-to-face.[14]

Consumer-created Web sites such as Amanda's Home Page (www.avoiliknk.co.uk/amanda) can be a source of information and solace for many with chronic disease. Health care organizations can address these same e-patient needs by developing supported and monitored communities that carry accurate and timely medical information and are created and managed by health professionals. At the very least, health professionals should visit consumer sites regularly and sanction specific ones for their e-patients.

For example, the American Cancer Society has taken action to support consumers by establishing a unique on-line community of cancer survivors (www.cancersurvivorsnetwork.org) that is available across the country through interactive voice response technology and the Web. This on-line community allows a consumer to select a picture of "someone like you" and then navigate information about how a person and his or her family coped with a life-threatening disease such as cancer.

PRESCRIPTION FOR SUCCESS: DRUG MANUFACTURERS CORRAL E-CUSTOMERS ON LINE

Pharmaceutical companies are positioned way ahead of most health systems and health plans when it comes to offering health information to e-customers, and the amount of information available on their Web services continues to grow very quickly. Drug companies recognize that e-consumers and e-patients want faster and better on-line self-service. The companies have focused their efforts on these savvy customers and have found it profitable. Of the estimated $265 million pharmaceutical companies plan to spend on advertising by 2002 (total health and medical advertising by 2002 is estimated at $10.3 billion), 50 percent will be direct-to-consumer.[15]

Clearly, the Web is a standard part of pharmaceutical companies' marketing mix in communicating and supporting their products. Companies realize the e-customer's desire to access health information and have capitalized on it. (Consider, for instance, the ubiquitous Claritin ads—on line, on television, on airline name tags, and everywhere else.)

Many times a pharmaceutical company's first investment in Internet marketing is a Web site dedicated to just one product such as Excedrin (www.excedrin.com) or Vivarin (www.vivarin.com). The primary focus of most of these drug- or condition-specific Web sites is consumer outreach. The Excedrin Headache Resource Center delivers valuable consumer self-care information about headaches and how to manage them. Registered users receive free Excedrin samples. The site includes a headache workbook for assessing headaches and a headache diary to track occurrences of headache. Also available are quizzes, tips on stress relief, and advice on starting an exercise program. SmithKline Beecham's Vivarin Web site is fun and colorful. All features (e.g., the Vivarin (Spring) Break-Ability Index) are focused on the needs of people in their late teens and early twenties who are studying for their finals. Anyone hitting the Web site can receive a free sample.

Pharmaceutical companies realize the value of courting e-customers and have seized the opportunity to meet their needs. Each has taken a different approach to positioning their Web service—from aggressive marketing sites, based on a product name, that showcase products through educational information, to broader, more general health care Web sites. Some pharmaceutical companies have even launched comprehensive disease or condition-specific educational resources on line.

Reach outside of your health care organization and consider pharmaceutical companies as partners in your Web strategy. You can offer pharmaceutical companies your e-patients' attention as well as your own, since you are responsible for recommending their product to consumers. They can provide needed sponsorship underwriting to give your medical Web service a boost. You can also use the interactive tactics and diagnosis-specific tactics as examples as you offer e-patients an interactive experience on your Web service. Take time to ask e-consumers if they are open to receiving money-saving offers from sponsors. With the consumers approval, there is the opportunity for on-line promotions.

OPEN 24 HOURS A DAY, ON LINE

Empowered e-customers can purchase thousands of prescription and over-the-counter drugs 24 hours a day, 7 days a week, on the Internet. During 1999, there were many well-capitalized on-line drugstore start-ups that promised delivery to the customers' doorstep and discount prices. The first major player, Soma.com, launched in January, and drugstore.com (Figure 3–5) followed shortly in February. With a name that was easier to remember and the announcement that Amazon.com was a major investor, drugstore.com got a lot of press. Soma.com was quickly bought for $30 million by CVS.

Caution. Regional health systems and physicians could likely lose revenues from pharmaceutical services if on-line drugstores offer more convenient service at a lower cost. Do not let over-the-counter and prescription sales be snapped up by national on-line retail outlets. Offer the convenience of on-line drug purchases within your own system, *on line,* and deliver prescriptions in an hour or the same day.

E-PATIENTS MANAGE THEIR OWN DISEASE

It is estimated that 15 percent to 20 percent of all physician and emergency room visits—and up to 35 percent of physician office visits by chronically ill patients—are inappropriate because of lack of information to the patient. What

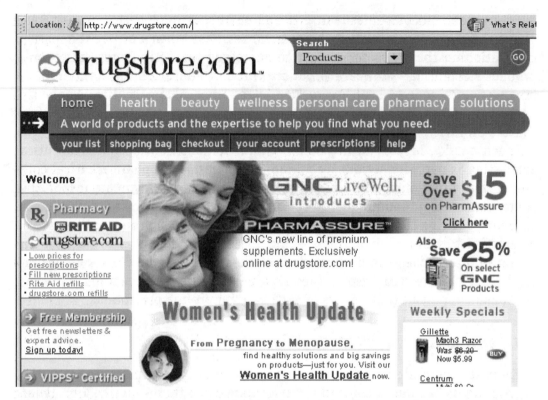

Figure 3–5 drugstore.com. *Source:* Reprinted with permission from www.drugstore.com, © 1999, drugstore.com.

if your health system and provider network could decrease this percentage by even 5 percent to 10 percent for at-risk populations using a variety of multimedia Internet and telephone-based interventions? That would mean a significant increase in the health of your customers and a decrease in costs. Continuous medical care, e-communication, supported self-service, and lower costs—that is what the Web can bring to medical care. E-care support revolutionizes medical care for those with conditions that need continuous monitoring. Diabetics and asthmatics, for example, must monitor their conditions on a regular basis, and until now, schedule frequent visits with their physician in person or through a broadband telemedicine connection into the home.

Web applications such as HelpDesk Online, by Patient Infosystems (www.healthdesk.com), give e-patients the ability to manage their condition at home. Save patient hassles, save money, save time; e-patients track their own health status and have access to diet and exercise information. Internet-based technology assists clinicians with oversight and management of their patient populations. The care support team generates on-line data, identifies patients who need attention, and modifies patient treatment plans on line. Consumers are communicated to via e-mail. Pharmaceutical companies such as Eli Lilly have also gotten into this approach. Lilly's on-line diabetes patient education program (http://diabetes.lilly.com), has a diabetes reference manual with information on diabetes and nutrition, a glossary, a patient log book, and educational video clips. There are basic facts on managing diabetes, preparing and injecting insulin, stages of care, controlling blood sugar, planning meals, exercising, foot care, and so on.

Home health will be revolutionized too, becoming home telemedicine. As information devices such as interactive telephones and WebTV connect the Internet via high-speed pipeline into the home, more and more patients will evolve into e-patients. The e-patient and provider sit "across" from each other and communicate over telephone modem or broadband cable, telephone, or electric company network. What beauty the Web can weave—patients obtain supported self-care and get regular e-visits from their physician or nurse, and self-management improves. Overall costs decrease, and e-patient wellness increases.

Get focused on specialty-specific and disease management services on line. Do physicians in your local community prefer to manage their own patients' disease or to hand off management to national cyberproviders? Partnering with existing interactive disease state management applications is a good way to use both cyberspace and air space. You will see a significant decrease in the overall costs of managing chronic conditions along with improved quality of life for the customer.

MANAGED CARE PLANS COMPETE FOR E-CONSUMERS AND E-PATIENTS

If your health system or medical practice has not embraced e-commerce and Web applications, take a lesson from insurers who have. HMO giant Kaiser Permanente (www.kaiserpermanente.org) jumped on line to offer members the opportunity to obtain free advice from a nurse or pharmacist, schedule an appointment, get a health risk assessment, and research health conditions and medications. Kaiser's focus on the e-customer is first rate, as the payer also offers health tip e-zines and on-line discussion groups. The members-only Web site for Kaiser is at www.kponline.com. Even if your organization is not a staff-model HMO, you could get many useful e-tips from the Kaiser site. It is not brochureware; it is designed to be an interactive encounter among e-patients, providers, and the health plan.

Meet the needs of your customers by creating interactive Web services that meet e-patient needs, integrate them with real-space transactions, and partner with your biggest payers. Offer e-patients daily transactions that go beyond mere information. Partnering with major health plans and others can provide e-consumers and e-patients a comprehensive, local-physician-sanctioned, one-stop shopping experience for e-consumers. It is all about service, convenience, and doing things that make people get better and live longer. Most important, it is about integrating information with quick and easy access to medical care services and self-care products.

REACHING THE NEW HEALTH CARE E-CONSUMER

What is your health care company doing to reach HMRs and chronic e-patients? If you are like many, your Web site was probably put up as a reaction and is a passive marketing presence. Most health care organizations' first-generation sites used brochureware—print content that was shoveled onto the Web site by graphic designers or computer jocks, who then dressed it up. First-generation Webmasters really did not understand the process of health care marketing and behavior change related to supporting better health.

But the days when on-line publishing and brochureware were acceptable are over. E-consumers expect much more from you. They want to do something—complete a transaction, interact with others. Your organization must deliver a flawless experience to e-customers and e-patients using this new, rapidly expanding, two-way medium. That means that every aspect of information, services, and transactions must be planned very carefully. Everything—from the number of page views required to reach critical points of the Web service, to fast and accurate fulfillment of product transactions or service interactions—must be nearly perfect.

Do not miss a beat. If e-consumers must wade through pages and pages of text before getting to what they want, they probably will not come back. If you do not update regularly, they will be bored. If it is not interactive, and e-consumers are left scrolling, they will get frustrated. And if you do not make it personal by addressing them directly, they will find that personalization somewhere else.

How do you develop a Web service that meets e-consumer needs? Simple. You ask them and get them involved through focus groups, volunteering, and other approaches.

Here is a good example. Bayfront Medical Center developed a premier on-line service—called Health Adventure (www.bayfront.org)—by asking patients what *they* wanted to see. Health Adventure provides both marketing and medical management to e-customers by empowering people to live healthier lives. Significant information about illnesses, disease, and injuries is served up as e-customers browse. Proactive Webcasting is based on an individual's needs and interests. E-patients have access to e-care delivery via information about local care centers, physicians, and other important caregivers. In 1997, Health Adventure was nominated for the Smithsonian ComputerWorld award for outstanding health care Web service design and content.

The result: Bayfront's interactive Web service, shown in Figure 3–6, has expanded the reach and effectiveness of its call centers and reduced the cost of health care by proactively providing proven preventive care and healthy living information. Health Adventure has become *the* on-line regional service for health—much like Digital City is AOL's on-line service for regional information. Its core features include 11 channels of evolving content and interactivity covering topics such as women's, men's, children's, and teens' health; specific diseases; alternative health care; and senior living.

Your local or regional company needs to follow Bayfront's lead and offer the recognized e-brands that consumers in your region trust. Why let them go to the competition when they can go to www.yourhospital.com or www.yourdoctor.com instead?

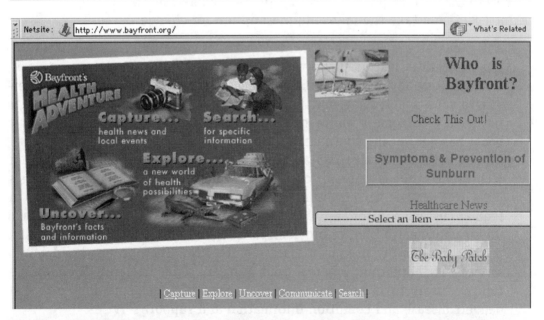

Figure 3–6 Bayfront Medical Center's Health Adventure. *Source:* Reprinted with permission from www. bayfront.org, © 1999, BayCare Health System.

BOW TO THE NEW HEALTH CARE E-CONSUMER AND E-PATIENT!

The Web revolution is only a few years old, but the message is clear: E-customers and e-patients want on-line support now. They want access to providers and health information on their own terms. It has to be convenient, it has to be personalized, and it better be just as user-friendly and comprehensive as HealthOnline.com, Medscape.com, Mediconsult.com, OnHealth.com, WebMD.com, and Disney.com.

National health Web portals today are not the complete solution to helping e-patients connect with care in their own community. The health care battle will be won locally, because that is where e-patients see their physicians. The experiences of national giants like Columbia HCA and now-defunct single specialty networks further illustrate this point. You cannot deliver medical care nationally. Health care is personal, between a patient and a provider, and *local*.

But taking an ostrich's approach is not the solution either. Your health care organization must capitalize on this new medium by becoming a recognized and convenient part of local e-customers' lives. In a world where health care content and tips are readily accessible (evidence the plethora of national Web portals pushing them), your health organization's competitive advantage is right in your backyard. In fact, it *is* your backyard.

Bow to the new, empowered health care e-consumer. Use the three Rs listed in Exhibit 3–4, and take the following prescription for change:

- **Ask e-customers what they want.** If patients come first and they want on-line health information support, then your health care organization can gain a competitive advantage by being a premier regional or national on-line service to your targeted segment. Do not put up a Web site only to find out it is not what e-customers want—or that few people use it because the on-line boom has not yet hit your market.
- **Do not build a one-size-fits-all Web service.** Build a consumer and patient Web service that is tailored, customized, and interactive. When consumers hit a Web service, it must address whether they are a first-time visitor or regular customer. After all, do you treat new members who have just signed up for your health plan or provider panel the same way that you treat that patient of record with known disease states? No. Then do not build a Web service like that either. Organize your Web service by delivering the information necessary for a new user as well as a private members-only area that delivers disease and condition information and support services.
- **Rally physicians around "your e-brand," and identify physician leaders.** Find willing, Web-enabled physicians. Test e-mail access with these willing

Exhibit 3–4 Focus on the 3 Rs

Relationship-Oriented: Build an e-brand that targets specific e-customers and e-patients and gives them what they want.

Retention-Oriented: Provide transactional opportunities—communication, e-zines, community, products—that bring e-customers back.

Really Easy: Build a presence that is easy for e-customers to locate and navigate. Do not go for the gusto right away—phase features in at a reasonable pace.

Source: Copyright © 1999, Douglas Goldstein.

providers and consumers. Determine how it can be rolled out, then launch the service, taking an aggressive position in the community. If your organization is first, it can gain a significant competitive advantage, using cyberspace to build air-space business.

- **Determine how your Web health service can develop its business model and facilitate mission-critical health care transactions.** Think information, services, products, appointment scheduling, eligibility checks. Your organization must develop comprehensive strategies and services to help consumers connect with their regional hospitals and physicians. A key goal is to be the premier on-line health resource in targeted markets. Various on-line initiatives can be self-funded through sponsorship, advertising, product sales, cross-selling of services, cost reductions, and numerous other mechanisms built into the business model.

- **Do not go for the gusto on day one.** Building a fully functional, transactional, and informational Web service is not as quick and easy as performing an appendectomy is for a surgeon. It takes time and planning. Phase in one or two elements at a time. Every Web service is a work in progress and must evolve based on the development of new technology and applications.

GO BEYOND INFORMATION TO WEB SERVICE

Empowered e-customers and e-patients are ready for health information, decision support, and medical care service delivery on line. The Internet-influenced market shift requires thinking about health care transactions, care delivery, information dissemination, and patient "power" in a whole new way. E-customers and e-patients are taking charge of their health. The distribution channel is changing. When providers and health care executives accept these facts, the opportunities for embracing e-patient needs are almost limitless.

Think services, transactions, and e-care delivery. Do it better, faster, cheaper—on line. Interact with e-customers and e-patients on the Web and focus on e-service, e-service, e-service. Follow this prescription, and you will revolutionize e-care delivery or whatever your current service or product in your markets.

REFERENCES

1. H. Taylor, "Explosive Growth of a New Breed of 'Cyberchondriacs,'" in *Executive Summary, The Harris Poll #11* (1999), 1.
2. "California Telehealth/Telemedicine Coordination Project Report" in *Smith Barney Analysis Report* (21 March 1997).
3. S. DeNelsky and M. Haspel, *e-Health: Getting Connected in a Digital Age* (ING Baring Furman Selz LLC), 2.
4. DeNelsky and Haspel, *e-Health*, 4.
5. "38 Million Americans Getting Wired," http://cyberatlas.internet.com/big_picture/demographics/mainstream.html (accessed 14 January 1999).
6. D. Rimer, P. Noglows, "Internet Appliances and Universal Access," http://www.iword.com/iword41/iword41.html (March 1999), accessed 24 August 1999.
7. United States Bureau of Labor Statistics, 1998.
8. "Females Lead Online Growth Spurt," http://www.cyberatlas.com/big_picture/demographics/nmr.html (21 June 1999).
9. *Consumerization of Healthcare* (Louis Harris & Associates, Inc., 1998), 1.
10. D. Bellandi, "Consumers First," *Modern Healthcare* (26 January 1998), 30.
11. "The Internet as a Driving Source of Social Change," in *New Voices, Consumerism in Health Care* (KPMG Peat Marwick Study, 1998), accessed 24 August 1999.
12. C. Martin, *Net Future: The 7 Cybertrends That Will Drive Your Business, Create New Wealth and Define Your Future* (McGraw-Hill, 1998), 91.
13. T. Ferguson and W. Kelly, "E-patients Prefer e-Groups to Doctors for Ten of Twelve Aspects of Health Care," *Ferguson Report 1*, no. 1 (1999): 1–3.
14. "The Internet as a Driving Force of Societal Change," http://www.intel.com/intel/e-health/internet.htm (1999), accessed 24 August 1999.
15. eHealth, inc., *Business Plan*, 22 March 1999, 24.

CHAPTER 4

The Explosion of Alternative Medicine Information and Products on the Web

S. Michael Ross and Pamela Tanton

ALTERNATIVE MEDICINE is a hot topic these days. People of all ages openly discuss their use of acupuncture, echinacea, St. John's wort, saw palmetto, and other "natural" remedies. Celebrities hawk ginkgo biloba on television, and natural supplements have become a multibillion-dollar business. Mainstream medical journals devote entire issues to alternative medicine. Larry King schedules Dr. Andrew Weil on his popular CNN prime-time television program, and the *New York Times* frequently covers alternative medicine topics in its Tuesday "Science Times" section. Tens of thousands of Web pages deliver tons of alternative health information—some good and some very questionable.

But what exactly is "alternative medicine?" The term has been defined as "medical interventions that are neither taught widely in U.S. medical schools or not generally available in U.S. hospitals."[1] As Figure 4–1 indicates, opinions about alternative medicine have become more positive in the past five years, and Americans have been turning to these therapies at such a rapidly increasing rate that the term *alternative therapy* is fast becoming a misnomer. Because of this, most experts now refer to treatment modalities such as acupuncture, biofeedback, chiropractic, homeopathy, naturopathy, massage therapy, and hypnotherapy as complementary therapies. Complementary and alternative medicine (CAM) and integrative medicine are new terms in the health care industry. In this chapter, we refer to alternative therapies as CAM.

There are two primary CAM topics that have found their way onto the Web. First are the CAM services themselves—acupuncture, chiropractic, and other holistic plans of treatment. E-consumers, e-practitioners, and others have posted information about these services across the international boundaries that make up cyberspace. Second, and probably more prevalent, are the herbs, tinctures, supplements, and holistic products that are touted by manufacturers and happy users. It is plain to see that there are significant dollars to be made selling these products on line—and no shortage of companies doing it.

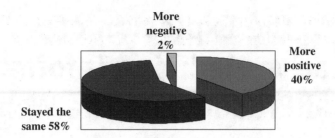

Figure 4–1 Opinions about Alternative Medicine—Change over the Past Five Years. *Source:* Data from Landmark Healthcare Survey of 1,300 Households, Landmark Healthcare, Inc., Sacramento, California.

This chapter introduces physicians, health care practitioners, and health system and plan executives to the CAM trends being driven by e-consumers and the pros and cons of e-information available on the Web. The consumer-driven trend toward CAM and integrative medicine cannot and should not be ignored. At the same time, however, health care providers and executives must realize that in their search for information about CAM on the Web, e-consumers can be led down a path of misinformation. Becoming informed, as well as listening to e-patients or e-beneficiaries, is a critical step for health care leaders, so they can assist e-consumers with ferreting out good CAM e-information from bad.

CASHING IN ON CAM SERVICES AND PRODUCTS

Demand for CAM services and natural products has exploded in recent years, and industry sources estimated out-of-pocket CAM expenditures of $27 billion in 1997. Exhibit 4–1 offers details about this growth. Much of this growth is being fueled by aging Baby Boomers' interest in healthier lifestyles, a national trend toward preventive medicine in response to rising health care costs, and a growing dissatisfaction with the effectiveness of conventional medicine in the treatment of many chronic conditions. In 1997, approximately 42 percent of consumers sought and used CAM products or services (up from 34 percent in 1990). These consumers scheduled approximately 629 million visits with CAM-related providers, versus an estimated 386 million visits to primary care physicians.

e-PREDICTION: *PATIENTS WILL BECOME MORE AND MORE DEPENDENT ON THE WEB FOR THEIR MEDICAL INFORMATION ABOUT CAM, AND PHYSICIANS WHO INQUIRE ABOUT PATIENTS' WEB USE AND*

ABOUT PATIENTS' USE OF CAM WILL BE MORE LIKELY TO FOSTER
SATISFACTION AND IMPROVED RELATIONSHIPS.

The market for dietary supplements is also growing at a rapid pace. Based on estimates by Packaged Facts, an independent consumer marketing research firm, the retail market for vitamins, minerals, and supplements has grown at a compound annual growth rate of 15 percent—from $3.7 billion in 1992 to $6.5 billion in 1996. Most of this growth has occurred in the sales of supplements, and primarily herbal products, which grew from $570 million in 1992 to $2.3 billion in 1996 (a 42 percent compound annual growth rate). Growth in this category has been driven by the popularity of such herbs as echinacea, garlic, ginseng, ginkgo biloba, and, more recently, saw palmetto and St. John's wort. Americans bought $100 million of St. John's wort and $126 million of ginkgo biloba in 1997, according to the American Botanical Council, the industry's main trade group. The Packaged Facts report forecasts that the supplements market will grow at a 25 percent compound annual growth rate through 2001, or twice the rate of the overall vitamin and mineral supplements category.

REASONS CONSUMERS LIKE CAM

While many physicians may view a patient's interest in alternative medicine as a sign of rejection, or perhaps a rejection of today's medical environment in general, one recent study indicates that dissatisfaction with physicians or man-

---

Exhibit 4–1 Alternative Medicine on the Rise

- The *Journal of the American Medical Association (JAMA)* devoted its November 1998 issue to alternative medicine.
- In 1997, 42.1 percent of consumers used at least 1 of 16 alternative therapies during the previous year (up from 33 percent in 1990).
- *Time* magazine's cover article for November 1998 featured alternative medicine.
- The *Los Angeles Times* ran a four-part series on alternative medicine in the summer and fall of 1998.
- Vitamins, supplements, herbal remedies, and other "alternative treatments" comprise a $27 billion dollar industry.
- Andrew Weil's Web page gets 3.5 million hits per month.

Source: Compiled by S. Michael Ross.

aged care appears to have little bearing on the use of alternative therapies.[2] Instead, nonconventional medicine seems to have an appeal because it complements people's values and beliefs about health and life. The study found that users of alternative therapies are typically well educated, suffer from specific conditions (including anxiety, back problems, chronic pain, and urinary tract problems), consider themselves committed to environmentalism or feminism, and hold an interest in spirituality and personal growth.[3] Exhibit 4–2 profiles the users of alternative medicine, according to this study.

One of the primary CAM demand drivers is widespread consumer frustration with conventional medicine's inability to treat chronic illness. Treatment success for conditions such as arthritis, asthma, and chronic fatigue syndrome—for which conventional medicine offers little relief—is often achieved using CAM therapies, more cost-effectively, and with fewer adverse side effects. Patients are also seeking a gentler, more natural approach to health care and disease prevention. They complain about the impersonal nature of conventional medicine and hurried interactions with physicians—which, according to some experts, have declined to an average of 9 to 12 minutes per encounter. Contrary to their dissatisfaction with rush-rush traditional physician visits, consumers indicate remarkable satisfaction with CAM services.

It is also important to consider the influence of the U.S. population's increasing diversity. America is no longer overwhelmingly Caucasian. The demographic makeup of young Americans aged 15 to 25 is one-third minority—African American, Hispanic, and Asian American. In fact, the minority populations of today will nearly be the majority in the year 2050. According to Census Bureau predic-

---

Exhibit 4–2 Profile of Alternative Medicine Users

- Well educated
- Poor health status
- Change in worldview due to a "transformational experience"
- Specific health problems (anxiety, back problems, chronic pain, urinary tract problems)
- Belonging to a cultural group characterized by commitment to environmentalism and/or feminism
- Interest in spirituality and personal growth psychology

Source: Adapted with permission from the *Journal of the American Medical Association*, Vol. 279, pp. 1548–1553, © 1998, American Medical Association.

tions, in 50 years, 47 percent of America will be composed of today's so-called minorities.[4]

It only makes sense then that the face of health care is changing as the American population diversifies. Asian Americans, for example, are used to receiving any number of Chinese herbs to cure what ails them. Hispanic populations too use natural products—it is part of their culture. American health care providers must have an understanding of international treatment regimes and herbs if they are to effectively treat their patients with an international heritage.

"NATURAL" PRODUCTS APPEAL TO AMERICAN CONSUMERS

Another allure of alternative remedies is that people view them as more "natural," which is consistent with the profile of people interested in the environment, in feminism, and in spirituality. Consider the example of Karen, an American consumer who is drawn to alternative therapies.

Karen is a 33-year-old American mother of a five-month-old infant. She has a master's degree in biology and describes herself as a feminist. While talking with a friend who had returned from Germany to visit a nephew, Karen discovered that, for inconsolable crying, the pediatrician of the German infant prescribed a chamomile suppository and recommended wrapping the infant in a heated blanket sprinkled with lavender drops. Not a typical American approach.

To Karen, this treatment sounded wonderful. She viewed it as a natural, gentle way to comfort her infant. But did she talk to her infant's pediatrician about this type of treatment? No. She turned to the Web to see what she could find. According to Eisenberg, more than 60 percent of consumers of alternative therapies do not talk with their physicians about alternative medicine.[5] They know that medical professionals are often reluctant to promote, endorse, or suggest alternative therapies, and they may fear being judged negatively or being told to stop the treatment. They may also not want their physicians to think they are rejecting their approach to medicine. So they turn to other sources for information and guidance. And because of the profile of these consumers, it is safe to assume that one of their main sources of information is the Internet.

THE PHENOMENON OF DR. ANDREW WEIL

Any discussion of CAM would be incomplete without mention of Dr. Andrew Weil.

Harvard-educated Dr. Weil is widely known for his push to integrate alternative therapies into traditional treatment regimes. Consumers view him as "the people's physician" because of his support of patient empowerment and rejection of the prevailing medical paradigm of the passive patient.

Enter the Web. If an e-consumer is even the slightest bit interested in alternative medicine, chances are that he or she has visited Dr. Weil's site, Ask Dr. Weil (www.pathfinder.com/drweil/). One of the most popular alternative medicine destinations, Ask Dr. Weil receives about 3.5 million hits per month, according to its Web staff. Dr. Weil has smartly capitalized on his own personal brand-name awareness with this Web service. His patient-friendly approach is appreciated by his e-audience, and the information provided is balanced and moderate.

Far and away the most popular CAM site, Ask Dr. Weil sports the recognizable brand name of renowned CAM physician Andrew Weil, MD. Ask Dr. Weil is an interactive site where visitors can submit questions about alternative therapies, search for a local practitioner, and gain tips and information about a variety of holistic remedies. Supplements are available for sale, and the site is also supported by advertisers. Ask Dr. Weil gets high marks for its ability to provide practical information that e-consumers easily understand.

Alternative treatment e-information on Ask Dr. Weil is backed up with evidence from recent studies, and it is frequently recommended that e-patients stay with their traditional regimen—and consider complementing it, not replacing it, with an alternative therapy. In fact, this is the method most consumers prefer, according to a Landmark Healthcare study, the results of which are shown in Figure 4–2. Ask Dr. Weil features links to places to purchase items, such as the Vitamin Shoppe, an on-line bookstore, and a monthly e-newsletter, *Self-Healing*. Visitors can search for a local holistic healer, participate in an interactive poll that asks questions such as "Have you ever bought vitamins through the Web?", and conduct a keyword search for alternative health topics.

CAM GOES MAINSTREAM

In addition to getting high marks from consumers, alternative medicine has been inching its way into mainstream medical organizations. Bastions of medical conservatism—including prestigious academic medical centers such as Harvard, Duke, Stanford, and Columbia—have begun exploring how to integrate alternative therapies into courses of treatment. In addition, each year more medical schools add CAM content to their standard curriculum.

In 1992, the National Institutes of Health (NIH) established the Office of Alternative Medicine (OAM) to facilitate the evaluation of alternative medical therapies and treatment modalities, to exchange information with the public about alternative medicine, to support research and training, and to prepare reports.

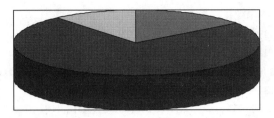

Figure 4–2 Combining Alternative and Traditional Care—Approach Preferred by Consumers Surveyed. *Source:* Data from "Combining Alternative and Traditional Care," Landmark Healthcare, Inc., Sacramento, California.

One of the study outcomes shows solid evidence that acupuncture is a useful treatment for postoperative and chemotherapy-induced nausea and vomiting, pregnancy-related nausea, and postoperative dental pain, and for a number of other pain-related conditions.[6]

Congress has increased OAM's budget each year. In 1997, the budget was $24 million. In November 1998, Congress promoted the OAM to NIH center status, ensuring a minimum appropriation of $50 million for 1998. Obviously, the NIH believes that OAM's work is worthwhile.

CAM SEEKERS GET EMPOWERED ON THE WEB

Clearly, consumers, health care organizations, and even some medical schools are very interested in CAM. But CAM information is still far from being widely distributed by the medical community. So where are consumers finding information about CAM? Put simply, they primarily find it on the Web. A report by Deloitte & Touche (Cyberatlas) and VHA, Inc., states that 17.5 million adults use the Web for health information, and these adults list alternative medicine as one of the topics for which they search. A report from Harris Interactive (www.HarrisInteractive.com) in 1997 indicated that 70 million Americans are going on line for their health information each year. With the easy access, and in the comfort of their own home, these e-consumers seek information that helps them make decisions about their own or their family's medical care.

The easy availability of CAM information on the Net has dovetailed with the increased interest in alternative medicine to create an e-consumer who is more informed (or misinformed, depending on the information accessed), more demanding about treatment, and more willing to go behind a physician's back for treatment. This shift has significantly affected the health care delivery system—and it is being driven by the lure of e-patient empowerment, convenience, accessibility, and self-service.

SUPERNET WOMAN LOGS ON

Recent statistics show that women make up an increasingly large number of Netizens. Cyberdialogue reports that 42 percent of on-line users in 1999 were women. The researcher also reports that one of the fastest-growing groups of Americans jumping on line is women over 50. Women on line seek health information and products for more than just themselves. A woman's diverse role as mother, head of household, or caregiver for an ailing parent or relative has driven SuperNet Woman to research health and CAM information for the whole family.

Power Surge is one site (www.dearest.com) that is capitalizing on this SuperNet Woman profile. Power Surge focuses on menopause and perimenopause and projects a tone that mirrors SuperNet Woman's attitude: "We're going to find our own solutions no matter what regimens our mainstream physicians want us to follow." Although the site is not officially an alternative medicine site, a quick review of chat room discussion topics reveals that the women who visit this site regularly and openly speak about dong quai, kava kava, black kohosh, and natural progesterone. These women know they are among other supporters of nontraditional regimes and are comfortable venting their frustrations. A comment from a woman on one message board asks, "Why, do you suppose, don't our physicians tell us about natural progesterone? Notice how quickly they provide free samples of prescription drugs by the mega-pharmaceutical houses?"

Visitors to the site clamor for alternatives to traditional hormone replacement therapy (HRT), and guests to the discussions include individuals such as Dr. Robert Atkins (www.power-surge.com/transcripts/atkins.htm), who during one discussion was promoting his most recent book, *Vita-Nutrient Solution*. Dr. Atkins says he wants to teach physicians about the "wonders of vita-nutrient therapy" and says that he is leery about HRT and suggests instead specific vitamin therapy. Power Surge urges visitors to talk with their physicians first before stopping prescribed treatments or beginning new ones, but it is easy to imagine many of the visitors to the site ignoring this advice, abandoning their HRT, and ordering supplies of products listed on the site.

Power Surge is a fairly typical CAM site—part commercial, part informational, using physicians and other highly credentialed professionals to support its claims. We wonder whether most mainstream gynecologists and health care executives are aware that Web sites like Power Surge exist and how they would respond if they did know. Would they discuss these issues with their patients? Would they try to dissuade them from going the alternative route? Would they explore opportunities to recommend treatments their patients are interested in?

OPENING PANDORA'S BOX

As many health care practitioners might expect, the Web continues to be a Pandora's box of CAM information. A general search for "alternative medicine" can turn up thousands upon thousands of matches. For example, a search on Excite (www.excite.com) turns up five directory matches and over 1 million site matches. The same search on AltaVista (www.altavista.com) returns over 58,000 matches, and on Infoseek (www.infoseek.com), 8,353,704. On Savvy Search (www.savvysearch.com), the result is a "meta-search" showing four pages of directory matches.

Although these searches can turn up some good information, clicking through many of the listed sites can easily lead down a road to holistic therapy for pets, tales of unidentified flying objects, offers for tarot readings, and discussions about urine therapy. Not to be outdone, manufacturers have purchased hundreds and hundreds of advertisements and other entreaties to buy vitamins, herbal products, homeopathic remedies, videos, and books. These advertisements are also culled by the search engines.

Another concern is that many alternative medicine Web sites are maintained by individuals who have personal experience with an alternative treatment or by product manufacturers—not by licensed, trained physicians or other practitioners. And because information about CAM products and services is unregulated, these sites may present biased or incomplete information.

Take the example of saw palmetto, an herbal remedy often used for treating prostate problems. Saw palmetto ranks sixth among top-selling herbal remedies and appears to be efficacious in reducing the symptoms of benign prostatic hypertrophy (enlargement of the prostate gland). If you want more on-line information about saw palmetto, you might type "www.sawpalmetto.com" into your browser and be taken to the Saw Palmetto Harvesting Company's Web site (www.sawpalmetto.com), where you can read all sorts of information about saw palmetto and its many benefits. But nowhere are any warnings or reported adverse side effects listed. Nowhere is the visitor warned that men taking saw palmetto for their prostate problems can actually have a reduced prostate-specific antigen level—which is an *indicator* of prostate cancer in early detection tests. If you are a physician or health care executive, this should be a wake-up call. Uninformed men who regularly take saw palmetto can mistakenly "pass" early detection tests—which means their cancer could go undiagnosed.

Another herbal remedy, St. John's wort, is a popular treatment for depression. Considered by many to be a natural alternative to drugs such as Prozac and Zoloft, St. John's wort is available in a variety of forms, including pills, foods, and even a transdemic patch. One popular site devoted to St. John's wort is My Personal St. John's Wort Pages, which is hosted and maintained by a man who has successfully taken St. John's wort to treat his depression. The good news is that although the Webmaster is not a practitioner, he does include a page about the herbal remedy's side effects as well as suggest that visitors consult their physician before taking the product.

When searching for vitamin, herb, and supplement information, e-consumers are more likely to find retail sites that are actually selling these products than information-only sites. And rarely do these sites mention side effects or offer other warnings—let alone an unbiased or clinical description of the remedy. In a search on AltaVista for St. John's wort, for example, 8 of the first 10 Web sites listed are commercial sites selling the product.

HEALTH PLANS OFFER CAM BENEFITS AND WEB SERVICES

If managed care is focused on preventing disease and keeping people well, integrating alternative therapies into managed care is smart. Managed care plans have found that more than 4 in 10 adults surveyed in late 1997 by Landmark Healthcare, a managed alternative care company based in Sacramento, California, had used alternative care within the past 12 months (Figure 4–3). Two-thirds of them said that availability of alternative care was an important factor in choosing a health plan. Health maintenance organizations (HMOs) understand the changing landscape, and they see alternative medicine as a way to differentiate themselves from the competition while controlling costs. It is a smart move.[7]

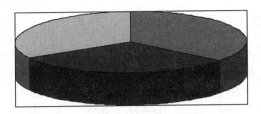

Figure 4–3 Importance of Availability of Alternative Care When Consumers Choose Health Plans, by Percentage of Consumers Surveyed. *Source:* Data from "Importance of Alternative Care when Choosing a Plan," Landmark Healthcare, Inc., Sacramento, California.

Since about 85 percent of our nation's health care dollars are spent on the treatment of chronic disease, managed care plans have become very interested in alternative therapies that can help minimize the cost of care for chronically ill people. The Centers for Disease Control and Prevention maintains that 37 percent of cancer, 49 percent of arteriosclerosis, 50 percent of cerebrovascular disease, and 54 percent of heart disease are preventable through lifestyle modification, so it is not surprising that 58 percent of HMOs surveyed by the National Association of Health Underwriters cover one or more alternative therapies. Among those that do, the top therapies used by their members are chiropractic, acupuncture, nutrition therapy, and osteopathic medicine.[8] Exhibit 4–3 lists the most frequently used alternative therapies.

Exhibit 4–3 Most Frequently Used Alternative Therapies

- Chiropractic
- Acupuncture
- Nutrition therapy
- Osteopathic medicine

Source: Data from J. Henderson, Mainstreaming Alternative Medicine: Survey of HMOs Regarding Alternative Therapies, *Health Insurance Underwriter*, pp. 24–25, © March 1998.

An increasing number of insurance companies and health plans are responding to this consumer demand and have begun to cover or explore coverage of CAM services. Currently, more than half of U.S. HMOs provide access to some form of it. The move to cover CAM services was in many ways precipitated by Washington State, which in 1995 passed legislation requiring all health plans to include CAM providers in their networks. Oxford Health Plans, based in Norwalk, Connecticut, was the first major HMO to add CAM coverage, which it began to offer in 1997, without a regulatory mandate.

Financial difficulties have stalled plans to enhance Oxford's offerings in this area, but the plan does offer a network of 2,800 alternative care providers—chiropractors, massage therapists, and acupuncturists—and nearly half of Oxford's 2 million enrollees use some form of alternative care. Oxford's Web site (Figure 4–4) has an alternative medicine page that gives members and providers answers to frequently asked questions, information about how to become a member of the provider network, and instructions about how to find a provider in a specific area. Articles about chiropractic care, homeopathy, Chinese Taoism, and other topics are also available on the site.

The move toward offering CAM benefits reaches coast to coast. In November of 1998, Denver-based Blue Cross and Blue Shield of Colorado began marketing an alternative care package to its Blue Advantage Medicare risk enrollees. Members are offered a blend of covered benefits. Kaiser Permanente of the mid-Atlantic states added alternative medicine to its roster of services in early 1999. Kaiser enrollees have access to a network of acupuncturists and chiropractors after obtaining a referral from their primary care physician.

e-Advice: If Health Plans Cover It, e-Patients Will Want It

Explore opportunities to add CAM services and/or information to your health system or health plan's Web service, as well as its menu of air-space workshops and services.

LEADING E-PATIENTS AND E-CONSUMERS TO CREDIBLE INFORMATION

CAM is not a passing fad, and neither is the Web. Health care practitioners and insurers who want to remain competitive and meet patient and beneficiary needs must understand what is going on in cyberspace and what e-consumers and e-patients are learning about alternative remedies. As a physician, wouldn't you want to know which alternative therapies your chronically and seriously ill patients are following, or herbal remedies they are taking? Most often this informa-

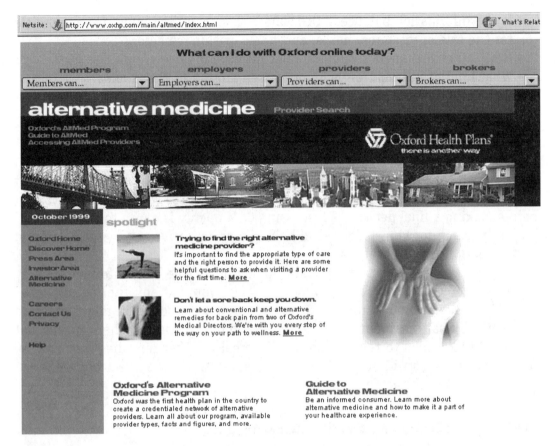

Figure 4-4 Oxford Health Plans. *Source:* Reprinted with permission from www.oxhp.com/altmed/main.htm, © 1999, Oxford Health Plans, Inc.

tion is not even asked about in the exam room—leaving a potential for drug interactions or worse.

Certainly there are a variety of benefits to CAM therapies. But it is critical that physicians and other providers recognize which CAM information on the Web is not reliable. The essential issues for physicians and other health care providers are twofold: be knowledgeable about alternative information on the Web, and *ask* patients about the CAM information they have found. Review it with them carefully, using the following series of questions:

- What is the sponsoring organization, and is it credible?
- Is it easy for the e-patient to discern what is reliable information and what is not?

- Is the information balanced? Or is the Web site nothing more than a vehicle for the sale of vitamins, herbs, and homeopathic remedies?
- How can e-consumers recognize sales pitches, if some are on the site?
- What kind of information is being passed around in chat rooms?
- If the site promotes the sale of products, does it also present unbiased information about other options?

Do not view alternative therapies, or Web information about them, as a threat to your practice. On the contrary, this is an opportunity to assist patients with assessing all their treatment options. Studies show that more than 90 percent of patients who find information on the Web want to share it with their physician before making a final decision.[9] Discussing CAM openly is a way to validate your patient's search for knowledge—and help him or her arrive at a medical decision that feels right for both of you.

How can you get e-patients to talk openly about the CAM information they have discovered on the Web? One way is to revise your patient information materials to include an invitation to discuss the topic with you. You might mention that you are aware that many people find useful information on the Web and that you would like them to tell you about all herbal or other remedies they may be following. Doing so will help patients understand that the subject of CAM is not taboo with their physician.

REVIEW CAM SITES USING SOUND CRITERIA

This chapter has already discussed some of the more popular CAM sites on the Web and pointed out the thousands of pages available for e-consumers on a search. But what really makes a CAM Web site good? Given the hundreds of thousands of sites about CAM on the Web and the fact that information served up by the major browsers is largely unregulated, how can physicians and other practitioners determine which sites are credible? It is time-consuming to click through the myriad of CAM sites—physicians and practitioners are busy enough just trying to see everyone on the schedule and get their claims out.

To assist busy professionals, we have compiled a list of characteristics that make a CAM site good. These guidelines are then used to evaluate a listing of CAM sites later in the chapter. They are:

- Truthful
- Unbiased
- Offering indepth information
- Easy to use

Trustworthiness and Reliability. What is the source of the site's content? Is the content provided by educational institutions (e.g., colleges, universities, medical schools), government reports or sources (e.g., NIH, Food and Drug Administration, Centers for Disease Control and Prevention), or licensed medical professionals? Does the site tell you how the content is deemed reliable (e.g., panel of experts, medical professional approval process)? How recent is the citation, and how sound was the study?

Lack of Bias. Is the site also selling alternative health products or services, such as vitamins, supplements, herbs, acupuncture, massage therapy, or aromatherapy products? Does the site try to steer you toward certain products or services? Does the site deliver pros and cons for product usage?

Depth of Services. How detailed is the Web site's information? Is the content varied, including articles, interviews, searchable information databases, message boards, and access to customer service people by telephone?

Ease of Use. Is the information clearly presented? How secure is the Web site for low-risk shopping? How easy is it to navigate the site? Is there a searchable database of information, and if so, is it easy to use?

Prominent Disclaimers. All medical sites should have disclaimers.

Focus on Service and Interaction. Are the information and products presented in a flat, buy-now way, or does the Web site deliver actual customer service features?

ALL ABOARD THE ALT.MED E-TOUR

Below is a listing of Web sites that are considered good based on the preceding criteria. As you visit each, understand that many Web sites can be chameleonlike. A good site today can be a completely different site next month—or even tomorrow—if the sponsor or Webmaster changes, or if the direction or vision of the organization changes. Maintain a sensitivity to hidden agendas, motivations, and sales goals in all the sites you visit. That said, you can typically assume that the tone and motivations of most sites are likely to remain fairly constant, without considerable change from one month, or even year, to the next.

A good general rule of thumb is that noncommercial sites often offer the most integrity. These include sites sponsored by government agencies such as NIH and sites sponsored by universities and other nonprofit organizations. Unfortunately, but probably predictably, many of these sites are not particularly amusing, diverting, or interactive. Because many of them are government or university based, they do not offer the quizzes and contests that a lot of commercial sites do.

Government- or university-sponsored sites are not the only organizations that produce credible e-information. Some commercial sites contain solid, useful tips and data for the e-consumer interested in alternatives to traditional medicine. And for pure fun, amusement, and interactivity, these commercial sites are the way to go. Win a prize, ask Dr. Weil a question, or get a certificate for a product discount—these are the lures that draw e-consumers to the commercial sites.

Using this list, readers who are new to CAM can further their understanding of this explosive growth area in the American health system. Review each site on your own and use it as a foundation for developing a list of sanctioned sites for the e-patients in your practice or health system. (Sites are listed alphabetically.)

Acupuncture.com

Acupuncture is an alternative treatment commonly sought by Westerners. This popular, distinctly non-Western site (www.acupuncture.com/experiences/exp.htm) offers a great deal of information about traditional Chinese medicine, a listing of acupuncturists worldwide, practitioner resources, descriptions of a typical first visit to an acupuncturist, and e-patient testimonials. The site clearly promotes acupuncture, but it does not pressure patients to buy products. It could also be viewed as a valuable introduction to the general topic of alternative medicine.

Alternative Health News Online

While it primarily serves up links to other alternative medicine sites on the Web, the Alternative Health News Online site (Figure 4–5) does begin with a full-page introduction to its method for selecting sites and offers guidelines for following the information presented. It says that its content meets criteria established by the National Center for Complementary and Alternative Medicine (NCCAM) at NIH. Particularly interesting here is the site's collection of recent articles published about alternative medicine.

There is great depth to the content offered on this site, and the site itself is easy to use. An unbiased, balanced perspective is evident in the offering of links not only to alternative medicine sites but to mainstream sites such as the *New*

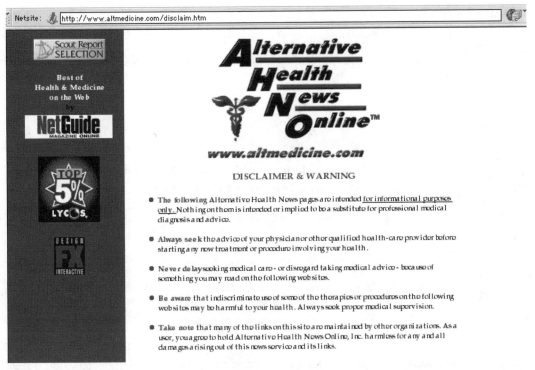

Figure 4–5 Alternative Health News Online. *Source:* Reprinted with permission from www.altmedicine.com/welcome.html, © 1999, Alternative Health News Online, Inc.

England Journal of Medicine and Quackwatch (Figure 4–6), a highly conservative, traditional site that could easily be characterized as against alternative medicine.

Alternative Medicine (from Yahoo! Search)

This site (dir.yahoo.com/health/alternative_medicine/) is a good example of the confusion that can arise when e-consumers do a simple search for "alternative medicine." While many of the links are sound, there are also such links as "urine therapy," "gemstone therapy," and "wiccan pages." Advertisers such as PlanetRX.com and "the eCenter™ for Alternative and Complementary Care" provide the banners. There is no question that there is a wealth of information here—it is simply a matter of knowing how to navigate the information overload. One of the site's better features is a searchable database and listing of treatment options for 114 diseases and conditions. Newbies be warned. For the nondiscerning e-consumer, this site may offer too much.

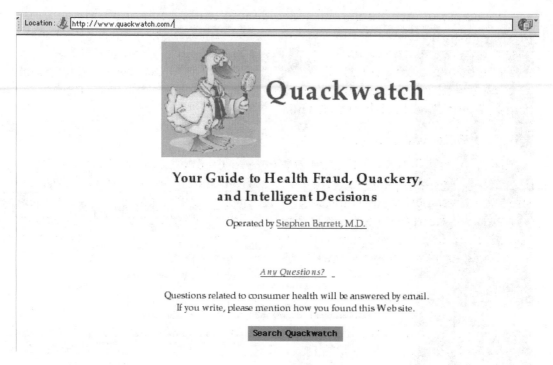

Figure 4–6 Quackwatch. *Source:* Reprinted with permission from www.quackwatch.com, © 1999, Quackwatch, Inc.

Alternative Medicine Connection

An extremely useful site (www.arxc.com/arxchome.htm) for laypeople and professionals, the Alternative Medicine Connection is a "jump station" that offers a listing of alternative medicine newsletters, community organizations, a directory of practitioners, a patient information exchange, and much more. Many of the listings lead to government and university sites, but there are also commercial sites that seem primarily interested in selling products—such as the Life Extension Foundation.

The Alternative Medicine Homepage

The Alternative Medicine Homepage (www.pitt.edu/cbw/altm.html) describes itself as a "jump station for sources of information on unconventional, unorthodox, unproven, or alternative, complementary, innovative, integrative therapies." It is a noncommercial site compiled by the Library of the Health Sciences at the University of Pittsburgh. Links include information on acquired immune deficiency syndrome (AIDS) and the human immunodeficiency virus (HIV), databases, Internet resources, mailing lists and newsgroups, government resources, and practitioners' directories. This site is useful for professionals and laypeople alike. A disclaimer responsibly states that the page itself "does not replace the care by a qualified health practitioner."

American Botanical Council

The American Botanical Council is a nonprofit educational and research organization whose Web page was created to answer basic questions about herbs. The site (www.herbalgram.org/directory.html) is understated and concise and seems to be geared more toward the professional than the lay individual, although the organization does hit e-consumers up for a tax-deductible donation. There is no searchable database on this site.

Chiro.org

The Chiro.org noncommercial site (www.chiro.org) is oriented toward professionals, but e-consumers and e-patients will find it informative too. Visitors can obtain a referral to a local practitioner via the site's database and learn about the history of chiropractic medicine. There is also a searchable database library and lots of links to other information.

HealthWorld Online

Describing its philosophy as one of "self-managed care," www.healthy.net (Figure 4–7) offers an abundance of material to laypeople, health professionals, journalists, and researchers. Free services include Medline search capability, a daily newsfeed, a global health calendar, a professional referral network, a speaker's network, and *Healthy Update,* an electronic newsletter. Visitors can search by selecting from a list of hundreds of diseases and conditions. Healthy.net is a commercial site, and consequently it has a health food store and a bookstore. It has interactive features too, like the discussion forum, in which individuals post queries about specific conditions or products, and anyone can post a response. The site is clearly designed and easy to navigate.

HealthWWWeb

Maintained by the Integrative Medical Arts Group, Inc., this Web site (www.healthwwweb.com) offers comprehensive, balanced, and useful information about natural health and alternative remedies for both e-consumers and medical professionals. HealthWWWeb promises development of an herb/drug/

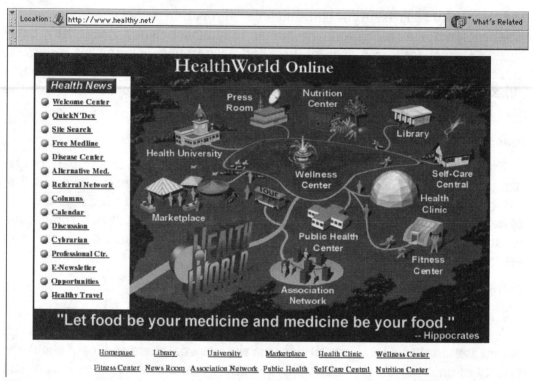

Figure 4–7 Healthy.net. *Source:* Reprinted with permission from www.healthy.net, © 1999, Healthy.net.

nutrients interactions database, which will present valuable information derived from the literature of medicine, pharmacology, clinical nutrition, and phytotherapy. In the meantime, this site offers in-depth information on alternative treatments, diet, and nutrition. It also provides information on health, wellness, and alternative resources on the Internet such as mailing lists, newsgroups, and networks.

The Herb Research Foundation

The Herb Research Foundation is a nonprofit organization "dedicated to responsible informed self-care with medicinal plants." The site (www.herbs.org) (Figure 4–8) delivers reliable and in-depth content and is straightforward and low-key. Its stated desire—to provide sound information about herbs to the public and to professionals—is believable.

The site is easy to use, but one major shortcoming is its lack of a searchable database. It does, however, list a variety of reliable databases where one can search for information.

The Herbal Information Center

The Herbal Information Center (www.kcweb.com/herb/welcome.htm) is an obviously commercial site that sells herbs and vitamins, but it does contain a lot of useful information on the more popular products, and there is a searchable database. It also offers a free newsletter and some interesting news updates. A bit disturbing, however, is the subtle push to encourage Web surfers to buy. For example, in one place on the site it says, "Take our Herb Poll. Find out what everybody is taking!" This tactic promotes use of products through a bit of peer pressure.

The Moss Reports

The Moss Reports site (www.ralphmoss.com) is a must for anyone interested in exploring alternatives to the standard treatments for cancer. In addition to pro-

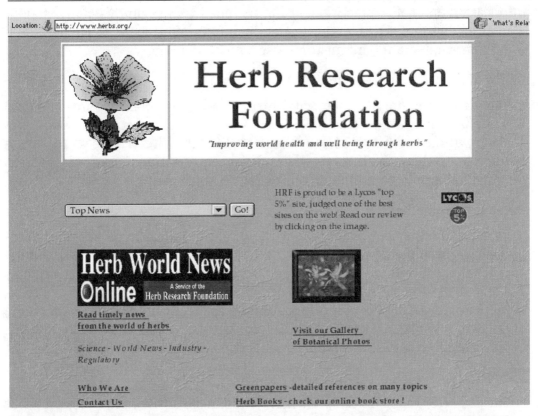

Figure 4–8 The Herb Research Foundation. *Source:* Reprinted with permission from www.herbs.org, © 1999, Herb Research Foundation.

viding in-depth information about all types of cancer and a searchable database, the site also continues the tradition of a printed newsletter called *Cancer Chronicles*.

The information on this site is provided "as a public service to patients and to all those who are interested in the development of more effective and humane ways of approaching the cancer problem."[10(p.16)] It contains 200 articles from back issues of the newsletter as well as new information about cancer treatment, prevention, and politics. This site is maintained by Ralph W. Moss, Ph.D., a member of the Cancer Advisory Panel of NIH and an advisor to the American Urological Association, the National Cancer Institute, the University of Texas, Columbia University, and the German Society of Oncology.

NCCAM

Organized under the director of NIH, NCCAM (http://altmed.od.nih.gov) conducts and supports basic and applied research and training and disseminates information on CAM to practitioners and the public. Links on this highly serious Web site (Figure 4–9) take the reader to information about CAM, news and events, research grants, information resources, and so on.

Office of Dietary Supplements

The Office of Dietary Supplements (http://dietary-supplements.info.nih.gov) is a federal organization established under the associate director for disease prevention within the office of the director, NIH. The site (Figure 4–10) has a searchable database and links to other relevant information. This site is research oriented and would be useful for the average e-consumer.

OsteopathOnline.Com

OsteopathOnline.Com (www.osteopathonline.com) aims to be the most comprehensive osteopathic resource on the World Wide Web. It features a general area for those interested in finding out more about osteopathy, and it explains the origins of osteopathy, the future of osteopathy, and the principles and techniques of osteopathy. There is information on becoming an osteopath, including details of schools in Europe, the United Kingdom, and the United States. OsteopathOnline.Com also contains a searchable database.

Vita-Web

This is one of the more comprehensive vitamin sites (www.vita-web.com), but people should remember that the site is maintained by Roche Laboratories. Although the site's information is decidedly comprehensive, Vita-Web does not

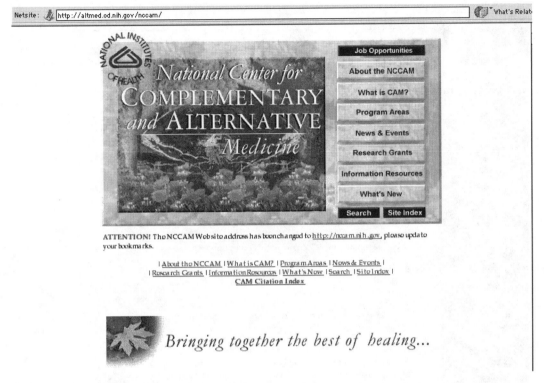

Figure 4–9 NCCAM. *Source:* Reprinted from www.altmed.od.nih.gov/nccam, 1999, National Center for Complementary and Alternative Medicine, National Institutes of Health.

score well when it comes to ease of use, since it requires a Flash2 plug-in to view the portion of the site intended for use by the general public.

e-Advice: Do Not Imagine That Your Patients Are Too Old or Too Traditional to Find These Sites on the Web

E-consumers are flocking to alternative health Web sites in droves. Review each of the previously listed sites to determine how *you* would rate them, based on your medical training or treatment philosophies. Then share your opinions with e-patients.

BEWARE OF LITTLE E-REGULATION

One of the biggest hurdles for e-consumers when it comes to alternative medicine—especially herbs, vitamins, and supplements—is the lack of standards and

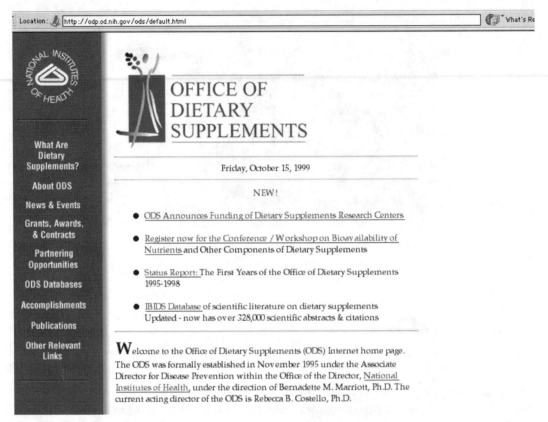

Figure 4–10 Office of Dietary Supplements. *Source:* Reprinted from http://odp.od.nih.gov/ods/default.htm, 1999, Office of Dietary Supplements, National Institutes of Health.

regulations. Vitamin, supplement, and herb manufacturers can make outrageous claims about their products, but there is little regulation and virtually no standardization in this market. And because of the growing popularity of these alternative treatments, some large pharmaceutical companies are starting to manufacture and distribute their own lines of alternative vitamins, herbs, and supplements. Warner-Lambert (www.herbalsupps.com), Bayer (www.bayercare.com), and American Home Products Corporation (www.ahp.com/ahp/products/consumer.htm) all have alternative herb and supplement product lines that are policed by virtually no one.

As these companies and others move into the CAM market, it is their responsibility to deliver reasonable, factual clinical studies and unbiased information, including information about dosages, side effects, and dangerous interactions.

At a minimum, consumers should be warned to always consult their physician before trying some type of alternative treatment. Without this discussion, there is an increasing danger of drug-herb and herb-herb interactions—such as was noted in a *20/20* segment about a patient who was on antidepressants and self-prescribed kava kava. The result: a temporary coma.

TAKE ALTERNATIVE E-ACTION IN YOUR PRACTICE OR HEALTH CARE ORGANIZATION

Chances are that if patients are interested in looking at alternatives to conventional treatment, they will pursue those alternatives with or without their physician's help. As more and more patients use over-the-counter herbs, botanicals, and supplements, it becomes increasingly important to discuss these practices—to protect their health, if nothing else.[11] Health care executives have a lot to gain if they provide simple educational programs that offer strategies and skills that help practitioners discuss alternative medicine with patients. Such discussion *is* possible, even for providers who do not feel particularly comfortable with the topic. Using the Web as a tool is one way for providers and patients to find common ground in this area, often a sensitive one. Here are some tips for getting started.

Open a Discussion about Alternative Therapies. Say something like "Many patients with symptoms like yours often use chiropractic, massage, herbs, vitamins, and so on." By starting out this way, you are giving patients "permission" to discuss a topic that they may previously had thought was unbroachable. Be careful not to refer to these therapies as "alternative," "complementary," or "unorthodox." Patients may view these terms as judgmental and will be less likely to want to continue the discussion. As a general rule, patients are often pleased when their physicians care enough to ask whether they use alternative therapies.[12]

Ask Patients If They Use the Web To Search for Alternative or Natural Remedies. This will provide an opportunity to see what kind of information the patient is getting and allow you to steer the patient toward the more reliable, less commercial sites. Additionally, this kind of dialogue will enhance trust.

Work with Patients to Determine the Right Course of Complementary Treatment. If a patient is interested in an alternative therapy for a condition for which conventional medicine has not been successful, it can be extremely helpful for you to discuss complementary treatments, their potential dangers, and success rates. Giving advice about choosing an appropriate practitioner, and perhaps referring to the listings on line, are also effective approaches.[13]

Distribute e-CAM Information Sanctioned by You and Your Partners. After surfing the CAM Web sites yourself, list those that you deem credible for the diagnoses you treat. If you are a health system executive, rally several progressive physicians to review the information and compile a recommended site list. Distribute this written information to e-patients; they will thank you for it.

Continually Educate Yourself. Opportunities for practitioners to learn about alternative medicine have increased greatly in the last few years. In the early 1990s, only 15 of 125 medical schools in the United States offered courses on alternative medicine. That number has risen to 60, and the list includes Columbia University, Harvard, Johns Hopkins, the University of California at Los Angeles, and Yale.[14]

In the winter of 2000, the University of Arizona's Program in Integrative Medicine in Tucson will begin offering a two-year, continuing medical education-accredited distance learning course for physicians and other health care providers who want to integrate alternative medicine into their practices. It is the first program of its kind in the world. The university also has been offering a two-year fellowship program on site, and eight fellows are admitted to the program each year.

Armed with computers and a sense of empowerment that did not exist until the end of this century, e-consumers and e-patients have complete confidence in their own ability to determine what kind of treatment is best for them. Like it or not, this often includes CAM therapies.

Shared decision making and open discussion about CAM and the information e-patients find on the Web will improve your relationship with patients. The steps help you to be able to assist e-consumers and e-patients in navigating their way through the as-yet-unregulated and overwhelming mass of alternative medicine information on line.

E-patients expect more treatment options and are discovering remedies on the Web that the traditional medical community has been silent about until now. Now that the cat's out of the bag, so to speak, it is up to physicians and other health care providers to address this issue with their patients. Using the power of the Net and working *with* e-consumers and e-patients to determine what their expectations are, to offer guidance, and to formulate treatment options will be healthy for everyone.

REFERENCES

1. D.M. Eisenberg, "Advising Patients Who Seek Alternative Medical Therapies," *Annals of Internal Medicine* 127 (1997): 61–69.
2. D.M. Eisenberg et al., "Trends in Alternative Medicine Use in the United States, 1990–1997," *JAMA* 280 (1998): 1569–1575.
3. Eisenberg et al., "Trends in Alternative Medicine Use."
4. U.S. Bureau of the Census, http://www.census.gov/population/www/projections/nasrh.html.
5. Eisenberg et al., "Trends in Alternative Medicine Use."
6. C. Rauber, "Open to Alternatives," *Modern Healthcare,* September 1998, 51–57.
7. Rauber, "Open to Alternatives."
8. J. Henderson, "Mainstreaming Alternative Medicine: Survey of HMOs Regarding Alternative Therapies," *Health Insurance Underwriter,* March 1998, 24–25.
9. "Intel Study on e-Health," http://www.intel.com/ehealth.
10. R.W. Moss, *Alternative Medicine Online: A Guide to Natural Remedies on the Internet* (Brooklyn, NY: Equinox Press, Inc., 1997), 16.
11. Eisenberg, "Advising Patients Who Seek Alternative Medical Therapies," 61–69.
12. Eisenberg, "Advising Patients."
13. Eisenberg, "Advising Patients."
14. Rauber, "Open to Alternatives."

CHAPTER 5

Yesterday's Medical Model Versus Today's Customer-Focused e-Care

Randy Dulin, Carroll Quinn, and Mark Garvey

A HEALTH CARE REVOLUTION

Remember "the good old days," when physicians were in solo practice and took their own calls 24 hours a day? When they met patients in the emergency room to check out a fever that had been around for two days and the insurance company paid the bill without question? When the physician kept handwritten notes to himself to enter into the patient's paper record the next time he was in the office? When no one knew or really cared that the cost of an elective surgery varied by 200 percent from one physician or geographical region to another? Revolution is hardly a strong enough word for the changes that have occurred in health care delivery!

As recently as 20 years ago, the major stakeholders in health decisions were patients and physicians. Care was delivered in a relatively unrestricted fee-for-service environment, and the physician was rarely questioned about clinical decisions. Medical recordkeeping was handwritten entries in hard-copy charts. In contrast, today's physicians are held accountable for following numerous guidelines and formularies and for participating in external evaluation processes. Recordkeeping and scheduling are often computerized, and many physicians routinely access medical information on the World Wide Web. The major stakeholders in health care now include employers, health plans, and the government. Along the way, strategies such as utilization review (UR) and case management, demand management, and disease management were instituted. Each has affected the way in which care is delivered and the relationship between the patient and the care providers. And each has pushed us closer to an e-care-supported delivery system that is fully integrated and customer focused.

The rules of the health care delivery game continue to change rapidly. The new players are primarily interested in reducing costs and increasing efficiency. Quality care is important but not assumed; it must be supported by quality improvement processes and documented through outcomes. Managed care organizations (MCOs) use e-technology to access, store, and analyze large amounts of information about the persons whose care they manage. With these data, they can identify industry trends in utilization patterns among the insured and in practice patterns among the providers. Electronic communication makes it possible for them to give providers and payers rapid feedback, with the expectation that the information is used to reduce variations in practice and improve overall quality and efficiency. E-technology also provides effective and efficient means for MCOs to document their achievement of operational standards set by accrediting and regulatory bodies.

An analogy can be drawn between the evolution of health care cost containment and the corporate restructuring that was common in the 1990s. While corporations at large cut budgets and instituted cost-reduction strategies such as outsourcing, the health care industry negotiated discounted payments to hospitals and physicians and created health maintenance organizations (HMOs) and other benefit redesign strategies that controlled expenses by reducing choice and shifting cost. Non–health care corporations restructured by downsizing management positions and laying off lower-tier workers; health care saw massive consolidations and mergers of hospitals, physician practices, and even HMOs, as well as layoffs among the rank-and-file care providers. Health care's equivalent of corporate decentralization and process improvement/quality initiatives was its attempt to develop integrated delivery systems (IDSs) to most efficiently and effectively manage specific disease populations and population risk factors.

SUPPLY-SIDE ECONOMICS

Much of the health care industry change was stimulated by a push during the 1980s to control runaway increases in health care costs. Initial cost containment efforts were initiated by insurers and employers and directed at the supply side of the equation in an attempt to control the amount of services provided and minimize the plans' medical loss ratios. Health plans increased employee deductibles, restricted services, and required second opinions. The UR nurse arrived on the scene. An employee of the insurance company, the UR nurse was charged with monitoring a patient's illness course and raising questions about the use of resources such as diagnostic and treatment options. These early efforts to control the supply of health services have evolved into increasingly sophisticated efforts to also control consumer demand for health care services. This evolution of managed care has been made possible by the surge of computer-based and now e-technology that makes data storage and rapid retrieval possible.

Utilization Review

Utilization review was introduced in the 1970s as a process for examining the necessity, efficiency, and appropriateness of the use of resources in all segments of the health care delivery system. It was particularly focused on reduction of excessive or unnecessary use of health services associated with acute hospitalization. Using historical claims data, the utilization reviewer advocated for the insurer by identifying physician prescribing or treatment orders that appeared to fall outside a norm. The reviewer then informed the physician and questioned the need for or the appropriateness of those orders. These initial attempts to restrict or control services were interpreted as highly intrusive and insulting to physicians. The process was perceived as one that drove a wedge between the physician and the patient. While the end result *may* have been beneficial for the patient, the primary intent was to cut the cost of care.

UR required access to data about norms related to particular conditions and diagnoses, including average length of stay, type and frequency of various diagnostic studies, and so on. The data were then applied to individual cases by a registered nurse who was an assertive, persistent communicator. Since UR was driven by national norms, the assumption underlying recommendations was that all patients ought to be "normal," and allowances for anything outside the norm were made difficult.

Case Management

Case management, introduced in the late 1970s, was a second generation UR process. Rather than focusing narrowly on specific procedures or number of days in the hospital, case management assessed resource utilization from the standpoint of the appropriateness of care for the individual patient involved. The second generation UR nurse was called the case manager. This nurse became a familiar presence, often walking the floors of the hospital with a laptop computer, scanning patient charts, and leaving mostly unwelcome reminders for physicians to consider discontinuing a daily lab study or discharging their patients just a bit sooner. The case manager's role was to ensure that, if a different and cheaper course of care was appropriate for a given patient, the transfer of services was made as efficiently as possible. In a sense, the case manager acted as a travel agent, helping the patient to navigate through the health care system and getting the appropriate care along the way.

An effective case manager had to know what was happening along the continuum of care; for example, what was available, how to access it, what it would cost. Good assessment skills allowed the case manager to identify the patient's needs and evaluate all the options. While the UR nurse almost solely represented the interests of the insurance company, case managers were patient advocates in that their goal was to make sure the patient received the most appropriate care at the time it was needed. Their advocacy role, however, was limited by the fact that they were employed by the insurance company or the hospital for the purpose of controlling costs.

Into the 1990s

The 1990s saw a proliferation of HMOs and rapid gains in HMO enrollment. Between 1992 and 1994, only a two-year period, HMO enrollment rose 23 percent, reaching 51.1 million across the country.[1] In many communities, hospitals and physicians collaborated to form physician–hospital organizations (PHOs), which were touted as vehicles for contracting with MCOs. Most of these PHOs sought to enter into fee-for-service arrangements with HMOs or preferred provider organizations, but negotiations also spawned a variety of risk-sharing agreements such as capitation and IDSs.

During this era, care providers became resigned to the use of formularies and an emphasis on increased productivity. In addition to initiatives designed to change physician behavior, strategies such as requiring precertification and second opinions were introduced to alter consumers' utilization patterns. But such requirements also increased the administrative aspects of plan management and made it more difficult for patients to receive the care they truly needed. Patients' opinions of these various provider arrangements were often negative; they believed they had less choice about which physicians and hospitals provided their care, and they experienced fragmentation and problems with accessibility. The primary goal was still to restrict services available to the customer. Decisions about appropriateness of care were based on the "normal" treatment of a "normal" patient with a "normal" disease course. The data necessary to look more closely at patient characteristics and needs in specific situations either were not available or were not readily accessible.

DEMAND MANAGEMENT

Demand management was one of the first attempts on the part of insurers and employers to address the demand side of the health care equation. Demand management is based on the principle that, given the right information and support, patients are the best managers of their health. Demand management strategies focused on providing education and support services that empowered people to manage minor health problems and make appropriate use of medical care. Self-care manuals that described common symptoms and problems walked the reader through an evaluation of the situation and suggested appropriate interventions. Similar assistance was offered by nurse-staffed call centers that provided access to registered nurses using computer-based triage protocols, 24 hours a day, seven days a week. These services were deliberately consumer focused and provided information and empowerment to consumers when and where they needed it. The services were also, however, narrowly focused on the episodic management of acute symptoms and based on "most likely" scenarios rather than true individualization of care. It was a convenience for Mrs. Smith to call the nurse triage line at 10 o'clock in the evening to talk with the nurse about her headache. It was a convenience to Mrs. Smith's physician that the triage nurse was able to determine that the headache could be safely managed without a late-evening call to the physician or a trip to the emergency department. But a truly individualized intervention—for a headache that, in the context of Mrs. Smith's current life situation, is closely related to her larger issue of adjusting to the loss of her spouse—couldn't occur, because the history or knowledge of the caller available to the triage nurse was minimal. The only follow-up to triage encounters was typically some type of communication with the primary care provider about the encounter and sometimes call-backs to the most seriously ill callers. In essence, demand management approaches lacked an emphasis on integration or continuity along the full spectrum of health care. Data were, and are, important to demand management, but primarily from a marketing perspective—to profile triage users and target market other health services. Rarely was information used to plan or improve the process of care delivery.

Disease Management

The concept of disease management was popularized in the early 1990s, although the Mayo Clinic began focusing management efforts on groups of patients with specific diseases in the late 1980s. Disease management took case management to another level by focusing efforts not on all or any hospitalized patients, but on groups of patients with the same diagnosis or health problem. Disease management is a comprehensive, integrated, systematic approach that improves medical management and reduces cost of care for a disease category by standardizing care. In disease management, the patient's care is customized and personalized from the standpoint that his or her caregiver fully understands and considers the life experiences and adjustments that are part of the experience of a specific chronic or unusual disease.

Disease management programs are highly data driven, computer databases and emerging e-technology have been a major factor in their success. Detailed baseline data are gathered and compared with outcomes as a measure of the success of the program. Clinical and financial parameters are monitored carefully as the patient moves through the program, and the data on these parameters are constantly fed back to the managers to use in their planning and decision making. As with case management, the patient has an advocate who interacts with him or her often and consistently to assist in the self-management of the disease. These interactions are typically by telephone and sometimes computer assisted. In fact, telephonic interactions may even be computer generated. InfoMedics, Inc.'s Telephone-Linked Care (TLC) system manages diabetic patients through automated telephone interviews. Using "branching logic," the TLC program asks a series of questions to which patients respond by pressing appropriate keys on the telephone keypad. TLC then responds with real-time feedback based on the information the caller provides, and if any of the values the patient enters into the program indicate the need for immediate attention, the TLC program notifies the primary caregiver at the end of the call.[2]

But disease management programs still focus on the disease rather than the patient. The customization falls short of individualization and care that is fully integrated around the holistic needs of the patient. Disease management programs are most effective for chronic conditions, and the people most likely to have chronic conditions are elderly people. In 1995, studies indicated that about 20 percent of persons 65 years and older had functional disabilities associated with chronic illnesses.[3] Most older persons have more than one chronic condition, and for these folks the continuity of care breaks down in disease management programs. Why? Because most disease management protocols and teaching processes are designed around single diseases only. If the patient happens to be enrolled in one disease management program for his diabetes and another for his chronic lung disease, he will likely experience overlap and redundancies or gaps in service, since neither program is designed to adequately address all issues arising from the secondary disease process.

EFFECTS OF HEALTH CARE EVOLUTION ON STAKEHOLDERS

At the beginning of the new millennium, health care delivery systems look dramatically different than they did 20 years ago. Many would argue that while there has been a great deal of change and frustration for major stakeholders, there has been little improvement in the quality of care that patients receive. Employers face continually increasing costs and more complex benefit designs. Insurers are operating in an increasingly competitive marketplace and being challenged over their supply-side controls and limits on services. Hospitals are experiencing reimbursement crises of overwhelming proportions, and physicians with years of education and specialty training are receiving unsolicited advice from multiple sources with alphabet soup names. Patients have experienced increased out-of-pocket expenses, difficulty accessing care, fragmentation of services, and a general disillusionment with their ability to control their own health care destiny. In general, the experiments of the past few decades have been less than totally successful. But with the growth of e-technology, we are on the brink of yet another revolution in the way care is managed and delivered. Our current capability to gather, store, analyze, and communicate information holds the key to true "mass customization" of care, to a focus on each customer served. The evolution to full customer-focused health management and e-care addresses the need for the "big picture" perspective on what is the best care choice for this particular patient at this point in time. This is the perspective that the primary care provider does or should have, and systematic, population-based programs must adopt this broader perspective in a way that early disease management programs did not. With the revolutionary capabilities of today's e-technology, this broad perspective is within reach.

A NEW PHASE—CUSTOMER-FOCUSED HEALTH MANAGEMENT

A new health care phase is emerging, one that promises a customized and individualized focus on the customer and patient. Picture this scenario: Dr. Robb starts his workday on his laptop at home. He accesses the Web and first scans an on-line newspaper that has been customized to send him news items pertinent to the general and clinical areas he has specified. He reads his e-mail, which includes the following:

- The best practices document he requested from the subscription research service offered through the IDS to which he and his practice partners belong.
- E-mail questions from two patients that he forwards to the nurse at the system's Contact Center. The nurse will outline an answer for Dr. Robb to send to the patients later in the day.
- A response to a request for information from a physician in Australia who

recently participated with Dr. Robb in an on-line roundtable discussion of rheumatologists from around the world.

- Copies of triage encounters between six of his patients and the Real-Time Center Nurse Triage Service during the night. This same info has been automatically added to the patients' electronic records, and the Triage Service nurses scheduled two of the patients for office visits through the electronic scheduling system.

Dr. Robb then views a month's worth of one diabetic patient's fingerstick blood sugars that the patient has sent from his glucometer over the Internet. He sends the patient an e-mail congratulating her on her compliance with the testing and the good blood sugar control she is maintaining. He then examines the brain scan of a patient who had a stroke and was admitted through the emergency department last night. Finally, he conducts an on-line telemonitoring assessment visit of a patient with unstable congestive heart failure. In response to the patient's request, Dr. Robb e-mails him a customized educational paper on the use of alternative therapies in heart disease, obtained through the system's electronic consumer health library. Then he leaves for work!

In this new era of health e-care delivery, the emphasis is on the demand side of the equation. The perspective has broadened beyond managing a disease to supporting the health of individuals, some of whom just happen to have chronic illnesses. This new phase of customer-focused health management and e-care uses Web technology to increase efficiency and customization and leverages Web technology to address the needs of consumers as well as providers and payers. Data from multiple sources are readily available to providers and payers over the Web, including results of lab tests, computerized scans, or X-rays to help providers design the best health management program for a specific patient. The ability to customize means that a program will look very different for a well-educated patient who is self-confident and ready to change than it will for someone who is poorly educated, in denial, and has limited money or social support systems. In an e-environment, educational materials and interventions can be tailored to the needs of each of these individuals and made quickly accessible to them through e-mail, voice mail box, fax, live interaction with a health professional via a 24-hour, seven-day-a-week real-time call center, specialty-oriented discussion groups on the Web, or telemedicine hook-up.

Health care consumers are no longer content to passively adapt to delivery system changes that do not work for them. It is no secret that consumers are taking a more active role in their own health management decisions, demanding more information and greater convenience. They know the convenience and flexibility of using the Internet, and they use the Web to access what the more traditional health care system does not provide for them. For instance, http://acupuncture.com/htm provides information on the use of acupuncture for common ailments, a treatment option many physicians dismiss as invalid. Sites such as http://www.homeopathic.com/danba/index.html/ and http://www.vegan-society.com/index.html give consumers information about homeopathic, herbal, and other alternative approaches that Americans spend billions of dollars for each year but which physicians know little about and do not believe in. Certainly, supply-side health management will not disappear. But designing delivery mechanisms from the demand side—using Web-enabled e-care technologies—can result in the benefits of cost control, better customer satisfaction, and improved quality of life.

An increase in information access on the Web is of great benefit to insurers and providers as well. Few would disagree that the consumer who understands simple symptom management can reduce emergency department visits. It makes sense then that the e-consumer who surfs the Web for medical information before coming to the physician's office can make more informed decisions about aggressive or experimental therapies for life-threatening illnesses. Insurers and employers are turning to Web-based strategies that provide them with linkages that allow the quality and value of the services they purchase to be monitored. Integrated delivery systems are building Web-linkages among disparate hospitals, medical offices, and other facilities to maximize the efficiency of service delivery across the continuum. Individual providers are accessing the Web to link with patients and to obtain the latest and best evidence upon which to base practice decisions. As all of these components of the health care delivery system come together through Web-enabled technology, the potential for further customizing and delivery of e-care is enormous.

One example of highly customized e-care is interactive telemonitoring. Interactive telemonitoring technology places the provider in the patient's home to assess symptoms, adjust medications and treatments, meet immediate needs for information, and help the patient avoid hospitalization. One small-scale telemonitoring pilot project conducted by Mercy Health Partners in Cincinnati, Ohio, averted 40 readmissions in a five-month period in a group of patients with congestive heart failure, representing a savings in excess of $200,000. Forty percent of these patients improved one severity level on the New York Heart Association Classification of Heart Failure, and 12 percent improved two severity levels. Patients who did have readmissions had shorter lengths of stay and more improved functional status compared to previous admissions.

WHAT EXACTLY IS CUSTOMER-FOCUSED HEALTH MANAGEMENT?

Customer-focused health management delivered through e-care technology is the next generation of disease management. It is a comprehensive, integrated, coordinated, information-based approach to health care with the objective of continuously improving the quality/cost ratio (value) of patient care with multimedia interventions. Over the past several years, disease management has become almost a household word in the health care industry, as health care organizations strive to achieve a new generation of value and accountability in a rapidly changing environment. The goal of disease management is to provide the most effective and efficient care regardless of treatment setting or source of reimbursement. Ideally, disease management prevents acute exacerbations of the illness or condition that result in the use of expensive resources. This is accomplished by proactively engaging patients in their own self-management and stressing prevention and risk reduction. Customer-focused health management broadens the management perspective beyond a single disease. It puts the consumer in the driver's seat by making health information and access to care providers as close as their computers or telephones.

Technology is the Key

One feature of early disease management is the standardization and close monitoring of medical management regimens. Based on research literature review and panels of experts in the specific disease area, medical management protocols are established and applied to all patients being managed within the program. The resulting reduction in physician practice variation and increase in patient compliance yield major benefits such as reduced cost and improved quality of life. One of the challenges of early disease management programs was that these protocols were most often provided to physicians in hard-copy format. A single physician was likely to be caring for patients from several insurers, each of which had a slightly different set of protocols for managing the same disease. In reality, many of the protocols wound up filed on a shelf while the physician struggled to figure out ways to remember who was to receive which medication when. Retrieval of patient information to document practice patterns was often cumbersome and time-consuming. Another challenge for physician providers was that, even though they "knew" from their clinical expertise that the best management decision for a given patient at a given time would fall outside the standard protocols, they had neither the time nor the access to research literature to support their sense of best practice. Thanks to evolving technology, that is no longer the case. First of all, electronic linkages allow providers to access the patient's record and the management protocol being used for disease management simultaneously. The physician receives electronic prompts reminding him or her of tests or treatments needed. Patients receive electronically generated notices via e-mail or telephone alerting them to access the physician's scheduling system and make an appointment for their next checkup. Telemedicine via telephone lines or the Web enables the provider to check the patient's blood pressure and pulse, listen to heart and breath sounds, adjust the dosage of an intravenous medication, or download stored physiological data such as electrocardiographic tracings or blood sugar readings from the past 24 hours. In addition, the provider has access through the Web to up-to-the-minute decision-support systems, such as the Cochrane Library (http://www.update-software.com/cochrane.htm) and other research centers that review, synthesize, and publish best practices information from throughout the world. All of this happens with the physician at his or her office personal computer (PC) and without the patient having to leave home.

The ability to communicate electronically with the patient moves disease management to another level. Using the Web and best practices research, a patient's care can be more closely and accurately monitored and individualized than ever before. The barriers to patient compliance can be better identified and addressed, and educational efforts can be more closely customized to meet the particular patient's needs.

Dr. Edwards has two patients with congestive heart failure who are being managed in the same disease management program. The electronic profiles of these patients tell the physician that Mrs. A is 75 years old, of Italian descent, does her own cooking and grocery shopping, has had two years of college, was last hospitalized two months ago for two days, then had a home care nurse for three postdischarge visits, and was seen in the office one week ago. Mrs. A has her own PC, accesses the Web for consumer health information and to send e-mail messages to Dr. Edwards, and belongs to a seniors chat service/support group on line.

Mrs. B is 86 years old and has diabetes in addition to congestive heart failure. She is of Latino descent and speaks English as a second language. She has had eight years of formal education, lives with a son and daughter-in-law who do the cooking and grocery shopping for her, and has not been hospitalized for 18 months. The family does not have a PC, but Mrs. B's daughter communicates vital information about Mrs. B's diabetes control to the health management nurse via interactive telephone every two weeks. Her most recent information reveals that Mrs. B has gained five pounds in a two-week period.

The information in these profiles has been customized based on the critical data Dr. Edwards wants about each of her patients. She can, for instance, select consumer health information about diet restrictions targeted to the immediate needs and characteristics of these two patients—easy-to-read Spanish language information about how to limit sodium in typical Latino menus in a printed or audio format for Mrs. B.; and, for Mrs. A, higher-level English language material sent via e-mail that includes "rehab" recipes for low-fat, low-sodium pasta dishes and contains a hyperlink to DietCity.com for additional information and diet planning if she is interested. Dr. Edwards may be following the same medical protocol guidelines for medications with these two patients and gathering the same physiological information about their congestive heart failure on a regular basis—that is, she is following the same medical management protocols—but the care she provides is individualized to each patient's specific needs. This degree of individualization is possible because the physician has the ability to pull data from many sources and tweak it to fit the situation. This would not be possible without the sophistication of e-technology delivered via the Internet or telephone, thus achieving e-care.

The Full Circle of Health Care

A hallmark of good health management and patient support is the "full circle" approach to health care (Figure 5–1). From this perspective, it is just as important to interact with individuals and monitor their health status during "wellness episodes" as it is during illness. Management is not episodic but continuous and occurs at each and every encounter along the continuum of needs and service delivery points. Consumer education is paramount; educational needs are constantly assessed and used as the basis for interventions in the context of that person's life situation, not just within the narrower context of the immediate situation or problem. In contrast, in a traditional medical approach, the individual's initial encounter with the health care delivery system is centered around an episode of acute illness, and interactions are focused on primary, secondary, or tertiary treatment of the episode. There may be some aftercare and continued monitoring, but it is usually minimal. Whatever consumer education or early detection occurs is disjointed from this episodic care; patients may have their cholesterol or blood pressure checked at the senior center or the workplace, but the physician is unaware that this has occurred and rarely sees the results. The majority of resources are spent on high-cost inpatient stabilization and immediate posthospitalization care. While providers in all settings try to provide

Health management's full circle approach to health care

```
        ┌──────────────────────────────┐
        │→   Consumer education      ←─┐
        │          ⇩                   │
        │        Prevention            │
        │          ⇩                   │
        │        Screening             │
        │          ⇩                   │
        │     Identification of        │
        │   "high risk" consumers   ───┘
        │          ⇩
        │      Early diagnosis
        │          ⇩
        │    Patient education -     ←─┐
        │     self care skills         │
        │          ⇩                   │
        │  Coordinated primary,        │
        │    secondary and             │
        │  peripheral treatment        │
        │          ⇩                   │
        │ Monitoring of compliance  ───┘
        │    and outcomes
        │          ⇩
        └── Aftercare and continued
              monitoring
```

Figure 5–1 Customer-Focused Health Management.

cost-effective care, typically no one takes the big-picture, long-term perspective on the cost and effectiveness of care across settings.

Patient Involvement and Empowerment

While traditional medical care focuses on *resolving* acute exacerbations of an illness or chronic disorder, the majority of existing disease management resources are concentrated on *preventing* the acute exacerbation and hospitalization in the first place. Patients are encouraged to take an active role in the management of their disease. They are given in-depth education about their disease and treatment and are taught how to recognize and report early signs and symptoms of trouble. But the focus of interactions with that patient stays on the primary disease and its control. Customer-focused care, on the other hand, forces the players in the system to look beyond the one-disease focus of early disease management programs and to discern how that one disease fits into the whole picture of the individual patient's situation. The patient and family are always considered the primary "managers" of health and symptoms. The role of providers is to equip the patient and family with the education and coordinated services they need to reduce risk factors and manage their own symptoms.

Customer-focused health management builds on best clinical practices to broaden the provider perspective on clinical practice to include not only traditional medical management approaches but also to consider what works best for the patients. This could mean listening to patients' requests and testimonials about alternative therapies and maybe even adopting selected therapies that have scientific support. Keep in mind that e-care consumers are sophisticated; they believe in the effectiveness of alternative therapies and they spend a portion of the millions of dollars spent each year in the United States for these therapies. They know about and visit the numerous Web sites devoted to nonmainstream approaches to health, sites such as Dr. Andrew Weil's www.drweil.com and the National Center for Complementary and Alternative Medicine at nccam.nih.gov/nccam/clearinghouse/.

Consumers are ready for new approaches to communicating and interacting with providers. They are more interested in actively participating in their care management and they are dissatisfied with the current state of health care delivery. They are more sophisticated and less passive than patients of the past, and they are forcing the provider and payer networks to acknowledge that patients/consumers have a key role to play in managing the cost and quality of their own care.

Cost Savings

The financial advantage of this "front-end" approach to care management is obvious (Figure 5–2). Along the full spectrum of care, the care management services needed for acute episodic treatment that are traditionally provided in tertiary and long-term care settings are also the most expensive. But a stable chronic illness can be very effectively maintained by good treatment compliance and preventive strategies carried out by patients in their own environments, monitored by their primary care physician or advanced practice nurse. Put quite simply, it is cheaper to keep people healthy than it is to get them well once they have become sick. Prevention and the integration of health promotion are not only cheaper but they result in an improved quality of life for patients.

A Team Effort

Conceptually, disease and health management integrate much more than medical interventions (Figure 5–3). Successful health management requires

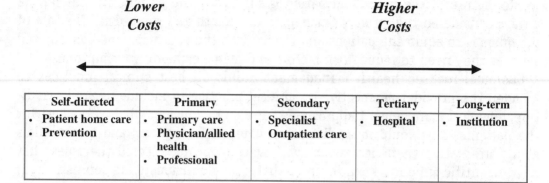

Figure 5–2 Spectrum of Care.

multidisciplinary teamwork and includes the patient and family members as critical members of the care management team. Communication and information-sharing among all participating parties are critical. This degree of integration and customization is made possible through e-technology. Unless the information and data comprising each of the conceptual components of health management

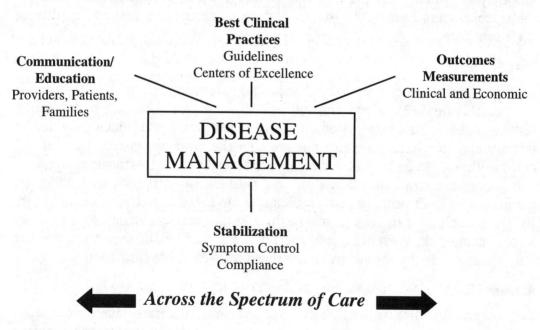

Figure 5–3 Disease Management.

are readily accessible and manipulable by all members of the team, truly integrated, customer-focused health management would remain nothing more than a good idea.

Outcomes Based

An important feature of disease management, from its inception, was the emphasis on outcomes measurement. Medical management protocols are based on treatment outcomes documented through clinical research. As patients are managed under these protocols, their clinical and functional outcomes are continuously tracked, evaluated, and used as the basis for improvements in treatment protocols. This constant feedback loop facilitates continuous improvement in the way care is provided and in the clinical and financial outcomes that are attained. The emphasis on clinical outcomes rather than care delivery processes keeps the patient's status and quality of life at the center of the equation; in other words, the fact that the patient received a treatment or took a medication is less important than what effect either of those had on how the patient felt or how well the patient's disease was controlled. The evolution from disease management to customer-focused health management and support further emphasizes the focus on patient status as the measure of success. With e-technology to support customization of care—as in the example of Dr. Edwards' patients' needs for educational materials—quality-of-life outcomes can be addressed and measured.

Customer-focused health management integrates a variety of innovative approaches into disease management (Figure 5–4). Wellness, health promotion, and prevention play a minimal role in traditional medical care, but they are a major emphasis in health management programs. Continuity of care across the continuum of settings and providers requires creative approaches to outreach services and a willingness to do things a bit differently. For example, traditionally managed patients typically receive verbal instructions and printed handouts as part of the hospital discharge process. The patient in a customer-focused health management program, on the other hand, may receive books, videos, telephone instruction and/or access to a Web site targeted to enrollees in the program. A health management specialist recognizes that learning styles vary and that the most effective and efficient patient education tailors the teaching format and approach to the style of the learner.

CUSTOMER-FOCUSED HEALTH MANAGEMENT IS NEEDED MORE THAN EVER

A number of social and financial factors have converged to set the stage for this new approach to health management. An aging population, the rising cost of

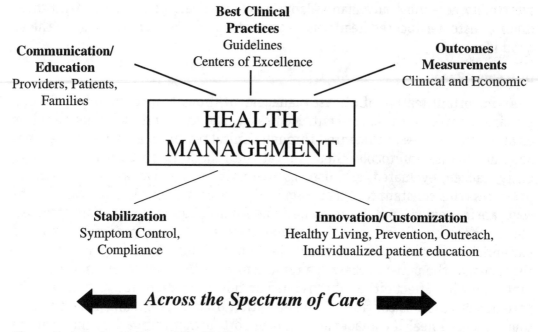

Figure 5–4 Customer-Focused Health Management.

improper utilization of services, and the fragmentation of care are all contributors to the need for a revision in our disease-focused care delivery strategy.

An Aging American Population

The health care impact of the aging American population is only beginning to manifest itself. As the baby boomers reach midlife and experience the physical symptoms of aging and the onset of chronic problems associated with aging, the potential implications of having large numbers of elderly people in the population become very clear. Predictions are that by the year 2030, approximately 20 percent of the population will be over 65 years of age and the proportion of persons over age 85 will more than triple.[4] While it is not the only factor, the aging of the American population is a major contributor to the rising cost of health care in this country. Typically, older people have more chronic health problems, so the push of the baby boomer generation through the American health care system will increase the ranks of the estimated 100 million people in the United States (45 percent of the noninstitutionalized population) with one or more chronic illnesses. And management of these chronic conditions is expensive. On average, health care costs for individuals with chronic illnesses are three times the costs of care delivered to others.[5]

The High Cost of Care

It is acknowledged that 20 percent of the population uses 80 percent of the health care dollars. Costs are increased by inappropriate or unnecessary utilization of services such as the emergency department. Unhealthy lifestyle choices increase the incidence of various illnesses, thus driving the cost of care higher. In one large study, smokers had 18 percent higher medical claims and were 43 percent more likely than nonsmokers to miss one week of work each year.[6]

Advances in health care technology also contribute to the increased cost of health care and are another reason why health management systems are needed today. Over the past 30 years, the introduction of sophisticated new diagnostic and treatment techniques, equipment, and pharmaceuticals has seduced patients and providers alike into believing that "more is better." Decisions regarding the use of these technologies are often based on patient demand, physician preference, or litigation concerns, rather than sound clinical research evidence.

Fragmentation of Care

The fragmented nature of the health care system is hard to deny. The traditional medical model delivers segments of care through disconnected points of service, such as the hospital, the physician's office, the home health agency, or the hospice. There are few incentives for the various provider entities to cooperate with one another. The primary care provider is assumed to have the big picture in terms of overall provision of services for a given patient, but often this is not the case. Physicians struggle with the lack of timely access to new information about drugs, treatments, and procedures; matters are further complicated by poor communication among specialists, insurers, and other providers. Information systems that don't interface and a lack of connectivity within the medical community both prevent timely data sharing and proper measurement and outcome analysis. The result is frequent duplication of tests and an inconsistency in treatment plans for the same diagnosis. Research further shows that there is wide variation in the way physicians practice and that patients' treatment and care costs are linked more closely with where they live than with what their diagnosis is. For example, in 1994 and 1995, Medicare residents of the St. Petersburg, Florida, hospital referral region underwent carotid endarterectomy at a rate that was twice the national average. And the price-adjusted reimbursement per Medicare enrollee for hospital care during the last six months of life in Manhattan was 2.8 times that of enrollees living in Bend, Oregon.[7]

So what does all this have to do with customer-focused health management? Plenty! Successful demand management programs have demonstrated that an educated consumer makes better choices about what services to seek and therefore is a better user of care, specifically in terms of not using the emergency department or the physician's office unnecessarily. Successful disease management programs have demonstrated that sound, research-based approaches to management of chronic diseases can reduce the cost of care by standardizing care and reducing variation in practice. The physician's use of researched best practices to make clinical decisions helps to educate patients about the appropriateness of diagnostic studies or medications they may think they need. The use of decision-support systems also protects the physician from litigation stemming from decisions not to offer expensive services, since that physician can demonstrate that her clinical decisions are consistent with state-of-the-art research. And customer-focused health management emphasizes the health promotion and behavior change that will reduce the number of chronic illnesses and deaths caused by lifestyle choices.

ACTION STEPS FOR SUCCESSFUL CUSTOMER-FOCUSED HEALTH MANAGEMENT

The need for a new approach to care management is apparent, and change is being driven by customer demand and new technological possibilities. What do you do now? Positioning for success in today's rapidly changing health care environment requires a new set of components, attitudes, and skills.

Get Your Arms around the Data

Outcomes tracking, data collection, and data analysis are integral to the success of customer-focused health management and practice improvement. One shortcoming of current practice is the lack of true outcomes data to drive best practice decisions. This results from a historical emphasis on process rather than outcomes and a lack of comprehensive information systems to gather, house, and analyze clinical data in particular. Yet the continuous improvement of clinical decision making is impossible without the proper data. The process of improvement begins with knowing, first of all, which data you have and which data you do not have. Next, the data you *have* should be made available so they can be used for making decisions and taking action. If important information has not yet been collected, mechanisms should be put in place to capture it. (Conversely, don't spend time gathering data you will not use—clarify the focus of your data-gathering effort.) The technology exists to gather large volumes of helpful information, to customize interactions with patients, and to track those interactions, almost in real time.

Invest in Computer Technology

Good health management programs cannot happen without information technology. Many highly successful programs are conducted almost exclusively through e-technology. At Cardiac Solutions regional center in Chicago, for instance, specially trained registered nurses use desktop computers and a telephone, in conjunction with electronically based interaction protocols, to teach patients and monitor their compliance. The nurses record their findings and interactions on an electronic patient record, communicate with the primary care physician through multiple media, including fax or e-mail, and generate a variety of quality-monitoring reports via sophisticated software programs. With minor additional investment, those nurses could send their patients customized educational materials via e-mail, on-line chat, or instruct patients to access a particular Web service to register for a class or to set up their next physician's appointment.

Keep Finance Involved from the Start

Financial representatives should be key players in any initial efforts to develop a customer-focused health management program. They can provide the hard data that turn clinical treatment decisions into dollars and cents. For clinicians who have traditionally not thought in financial terms, the financial data, coupled with good research to support an alternative treatment approach, may be a real eye opener and motivation enough to buy into the medical protocols with a health management program, even though the protocols may require a different approach to medical treatment.

Set Priorities

Tempting as it might be to try, you cannot do everything at once. Instead of attempting to manage every high-risk patient in every disease category, it is best to target carefully. In light of what the data are telling you, what are your biggest areas of risk, in terms of either disease states or patient populations? For some, it will be congestive heart failure patients or patients with diabetes. Others will find their greatest risk lies with the indigent patient population or perhaps with Medicare patients. Careful consideration and weighing of risks will guide you in setting priorities and will simplify your implementation of customer-focused health management.

Match the Program to the Patient

Customer-focused health management, as the name implies, is a patient-centered philosophy. As they should, patients themselves will decide when and how to access the health care system. They will also decide whether to comply with the diet, exercise, medications, screenings, and follow-up appointments you give them. When they do not do these things, it is most often from lack of knowledge about consequences, lack of self-management skills, or other social, financial, psychological, or religious barriers. The most successful health management is personalized in a way that attends to these areas from the patient's perspective. Programs for individual patients, even though different patients may share a diagnosis, will—and should—differ significantly from one another. Technology now provides the tools we need to understand and categorize health care consumers based on a wide variety of social and emotional criteria—not just disease states. Accounting for educational levels, functional status, and patient readiness to change will allow for further customization of approach, giving each patient the help he or she needs in the form in which he or she is best able to understand and apply it. Patients who are having a difficult time accepting and dealing with their illness, for instance, might be helped by a program of fairly frequent interventions. Before the technology boom, the opportunities for interactions with such patients were limited. Today, with the multiplicity of telephonic and networked Internet-based connections linking patients to caregivers, contacts (some of them automated) can be made as often as necessary, even daily.

Meet the Staffing Challenge

Tapping the resources of patient-supported self-management calls for a professional staff of nurses, social workers, or other specially trained individuals with a different set of skills. These individuals need a holistic perspective from which to assess patient needs and plan care. They should be comfortable with the patient and family as the key care managers and the home as the focal point of care. Health managers think "systems" and "continuum" and are effective at teaching patients how to navigate the system in order to get the right match of service to meet their needs. Health managers are data savvy and totally wired: they recognize the potential of the Web to support e-care, and they use e-technology to build relationships and customize their services to the individual patients they manage. Catholic Healthcare Partners in Cincinnati, Ohio, has a health management program in which the care managers are called personal health partners. These health partners attend an initial five-day training session to study the holistic interpretation of health, the integration of alternative therapies with mainstream medical practice, and how to assess the patient's readiness to change. They learn motivational and goal-setting techniques and, through the use of electronic databases, telephone, and Web interfaces, they customize their interactions to suit the needs and interests of the patients. This is a first-generation e-care program. As e-technology evolves, so will the approaches to support telemedicine in the home.

Aim for an Early Success

Initial implementations of the customer-focused health management model should be chosen on the basis of their likelihood of succeeding. Health promotion and risk reduction are important components of the model—but the return on investment is long term, and it is not likely that significant changes will occur in a six- to eight-month pilot project. The quickest and most dramatic cost savings and functional status changes are achieved by managing and stabilizing acute episodes of chronic diseases. This may seem like just another disease management program; what makes the model different is the customization of the program to fit more closely with the unique needs and circumstances of each patient. Unlike typical disease management programs, the more holistic approach provides a structure for the long-term monitoring of health behavior and compliance that is important to the success of chronic disease management in a capitated system.

E-TECHNOLOGY IS THE KEY

Early case management and disease management programs did not have the broad, big-picture perspective because they did not have access to the necessary data. Good health management programs are grounded in good data—adequate baseline information, good tracking mechanisms, and real-time feedback. The better the data, the better the care that is based on them, and ultimately the better the outcomes. Web technology improves access to data and the ability to analyze, share, and apply those data. Advances in information technology management increase the ability to gather, store, and analyze data so that findings from research and program evaluations can be quickly applied to the improvement of processes of care. And advances in communication technology provide exciting new channels for interactions between providers and patients.

Web technology has greatly improved our ability to communicate with e-patients. The education that is a key component of health management programs can be even more effective because technology-based education can be customized/personalized to the patient's needs and it allows the patient to participate more actively in the learning process through interactive Web applications. Ultimately, e-care health management programs will routinely include a video component, enabling the patient and the health management nurse to interact visually even though they may be widely separated geographically. To use the technology optimally for the benefit of the patients, all systems need to be fully integrated.

COMING FULL CIRCLE, WITH A DIFFERENCE

The evolution from independent, full fee-for-service medical practice to customer-focused health management delivered through e-technology has seen the focus of care decisions shift from

- the physician and a single patient at the bedside, to
- that "case" being compared to national norms by a UR nurse removed from the specifics, to
- the case manager's focus on getting individual patients into less expensive care, to
- the demand management triage nurse's focus on one patient's symptoms, and
- the customer-focused health management view of patients as unique persons with multiple health concerns/problems, all of which need to be taken into account when making cost-effective care decisions, as communication through e-technology.

The irony of this movement back to the patient-specific decision is that there may be a return to some of the UR and case management approaches, albeit for different reasons. All of these approaches to decision making and care management were born of the desire to cut costs and were based on the assumption that the most effective way to do that was to restrict services. Data on average lengths of stay for given procedures, or formularies, or medical practice guidelines were used to convince care providers that even though they were cutting costs by practicing in a different way, the quality of care would not be adversely affected. Providers and patients alike are now beginning to see these data as decision-support systems, not simply ways to justify cost reductions. Web and e-technology has made it possible for providers to readily access data where they practice, and the information that was once used by the insurance companies to tell physicians what they had to do is now being used by physicians to help make evidence-based practice decisions. There is a strong foundation of science and e-technology being applied to meet the challenges of e-patients to get their care better and faster through e-care.

REFERENCES

1. P.D. Fox, "An Overview of Managed Care," in *The Managed Health Care Handbook,* 3d ed., ed. P.R. Kongstvedt (Gaithersburg, MD: Aspen Publishers, Inc., 1996).
2. "InfoMedics Claims Savings Based on Diabetes Pilot," *Disease Management News* 3, no. 19 (1998): 6.
3. C. Evashwick, *The Continuum of Long-Term Care* (Albany, NY: Delmar Publishers, 1996), 18.
4. U.S. Department of Health and Human Services, *Aging America: Trends and Projections* (Washington, DC: 1991).
5. J. Christianson et al., *Restructuring Chronic Illness Management* (San Francisco, CA: Jossey-Bass Publishers, 1998).
6. S. Brink, *Health Risks and Behavior: The Impact on Medical Costs* (Milwaukee, WI: Milliman & Robertson, 1987).
7. Dartmouth Medical School, Center for the Evaluative Clinical Sciences, *The Dartmouth Atlas of Health Care* (Chicago: American Hospital Publishing, 1998), 67, 92.

e-Communications and Interactive e-Care: The Next Generation of Disease Management

Neal Sofian, Daniel Newton, and Joan DeClaire

IF YOU ARE READING this chapter to learn about the latest disease management model, set forth by experts who advocate new ways for providers and health systems to manage patients with a particular disease state or chronic condition, you are in for a surprise. This chapter is about a new generation of disease management. It does not cover any models that focus on providers or health systems. Instead, it suggests opportunities to really manage disease—using consumer-focused supported self-care and health behavior change tools that incorporate interactive technologies such as the Web, audio and video streaming, and interactive telephony. This is not a traditional disease management chapter.

The first time the three of us attended a disease management conference, we expected to hear a great deal of talk about the most effective ways to help people manage their disease states and the health risks that affect those disease states. We expected to hear about effective protocols for influencing behavior, tying behavior to drug compliance, and sustaining patient compliance when the patient is far away from the care delivery system. Because we come from a mixture of public health, behavior change, health risk, and marketing backgrounds, this seemed to us an obvious constellation of subjects for the conference.

As it turned out, our assumptions were off the mark. As far as we could tell, the concept of the individual being at the center of care was never mentioned—let alone seriously explored. Health behavior was considered irrelevant, and "management" referred only to the best way to manage the health care delivery system or the pricing of pharmaceuticals. It was a rude awakening and showed clearly what is considered state-of-the-art disease management in the American health care system.

Since that conference, there has been some progress, but by and large, disease management has remained the province of critical care pathway designers, prescription guidelines, and health systems engineers. In short, the focus is primarily on the health care system. The central assumption is that if the behavior of physicians and the health system can be modified, patients will be affected and will experience improved outcomes.

Although some of this work may be valuable, Figure 6–1 shows our belief that the focus of disease management should be on the patient—the customer. Patients must be the core of any change process, and the health care delivery system must be built around them. The role of the physician and the care delivery system is to serve the client, not the other way around.

The good news is that advances in information and communications technologies, coupled with a growing interest in how people change health behaviors, are revolutionizing the way we can prevent illness and manage disease. For this revolution to truly occur, however, health care executives and physicians need to re-think the concept of the care process itself—and the roles of the patient, physician, and delivery system in that process. The key is to move beyond using technology simply to accomplish health and medical care tasks faster, and instead to fundamentally re-think the core approaches used in the delivery of health and medical care.

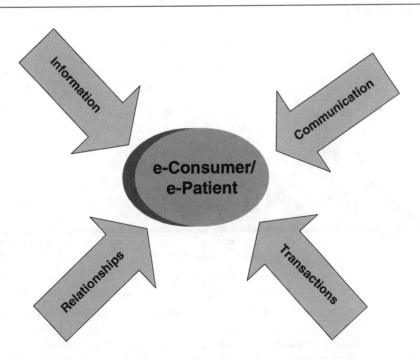

Figure 6–1 A New Perspective of Care. Courtesy of The NewSof Group, Inc., 1999, Redmond, Washington.

EMBRACE THE WAVES OF CHANGE

Figure 6–2 depicts the waves of change occurring in the health care system. We have moved from increasing patient access to care, to managing patient utilization of the care system, to the emergence of a time where the customer is beginning to drive the care delivery system. Physicians are finding themselves in a partnership with consumers who often have more up-to-date information than they have had in the past.

Equally important, the nature of care itself is changing. The behavior of the consumer is at the core of the care process and the outcomes that will occur. As behavior becomes more central to the care process, a core competency of the delivery system will be how to create relationships with the consumer that foster and support the behavior change process. Increasingly, it will become essential that the health care delivery system build a community of support around the individual to facilitate personal change and compliance. The question is not whether this process is going to be a central element of the future, but how it will happen. The nature of new communications technologies and a growing understanding of how to change individuals and communities will be at the heart of this disease management process.

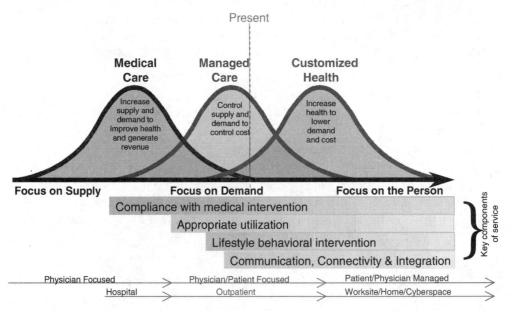

Figure 6–2 From Medical Care to Customized Health. Courtesy of The NewSof Group, Inc., 1999, Redmond, Washington.

CONNECTING PROVIDERS AND PATIENTS

The development of computer hardware and software has spawned tremendous progress in the ability to integrate, manage, and manipulate enormous amounts of health and medical information. While the speed of computing doubles every 12 to 18 months, the cost of hardware declines by half.[1] Advances in the development of sophisticated rule-based programming (also called artificial intelligence) allow us to instantly and automatically find, tailor, and deliver very specific pieces of information to individual providers and patients—information that can make a critical difference in patient care. The implications of this growth of information are stunning. Even the means of transmission of this intelligence is changing dramatically.

One company has developed a working prototype that can translate brain waves into digital content and transmit this content as e-mail through an Internet Service Provider. In other words, we can literally do e-mail in our heads. Although not yet commercially viable, this prototype shows how advanced communication technologies are becoming. What most of us believe is the future is already here.

But the integration of e-care delivery will require health care professionals to stretch their thinking tremendously. Technology changes are creating a growing discontinuity between where we are now and where health care delivery and technologies are moving. The market will be huge for these changes. According to a January 1999 Hambrecht & Quist Institutional Research report, the "health.net" industry—including e-commerce, disease management, and system connectivity—could total hundreds of billions of dollars per year by early in the next century. Whether you are a health care administrator or a professional, you will be slung into this next technology phase; you should be prepared to handle it.

Concurrent with these technological advances, our society is growing in its awareness that health behaviors play a significant role in the ability to prevent, heal, and manage illness. We now know, for example, that half of all deaths with known causes can be linked to lifestyle factors. We also know that more than 70 percent of all potential years of life lost in the United States before age 65 are linked to preventable causes. Of these years, 75 percent can be linked to tobacco use, hypertension, and being overweight.[2]

Such evidence is changing providers' ideas about disease management. Rather than seeing it as something our health care systems must "do" to patients during the limited time the patients spend in a clinic or hospital, providers are acknowledging that disease management happens, in large part, as a result of the choices patients make on their own time, in their own environments. This includes patients' everyday decisions regarding drug compliance, social support, and lifestyle issues such as exercise, nutrition, smoking, and stress management.

If physicians and other providers hope to influence such decisions, they must approach patients with an understanding of how and why people change health behaviors. They must see health decisions from the patient's perspective. They must pay attention to factors such as the individual patient's motivations, barriers, health beliefs, learning style, preferences, and readiness to change. And in order to affect large populations, health care systems must find cost-efficient ways to deliver behaviorally based disease management interventions to large populations, *one person at a time*.

Figure 6-3 outlines the complexity of this approach. To generate value for both consumers and providers of care, a web of information will have to be integrated that looks at the interplay of current and projected health care costs, health risk and status, personal health behaviors and motivations. This information can then generate e-care strategies (face-to-face, print, telephonic, Internet, etc.) to reach and affect consumers and their providers and ultimately to optimize interventions.

Fortunately, the technologies and emerging behavioral strategies that allow individual customization of disease management programs are available today. The remainder of this chapter describes 10 ways these interactive and e-tools can and will be used to improve health outcomes.

1. THE ABILITY TO MORE ACCURATELY PREDICT UTILIZATION AND COSTS

For decades, proponents of preventive care and disease management have postulated that payers could reduce health care utilization and costs through interventions that address individual lifestyle issues such as drug compliance, exercise, diet, and smoking. But it was not until the past decade, through the power of advanced data integration, that institutions were able to predict accurately how their efforts might affect future health care utilization and costs for populations and for individuals within those populations.

Health organizations now have access to computers powerful enough to combine data from many sources—including medical claims, pharmacy claims, health risk appraisals, personal medical records, and even employee absenteeism and health programming records. This information allows them to create individual and population profiles, and then to stratify populations on the basis of expected outcomes and costs. Such stratification enables organizations to be more strategic in determining approaches to intervention at population and in-

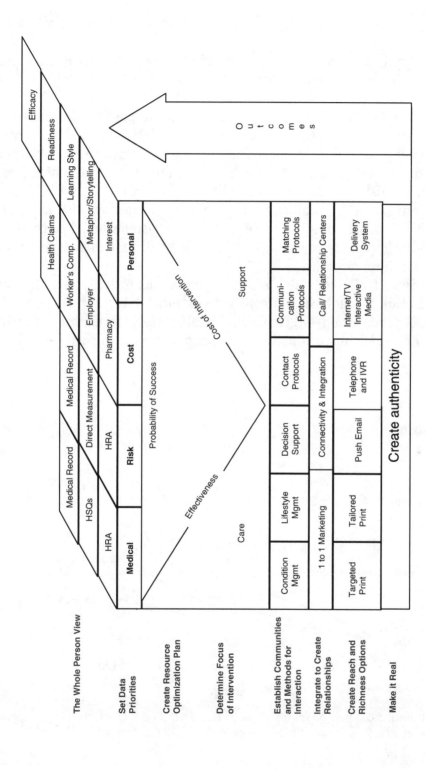

Figure 6–3 Creating *Communities of Care* and Managing Populations. Courtesy of The NewSof Group, Inc., 1999, Redmond, Washington.

dividual levels. These organizations can also look back and see what worked and what didn't work.

Dr. Dee Edington, dean of the University of Michigan's Health Management Research Center, has done landmark work in this area, developing highly refined stratification models that use algorithms to identify potential high utilizers on the basis of lifestyle-related data.[3] Such tools make it possible for payers to assign health care cost trends to each person in a population, then design intervention strategies based on future needs and expenses. As can be seen in Figure 6–4, the traditional health care cost curve is further refined to represent the cost of people with low risk, low dangerous conditions (LR-LDC), low risk, high dangerous conditions (LR-HDC), high risk, low dangerous conditions (HR-LDC), and high risk, high dangerous conditions (HR-HDC). Such systems help health plans, employers, and others monitor, plan, and implement disease management and health promotion interventions.

Today's computer technology also allows organizations to analyze health care costs and utilization through comparisons with external databases. For example, through the Medstat Group—a Thompson Healthcare Information Company based in Ann Arbor, Michigan—institutions can gain access to cost and utiliza-

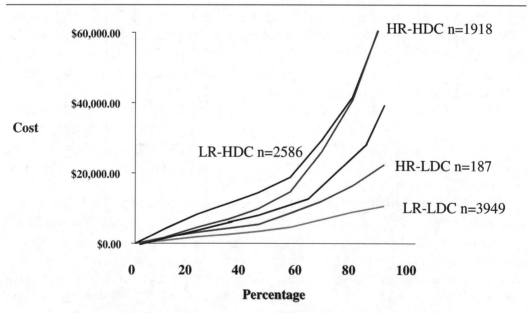

Figure 6–4 Distribution Comparison for Nondiseased Men Ages 55–65. Courtesy of Dee Edington, Health Management Research Center, University of Michigan, 1998, Ann Arbor, Michigan.

tion information from enormous data warehouses.[4] One of the Medstat Group's products allows clients entry to a database that represents inpatient and outpatient health care services for more than 7 million persons.[5] Such information can help Medstat's clients develop better strategies for monitoring outcomes, and managing and forecasting the utilization and cost of various treatments.

2. IMPROVED CASE MANAGEMENT

Having the right information in the right place at the right time has always been essential to good case management. With today's health care systems growing in size and complexity, that challenge becomes even greater. Fortunately, progressive organizations are building information systems that use advanced data integration and artificial intelligence to cut through the complexity and deliver the right information to providers and patients when they need it. An example is UniHealth, an integrated health delivery system in Southern California that partnered with Monsanto Company to build a better information architecture for its Medicare population.

One of the challenges facing UniHealth was to coordinate the efforts of all the various entities that conduct disease management programs for Medicare beneficiaries in its facilities. Officials predict that the number of discrete protocols— including those sponsored by various health plans, pharmaceutical companies, and providers associated with UniHealth—may eventually be in the hundreds.[6] By working with a highly integrated information system that encompasses the entire population, rather than subsets of its population, UniHealth can coordinate its efforts on behalf of these various disease management programs while eliminating duplication of effort and improving quality of care.

Coordination includes pulling all the disparate data streams into one unified database. It also means creating a system for identifying and stratifying patients by particular risks. And finally, it means creating a system that can regularly monitor all the information collected on individual patients and raise flags when particular interventions are needed.

Rather than doing weekly or monthly retrospective data searches to flag high-risk individuals—the method used in most current disease management settings—UniHealth's system monitors information about its entire Medicare population every day. This means that the appropriate case manager knows if a patient's status has changed in a way that requires intervention. The case manager knows, for example, if a patient has a prescription for a new drug, has had a particular set of lab tests, or has been admitted to a hospital. Such a system can tell a case manager not only that a diabetic patient is in the hospital for surgery, but that the patient lives alone, has congestive heart disease, filled three new drug prescriptions, and has not been authorized for home health care.

Stored separately, these pieces of information might not signal a case manager to consider taking a specific action. But when the information is collected and interpreted using a rules-based information system ("if x, y, and z happen, do n"), the system can alert trained coordination specialists that specific steps may be needed. The system does not replace the clinical judgment of providers or case managers, of course, but it can ensure that the right professional is getting all the relevant information and guidance when it is needed. A number of companies are attempting to create the next generation of these types of services, including Abaton.com (Figure 6–5), Lifemasters.net, and Healtheon.com.

Efforts to build more highly integrated and intelligent information systems can certainly enhance today's disease management programs as we know them, but we can also look forward to the day when such systems are expanded to include information about the prevention of disease as well as the management of it. In other words, we predict that progressive health-related organizations will soon benefit from including lifestyle information related to issues such as stress, weight management, exercise, and smoking in their databases. This will

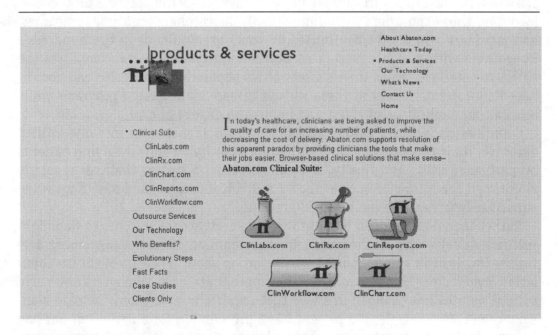

Figure 6–5 Abaton's Clinical Suite Integrates Data Sources. *Source:* Abaton.com, Inc. © 1999. Reproduced by permission.

give organizations better information with which to plan, implement, and monitor population-based and individual interventions. These systems will require the integration of algorithms such as those used by the University of Michigan with the management protocols and software tools of both health risk vendors such as WellMed and disease managers such as Lifemasters. Creating these systems will also require the continued focus on the patient as an integral provider in his or her own health management. To that end, new tools, such as personal health records, are now available to help consumers and patients manage their health information.

3. IMPROVED INTERVENTION BY TARGETING SEGMENTED POPULATIONS

Using a combination of computer technology and behavior change theories, disease management programs can now segment populations on the basis of any number of characteristics—including risk level, demographics, or psychodemographic traits such as health beliefs, readiness to change, or learning style. Such segmentation enables health care organizations to be more strategic in the way they design interventions. It is a technique that advertisers and marketers in other industries have used for some time. Rather than simply look at traditional demographic segments, UniHealth has also explored psychodemographic states that match traditional splits of the population. The company has consistently aimed to learn more about individuals, beyond the specifics of their consumption of a given product. The hope is to garner clues about these peoples' motivations in general, so that they can be applied to specific transactions.

Consider, for example, the way tobacco advertisers segment by psychodemographic characteristics. Knowing that a high percentage of young women want to look thin and feel more powerful, Virginia Slims populates its cigarette ads with very thin and highly assertive women. For young men who seek a virile, rebellious identity, the tobacco industry has offered images such as the Marlboro cowboy and Joe Camel. Tobacco advertisers also know they'll get the biggest return on their advertising dollars by designing ads and promotions that appeal to the people most likely to pick up the habit—youngsters. Thus, we see young-looking people in their ads. At the same time, tobacco companies create highly targeted publications, games, incentives, and events designed to reach discrete populations in various psychodemographic categories—which results in a world of tobacco promotion that is virtually hidden to people outside their target markets.

The same kinds of segmentation strategies are beginning to be used to promote healthy behaviors. Several health-related organizations, for example, have been experimenting with segmenting populations according to people's readiness to change problem behaviors such as smoking or poor eating habits. These efforts are based on the transtheoretical model of behavior change proposed by James O. Prochaska and Carlo C. DiClemente,[7] a theory that places people into one of five categories:

- Precontemplation (no awareness of the problem; no intention to change)
- Contemplation (awareness of the problem; considering change)
- Preparation (actively planning to make a change in the next 30 days)
- Action (practicing new behaviors)
- Maintenance (continuing changed behaviors over time)

Segmenting populations this way allows organizations to optimize their resources by investing the most in those people most likely to benefit from the opportunity. BJC Health Systems in St. Louis, for example, uses this segmentation strategy for its employee smoking cessation program. BJC offers all interested employees a tailored newsletter that addresses issues such as their unique risks, motivations, and barriers to quitting smoking. But the organization makes a larger investment in a subset of smokers—those who are assessed as being in the "preparation" stage or further along. These smokers have access to telephone-based personal health facilitators who are specially trained in behavior-change counseling. Facilitators regularly telephone this subset of BJC smokers to counsel them, and send self-help print materials aimed at helping them through the process of quitting.

By integrating these two technologies—a telephone call center and a tailored newsletter program—BJC provides the most appropriate care to its employees based on their stage of change, and at the lowest possible cost. Intervention segmentation will become even more complex as on-line options allow the company to deliver programming to the employee's desk, virtually eliminating the cost of delivery of intervention for low-probability quitters.

Although it is still too early to measure the effectiveness of BJC's approach, Prochaska's studies show that designing smoking cessation interventions according to stage of change can double quit rates over standard approaches.[8]

Segmenting on the basis of readiness to change is just one, fairly limited option. Another is to segment on the basis of risk. For example, an organization might try different intervention approaches with its high-risk and low-risk smokers. Low-risk smokers might simply receive brief telephone counseling or on-line interventions. High-risk smokers, on the other hand, might get the drug buproprion (Zyban) as well as telephone counseling. This same process could be applied to any risk factor or chronic disease state—for example, segmenting individuals with a moderately high fasting level of glucose versus diagnosed diabetics.

As organizations begin to take advantage of the variety of e-care media available, they may choose to segment their populations on the basis of factors such as learning style or media preference. Those who learn best by reading, for example, will get self-help booklets, while those who are auditory learners will get their instruction via a telephonic audio library. And those who learn best by hands-on activities will get a highly interactive CD-ROM or connect to an on-line Web module.

As we described earlier, organizations may choose to segment their populations on the basis of expected utilization and costs. Stratification tools such as the one developed by Dr. Dee Edington—which allows organizations to predict future utilization and costs on an individual basis—make decisions of this kind easier. Without these tools, such determinations would be guesswork based on what *might* be known about individuals or the segments to which they belong. Now, however, stratification can be done focusing on individual data within a segment. Research firms such as the Sachs Group (www.sachs.com), based in Evanston, Illinois, specialize in helping health care organizations develop and implement segmentation strategies.

4. USE OF TAILORING TO DELIVER HIGHLY INDIVIDUALIZED INTERVENTIONS

Once a population has been segmented according to risk, expected utilization, readiness to change, or any other factors, organizations can provide interventions targeted to fit that group. Tailoring takes this concept even further to create "segments of one," that is, designing interventions to fit each person's unique set of characteristics and needs.

In Figure 6–3, we showed a variety of ways to look at the individual, from risk or cost information, to the person's learning style and sense of self-efficacy to make change, to the kinds of metaphors the person finds meaningful. Two things are accomplished with this approach. First, messages are created that specifically match the needs of that individual, which facilitates a much greater opportunity for change. Second, and equally important, the process of creating a high degree of tailoring helps the person feel more comfortable with the care he or she is receiving. The patient does not experience as much of the discomfort associated with having to bend to the limitations of the intervention's approach. When the message and the medium are appropriate, the person is not being asked to do things outside of his or her comfort zone. This approach is the next best thing to the consumer perspective of the best change being no change at all.

In the past, highly individualized intervention could only be designed and delivered via intensive one-on-one counseling, an expensive proposition and one that many consumers do not care for. But now, computerized tailoring engines can use rules-based programming to automatically mix and match messages and mediums to fit an individual profile. Such tailored interventions can be delivered using a variety of media, including telephonic interactive voice response (IVR) systems or individually generated Web pages or newsletters.

The effectiveness of tailored interventions has been demonstrated in a number of studies, including those designed to encourage smoking cessation,[9] breast cancer screening,[10] dietary change,[11] and exercise.[12] In a study of smokers who received personally tailored newsletters that zeroed in on factors such as cigarette consumption, interest in quitting, and perceived benefits and barriers to quitting, health psychologists Dr. Victor Strecher and Dr. Matthew Kreuter showed impressive results. After six months, 30.7 percent of moderate to light smokers who received tailored newsletters had quit smoking, compared with 7.1 percent in a control group who received a generic stop-smoking newsletter.[13]

The Health Communications Research Laboratory at Saint Louis University, under the direction of Dr. Kreuter, has developed some innovative uses for tailored messaging. One is a wall calendar for families of infants that features a picture of the baby along with the baby's immunization schedule and tailored safety and parenting advice (Figure 6-6).[14] In a study to determine the calendar's effectiveness among underserved families at public health centers in St. Louis, Kreuter found that at least 75 percent of the families who received the calendars complied with the recommended childhood immunization schedule. This compares with a citywide immunization rate among preschool children of just 40 percent.

Tailoring works because it allows patients to cut through today's information overload to find the content that is most related to their personal interests and priorities. "The sheer length of generic self-help manuals and pamphlets may discourage effective use of these materials," writes Strecher, "whereas tailored materials, which include only relevant information, can maximize vividness and persuasiveness. Tailoring also allows for the provision of more information concentrated on a few key topics rather than less information on a larger number of topics, as is typical with pamphlets or short self-help guides."[15]

Researchers at Brown University School of Medicine recently conducted the first prospective, randomized, controlled trial demonstrating the efficacy of an exercise intervention tailored to motivational stage.[16] In a study of 900 hospital

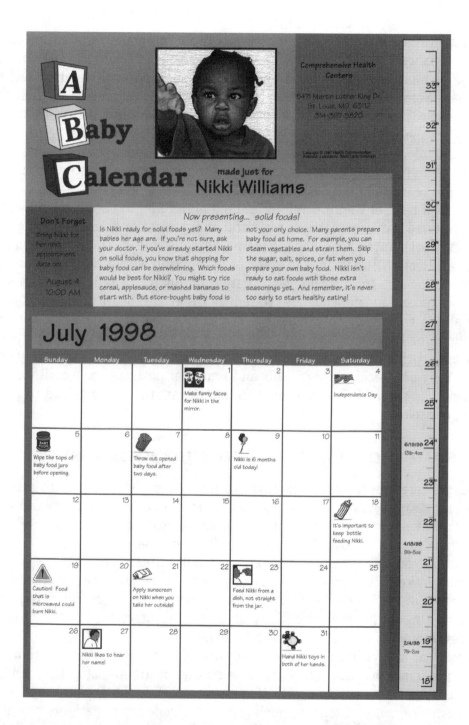

Figure 6–6 Example of a Tailored Prenatal Calendar. Courtesy of Matthew Kreuter, PhD, MPH, 1999, School of Public Health, Saint Louis University, St. Louis, Missouri.

workers enrolled in a workplace health-promotion program, results showed that participants who received tailored materials made greater progress along a continuum of motivational stages than did those who received standard self-help materials. Some 37 percent of those who got materials tailored to fit their stage of readiness (precontemplation, contemplation, preparation, action, or maintenance) progressed to a more advanced stage, compared with just 27 percent in the standard group. Furthermore, those who advanced in motivational stage started spending significantly more time exercising after the intervention than those who regressed or did not advance.

Although most of the research in tailored messaging to date has involved the use of tailored print newsletters, a handful of organizations are developing interventions to be integrated and delivered across a broad range of media. The American Heart Association, for example, is working with a North Carolina firm called Micromass, Inc., to deliver "Change of Heart," a tailored intervention aimed at making lifestyle changes to reduce the risk of heart disease.[17] The program allows consumers to complete a health risk and lifestyle assessment over the phone or the Web. Then, in addition to a printed kit tailored by stage of change, participants receive a highly tailored print or Web-based quarterly newsletter. They also receive phone calls and reminder postcards or e-mail messages based on the stage of change they were at the last time they talked to phone-based counselors.

5. INTEGRATED TECHNOLOGIES THAT OFFER BETTER ACCESS TO INTERVENTIONS

Using e-care multimedia technology to improve patients' access to interventions can mean a number of things, including expanding the times and places that services are available. It is not the Internet in particular, but the *integration* of any medium that most effectively matches the needs of the individual. This integration can help patients navigate through an increasingly large and confounding maze of information to quickly find the material that is relevant to their situation. This same onslaught of information also faces practicing physicians, who would have to essentially give up their practices to stay abreast of new developments and research in their fields.

Access has always been a challenge for disease management and patient education programs that use traditional one-on-one or group instruction in clinics and classrooms. One problem with these approaches is the expense of staff and facilities. Also, some studies have shown that a majority of patients find group programs unacceptable for reasons that range from inconvenient times and locations to discomfort with learning in a group setting.[18] According to a 1997 report from the Agency for Health Care Policy and Research, only 5 percent of smokers are willing to enroll in group programs.[19]

Teaching during clinic visits is also fraught with problems. Providers rarely have enough time to devote to even one effective lesson in smoking cessation, weight loss, medication compliance, or the like. And even when they do, one lesson is rarely enough to help people successfully change behaviors. In addition, studies show that material learned in one environment is best remembered in that same environment.[20,21] In other words, patients may be better prepared to practice healthy new behaviors if they learn those behaviors in their own living rooms, kitchens, and offices. Is it any wonder, then, that so many physicians' instructions are never carried out?

Some of these problems are being solved through the use of technologies such as real-time telephone call centers, IVR systems, and Web-enabled e-service applications. Not only do these solutions extend interventions beyond the limitations of geography and busy schedules, but they also allow delivery systems and physician practices to reach more people while producing better outcomes. As shown in Figure 6–7, achieving these outcomes requires a careful balancing of the ubiquity of technological reach with the richness of one-to-one interactions.

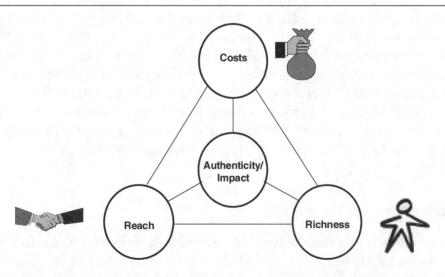

Figure 6–7 Balancing Technology and Authenticity. Courtesy of The NewSof Group, Inc., 1999, Redmond, Washington.

Some common examples of technology-centered approaches to care are discussed below.

Real-Time Telephone Call Centers

Real-time call centers, staffed by nurses for the purpose of demand management, have existed for more than 20 years. See Chapter 8 for more information on real-time call centers. These centers typically take calls from patients who need triage, advice, or information. Most large health plans offer some form of call center phone-based advice program to their members,[22] because studies show they can curtail unnecessary visits to emergency departments and physicians' offices.[23]

Call centers that make calls for the purposes of disease management and behavior change are a newer trend. Such services may be staffed by a variety of professionals—including nurses, counselors, or behavior-change facilitators—depending on the type of intervention needed. Staff members typically call patients at home or at work to monitor compliance with drug regimens; help them control chronic medical conditions such as diabetes, congestive heart failure, and asthma; or offer coaching and support for difficult behavior changes such as smoking cessation and weight management.

The power of call centers to effect behavior change was proven in 1986 in a National Cancer Institute study of Group Health Cooperative of Puget Sound's Free & Clear smoking intervention.[24] By placing four phone calls to each participant over 60 weeks, Free & Clear achieved 16-month abstinence rates of 23 percent. This compares with a national average of 11 to 12 percent for self-help cessation programs and 30 percent for high-quality group programs. By expanding the intervention to include six calls over a year, the program demonstrated 12-month quit rates of 34 percent.[25] Group Health Cooperative had done similar work in diabetes and asthma, using a mix of registered nurses, certified nurse educators, and health educators to provide different levels of intervention and counseling.

Interactive Voice Response (IVR)

Incorporating IVR technologies into real-time telephone call centers allows organizations to expand the reach of their interventions even further. Simply put, IVR involves combining telephone equipment with a computer. The phone receives a call and transfers it to the computer, where the caller then hears instructions prerecorded on the computer hard drive—typically a menu of options. The caller then enters data directly into the computer by pressing codes on the Touch-Tone pad or—if the system includes voice-recognition technology—simply by talking.

Health care organizations use IVR for a variety of purposes, including assessment, monitoring, and patient education. The system can be programmed, for example, to call a patient automatically, collect health risk assessment data, give immediate feedback, and deliver patient information to the patient's provider. The provider then can respond by recording feedback about the patient's health status. The system can also be programmed to call patients and remind them about medications, behavior-change goals, or appointments.

In addition, providers can use IVR to respond to their patients' queries with a series of the providers' own prerecorded messages. Using tailoring software, providers mix and match those messages to create speeches that are personally designed to fit a particular patient's situation at a particular time. The provider may also direct the patient to an audio library of longer prerecorded programs produced by outside vendors on a variety of health topics. Such audio libraries are becoming increasingly sophisticated.

A Seattle-based company called HealthTalk Interactive, for example, produces interactive telephone and Internet "talk shows" (Figure 6–8) featuring experts and lay people speaking on a variety of diseases, including asthma, headaches, multiple sclerosis, prostate cancer, and kidney disease.[26] Each show is created live and resembles a call-in radio talk show. Tapes of the show are then edited and stored by topic for other individuals to access via phone or computer. The shows provide opportunities for people to tell their own stories and listen to the stories of others. Patients can share information about how they have lived with a chronic illness or the challenges they have overcome to make significant changes in their health behaviors. This format provides an environment for the kind of personalized and intimate communication that can support life changes. At the same time, it can reach large numbers of people, leveraging an organization's initial investment in one show thousands of times.

Several studies have shown IVR to be useful in preventive care and disease management.[27–29] For example, internist Robert Friedman's work at Boston University Medical Center has shown IVR to be an effective tool for helping patients with hypertension and hypercholesterolemia comply with medication regimens and manage their conditions.[30]

Providers with experience in IVR emphasize that it should not be a barrier to the patient–provider relationship. Instead, they say, IVR can enhance patient

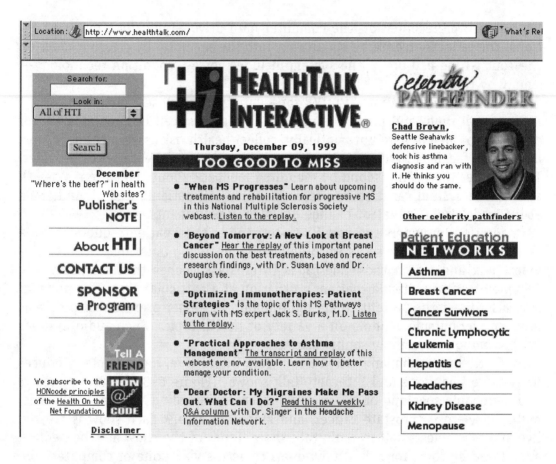

Figure 6–8 Audio Technology Enriches Communication for a Wide Audience. *Source:* Reprinted with permission from www.healthtalk.com, © 1999, Schorr Communications.

care because it allows health care organizations to share tailored information with their patients in a timely, consistent, and accurate way. Indeed, in some instances, IVR may encourage patients to communicate more honestly with providers. In a study of primary care patients with mental disorders, for example, Kenneth Kobak and his associates found that patients were willing to disclose more about sensitive behavioral information when they used an IVR assessment than when they were being interviewed by a clinician.[31] Patients using IVR in that study reported rates of alcohol abuse that were twice as high as the rates they reported to their physicians. IVR is another key tool in the emerging electronic care or e-care toolbox.

Web-Enabled e-Services Applications and CD-ROM

Just as the development of phone-based interventions increases patient access to disease management and behavior change programs, so does the development of CD-ROM and Web-enabled e-service interventions.

By connecting to the Internet, patients have free access to huge searchable databases of health and medical information. The U.S. National Library of Medicine's Grateful Med, for example, allows consumers to search more than 9 million citations from international biomedical literature dating back to 1966.

Having such a mass of data at their fingertips, however, does not necessarily mean that patients have access to material that is credible. And even the most credible information is not necessarily useful for changing health habits or controlling disease processes. Indeed, the effect can be just the opposite, as people become overwhelmed or confused by the sheer amount and complexity of data. The real challenge for e-patients is to find personally relevant content they can trust—a problem that can be solved through the use of an authoritative, computerized resource that can scan credible health information sources and then re-purpose them in the way that best fits each person's needs.

A handful of companies—including Micromass, Wellmed.com, and HealthOnLine—are currently developing behavior change and disease management interventions that will do just that. WellMed's "HQ" on-line product, for example, allows users to create their own personalized, action-oriented Web services that present content tailored to the individual's readiness to change, personal health beliefs, and other psychodemographic factors.

Studies have shown that patients use and appreciate computerized interventions. A systematic review of computerized patient education interventions was conducted by a group of researchers from medical schools at the University of Missouri-Columbia and the University of North Carolina.[32] After evaluating 13 instructional programs, 4 information-support networks, and 4 systems for health assessment and history taking, the group concluded, "Computerized educational interventions can lead to improved health status in several major areas of care." The group found that programs frequently helped patients with chronic diseases better understand their conditions. These programs also helped give them a greater sense of control and confidence in their ability to improve their own health. The patient's age did not seem to make a difference in the findings; patients of all ages were similarly satisfied. And, just as Kobak found among the mental health patients he studied, these groups generally seemed more willing to reveal sensitive or potentially embarrassing information to computers than to human interviewers.

While there is little doubt that people find computerized health interventions helpful, some health care professionals worry that access is limited because computers are too expensive and too complex for some patients to use. Others, however, look forward in the next few years to the widespread emergence of high-speed Internet and greater multimedia bandwidth. Once greater bandwidth to the home becomes widely available, Web-based audio/visual content is likely to become as ubiquitous as the telephone, allowing patients access in their homes to a flourishing array of computerized disease management and behavior-change resources.

This convergence of e-care communication mediums will be at the heart of the intervention process. As shown in Figure 6–9, creating disease management interventions will involve the selection and integration of various technologies applied to desired outcomes. Differentiating among phone, television, and the Web will seem arbitrary and irrelevant in the near future. All of the content loaded on an IVR system as described above could be Web enabled, with the addition of visual content and links to other telemedicine e-services. Consider the following possibility.

A person who has diabetes listens to an audio segment about the importance and timing of blood glucose monitoring, and about having his hemoglobin A1c checked twice a year. In the past, this patient may have called to make an appointment with his doctor for testing; more likely, he did nothing at all. However, the patient in our example has an iPhone® telephone, Internet television, and on-line computer system that run through one broadband connection, making them all accessible to the patient and to the health care delivery system in real time.

After hearing about the importance of what he needs to do, the patient clicks to be connected to a clinician via two-way audio on the Web, and talks to her to develop a plan for ongoing diabetes education, nutrition management, and glucose monitoring. The patient then connects to an e-commerce Web service, which has been recommended by his physician, to purchase a glucose monitor, strips, and any other supplies and educational materials he will need to manage his disease. Over the next 10 weeks, the patient completes an on-line education program that teaches him how to manage his diet and exercise, monitor blood sugar, check his feet, manage sick days, and quit smoking if necessary.

Each day, after using his glucose meter, the patient downloads the data through his computer to his physician's office. If at any time the readings are

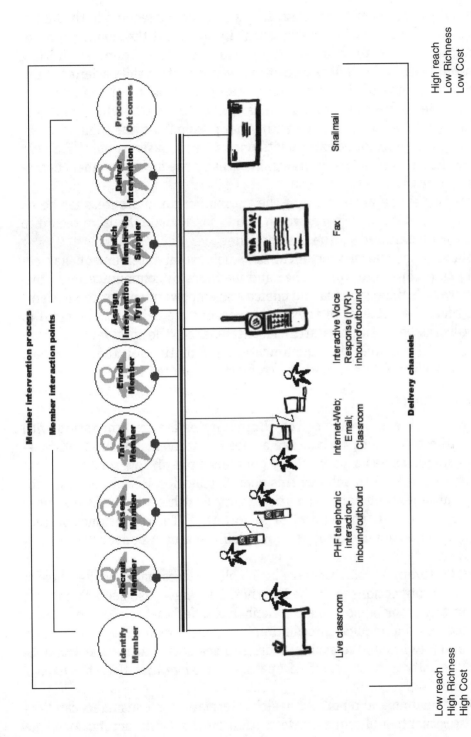

Figure 6–9 Assembling e-Care Technologies To Create Interventions. Courtesy of The NewSof Group, Inc., 1999, Redmond, Washington.

consistently out of compliance, a message is automatically sent to both the patient and the provider indicating that there is a problem. If the readings do not improve, a registered diabetes educator is notified to call the patient and initiate an intervention. Occasional, tailored print pieces are sent to the patient to support this process. In one of the print pieces, the patient is given the names of three other people with similar backgrounds and issues, all of whom have expressed an interest in being connected with other people "just like them" to form a support group. The support group meets on a regular basis as part of a chat room through their provider's Web service. Eventually the group members decide that they would like to meet in person.

Throughout this entire process, all of the transactions and progress are being stored in a common data repository, which allows for a comprehensive record to be developed and monitored by the care provider.

A comprehensive educational, clinical, and behavioral intervention has occurred, using many different approaches and mediums of communication, optimizing the provider's time and creating choice and empowerment for the patient. At the same time, the patterns of these interventions are being accumulated to "learn" what works best. Through artificial intelligence, the interventions continue to adapt to those areas of communication and motivation that work best for the patient. Welcome to the world of connected, tailored e-care.

A "Connected Community"

Many health organizations across the United States are experimenting with various types of e-technology to improve access to interventions and deliver e-care, but one stands out as a particularly good example of how several e-technologies can be integrated to achieve this goal. Celebration Health, an Orlando-based Disney subsidiary, operates a multispecialty health center in Celebration, Florida—Disney's planned "community of tomorrow."[33] The e-consumer portion of the system is a Web service designed for Celebration by a Denver-based company called HealthMagic.

Since 1997, Celebration residents have been able to access most of their health records via secure connections with the Internet. They have also been able to use their computers to book appointments, send messages to their doctors, view their billing records, and request information from an electronic health library. It is all part of a highly integrated system built into the core information architecture for the specialty center, which is operated by Adventist Health Systems' Florida Hospital.

In addition to reading and reporting health information, e-consumers can take health risk assessments and request information on their risk factors. Also, the system can routinely send e-consumers information based on their health needs. A person with seasonal allergies, for example, might get messages in May warning about fluctuating pollen counts and suggesting tips for symptom relief.

As we have come to expect with Disney-related projects, no innovation seems too fantastic. Celebration's future plans call for video links to homes so nurses can visually assess injuries or illnesses while the patient is still at home. Physicians and patients would be able to communicate "face-to-face" over the computer, thus address the principles of e-care—better outcomes, cost effectively.

6. REDUCED CYCLE TIME FOR CASE MANAGEMENT AND BEHAVIOR-CHANGE INTERVENTIONS

Because e-care technologies such as IVR and the Web allow patients and providers to instantly enter and retrieve information from integrated databases, processing time-lags are reduced. The pharmacy industry has used computers in this way for decades, checking prescription databases to prevent dangerous drug interactions or other serious medical problems before dispensing new medications. Now, as described in the earlier UniHealth scenario, providers can have immediate access to many different kinds of pertinent data about their patients, enabling them to make better decisions about that patient's care.

A case manager, for example, will not have to wait for monthly reports to learn that a particular patient has been diagnosed with diabetes and needs self-care instruction. Using the integrated information system that organizations such as Axololt.com, Abaton.com, and Healtheon.com are developing, the case manager knows very quickly that the patient has been newly diagnosed and needs support. These same systems will be able to refill prescriptions as needed through on-line pharmacies such as Drugstore.com and CVS.com.

E-care technology that provides instant access to pertinent information is also changing the way we conduct the classic, assessment-driven behavior-change interventions. In fact, e-technology can change the way patients perceive and respond to their own health risks. Until now, however, response time was protracted. For example, an overweight, middle-aged smoker hears that his favorite 1960s rock musician has just died of a sudden heart attack. Confronted at that moment with his own mortality, the smoker feels highly motivated to learn about his risks for heart disease and what he can do to reduce them.

If the man has access to a traditional wellness program through his health plan, he might call and request help, which would start with the completion of a paper-based health risk assessment (HRA). After waiting three days to get the HRA by mail, he completes it, sends it back, and then waits four weeks while it is being processed before he gets the results. Once he has the results, he may be invited to join a self-help intervention, so he waits another week before receiving a self-help booklet on smoking cessation, weight management, or exercise. By the time all this has happened, his rock 'n roll hero is long dead and buried and the "teaching moment" has passed. Indeed, the man may have forgotten the reason he called the wellness program in the first place. And even then, the material he gets will probably be written for a general audience. He will have to sift through a lot of irrelevant content to find information that is pertinent to his situation.

Compare that scenario with one in which the smoker has access to an on-line e-care health program.

Hearing that his hero has died, the man begins to worry about his own risk. He logs on to his computer or television, finds his health plan's Web site, and enters "heart attack" into its search mechanism. The man instantly gets information about the warning signs of a heart attack. Then he sees a link to an e-service that promises to tell him about his own risk for heart disease. He clicks on this link and begins to complete an online HRA. Within minutes he learns how his smoking, eating habits, and sedentary lifestyle are all putting him at high risk for his own cardiovascular event. He also gets recommendations on things he can do to reduce his risk, real time.

In addition, he finds interactive tools (tailored content, computerized tracking mechanisms, calorie counters, nutritional analysis, etc.) that can help him design and stick to his new healthy-lifestyle plan. And finally, he learns about his health plan's resources and support groups, and is offered a number of appointment options to discuss this issue with his personal physician.

Then he connects to a live on-line video chat, where people in the same situation are sharing their feelings about the rock hero's death and resolving to support one another in changing their ways. If our smoker is at high risk, his health plan may arrange for him to be contacted by a "personal health facilitator" from a real-time telephone call center. The facilitator may call him and set up a schedule of regular calls to coach him on ways to improve his health.

Once WebTV-like and iPhone® technology takes hold, this information exchange may happen even more automatically, more seamlessly. The rock fan will not have to log on to his home computer to interact with a health-related database. Instead, a computer prompt might appear as a small icon on his television screen during the news story about his hero's sudden death. If the viewer chooses to respond to the prompt, the news program could be reduced to a small window on the screen while the viewer does a quick assessment to see if he has the same risks as the rock star. That way, he can move from the "teaching moment" to the first part of an intervention without missing his TV broadcast.

In another e-care scenario, a viewer might receive a prompt to take an assessment during a one-minute commercial break from an afternoon soap opera. A patient with asthma, for example, might be asked to share information about her use of her inhaler, and then be given tips on the early symptoms of an asthma attack and the optimal time to use a beta agonist. In this same way, someone with a risk for heart disease might be asked to record how much time he exercises and then be given an encouraging word to become more physically active.

Finally, wireless satellite technology that links mobile communication devices to mainframe computers may allow instant data exchange independent of specific sites—an innovative approach for organizations that need to aggregate data collected over broad geographical areas. Examples might include large employers, delivery systems, or organizations such as independent practitioner associations that contract with thousands of doctors across a state or region.

The advantage of satellite technology is its ability to transmit computerized assessments, reports, and interventions in a matter of minutes, anywhere at any time. All these data are then aggregated so that any health plan, employer, or delivery system can determine what is happening to a population, regardless of the geographical expanse of that population. The technology also allows organizations to deliver consistent and proven interventions, while accounting for outcomes. Like cable and long distance phone providers, satellite technologies will soon offer integrated access to phones, computers, personal data assistants, and television, all through one signal, allowing an almost infinite number of combinations of intervention to be delivered anywhere in the world—even in locations that do not have the latest in fiber-optic or cable access. This capability will be significant for the delivery of disease management to rural and other underserved areas.

7. COMPUTERIZED DECISION-MAKING TOOLS EMPOWER PATIENTS TO TAKE A MORE ACTIVE ROLE

In addition to providing relevant information in a timely fashion, e-care technology applications are emerging that can give patients a solid framework for making difficult decisions about their health. This is a highly valued function, according to Regina Herzlinger, author of *Market-Driven Health Care*. Today's generation of patients is typically "time-bankrupt and decision-weary," she writes.[34] At the same time, they are fairly well educated and not prone to letting their physicians make important personal decisions for them. Instead, these patients show up in the clinic as "focused experts"—people who have a lot of information about their specific health problems, but who need health professionals to help them put that information in the proper context and give them a model for making choices.

That is where computerized decision-making tools can assist. Such tools help patients to weigh their treatment options in a thorough, systematic way, taking into account expert opinion, research, personal risks, preferences, and lifestyle issues.

Some health care organizations are finding that interactive video can help patients with tough decisions. Researchers at Duke University Medical Center, for example, discovered that an interactive video program helped patients with ischemic heart disease understand and choose from among three treatment options: medical therapy, angioplasty, and bypass surgery.[35] To help patients make their decisions, the program presents information from a physician narrator, testimonials, and empirically based, patient-specific outcome estimates of short-term complications and long-term survival. Patients who participated in the study said the video program was more helpful than all other decision aids, except for discussions with their physicians. They also expressed increased confidence in their treatment choice.

Comparable programs for men trying to decide whether or not to have surgery for benign prostate hyperplasia—a noncancerous enlargement of the prostate gland—have produced similar results.[36] In fact, a study of the prostate decision-making program conducted at Group Health Cooperative of Puget Sound and Kaiser Permanente of Colorado resulted in a 40 percent drop in surgery rates because fewer patients chose the elective surgery.[37]

In addition to videos on ischemic heart disease and prostate cancer, the Foundation for Informed Medical Decision Making at Dartmouth Medical School offers videos on breast cancer, hormone replacement therapy, benign uterine conditions, low back pain, hypertension, and advance directives.[38]

Researchers from the University of Wisconsin have also done landmark work in the areas of computerized patient decision making with the development of their Comprehensive Health Enhancement Support System (CHESS). Designed to help people facing health-related crises or concerns, CHESS combines decision-making software with information, referrals to providers, and social support. CHESS was originally a DOS-based product, but portions of the system are now being reprogrammed for the Web.[39] The University of Wisconsin licenses CHESS to health care providers, patient advocacy groups, and employers. Modules on breast cancer, human immunodeficiency virus (HIV)/acquired immune deficiency syndrome (AIDS), and caregiving for Alzheimer's disease went on line in mid-1998. An on-line module for heart disease, which includes tailored interventions for changing risky behaviors, launched in 1999.

CHESS helps patients make specific decisions—such as whether to have surgery for breast cancer and what type of surgery to have—by presenting insights from experts and brief personal stories from people who chose that option. Patients also can read criteria that other patients used to make their choices, and they can see what research has revealed regarding each option. In addition, CHESS helps users set action plans related to their options. It also solicits data from the patient on quality-of-life issues every seven days and, based on concerns that may surface in this assessment, CHESS refers the patient to specific content in a program. In the near future, these types of programs will not only support the decision-making process but will then connect patients to providers, products, and services.

CHESS has been well accepted by patients. A 1992 study of the breast cancer module, for example, revealed that it made participants feel empowered, supported, and understood.[40] When given the choice, 88 percent said they preferred CHESS over a cancer-care counselor because of CHESS's anonymity, its availability at any time, and the patient's ability to continue at her own pace and talk with many others through the system's support group. Another study revealed that the breast cancer module was just as appealing to women in an underserved, impoverished neighborhood as it was to women from middle and upper socioeconomic classes.[41]

An important aspect of CHESS's success is its ability to give people a greater sense of control over their health. This sense of control comes not only from the information and support the product provides, but also from the encouragement it gives patients to take action on their own behalf. Many on-line Web sites now provide highly accurate, thorough, and accessible libraries of consumer health information that are easy to find; the Mayo Clinic's Mayo Health Oasis (www.mayohealth.org) and Johns Hopkins' supported Intelihealth (www.intelihealth.com) are two such examples. But people need more than information to take action, especially when it comes to lifestyle-related behavior-change issues. Consequently, a growing number of organizations are developing e-care on-line interventions to help people move beyond awareness-building or contemplation into taking the concrete steps needed for health improvement. One solution may be to help people create their own personalized e-care pages on the Web, where they can go to plan and track their progress at behavior change. Organizations such as WellMed.com are building tools specifically for this purpose (Figure 6–10). When they use these tools, people move through a process of

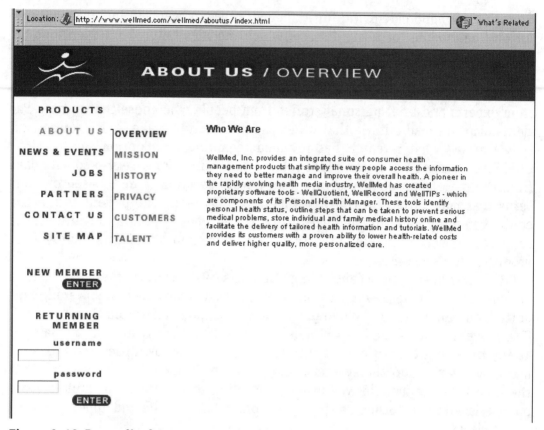

Figure 6–10 Personalized Assessment and Health Information Tool. *Source:* Reprinted with permission from www.wellmed.com, © 1999, WellMed, Inc.

self-discovery, learning what methods "work for me" and making health choices based on personal knowledge.

8. BETTER SOCIAL SUPPORT THROUGH E-COMMUNITIES

Disease management professionals have long recognized the value of support groups in helping patients to prevent and manage illness. It has been demonstrated, for example, that social support helps people in health crises feel a greater sense of control in their lives,[42] which in turn can help them cope with or adjust to health problems.[43] In addition, strong social support can reduce patients' feelings of anxiety and hopelessness.[44]

Today, as the health care industry becomes increasingly aware of the importance personal behaviors play in prevention and management of disease, social support takes on additional significance. Health care professionals are recognizing that physicians cannot do as much for their patients as the patients can do for themselves—especially with the help of a supportive community. Research shows that new e-technologies such as real-time call centers,[45] interactive voice response systems,[46] and Web-enabled bulletin boards[47,48] can effectively provide the kinds of social support once available only through group meetings and one-on-one counseling. In fact, e-support groups even offer advantages over traditional support groups. First, they are not limited by members' schedules or geographic location. And second, they allow participants to remain anonymous, which helps many feel freer to disclose more information about themselves.

The number of health-related Web services offering support groups in bulletin board and live-chat formats is increasing. The University of Wisconsin's CHESS programs provide an exceptional example of what can be accomplished in this medium. CHESS support groups differ from most groups on the Web in that access to each group is controlled and limited to the same 40 people over time. Without a constant infusion of new participants, members have a better opportunity to get to know one another, providing more personalized and in-depth support.

Also, the CHESS groups—like other high-quality health sites, such as Mediconsult (www.mediconsult.com)—are moderated by health professionals who respond to health-related questions and clarify issues from time to time. Many other Web sites are moderated only for inappropriate postings and may not be as much help to patients trying to make sense of complex, conflicting, or inaccurate information.

As the CHESS AIDS/HIV program demonstrated, computerized support groups can help reduce utilization and cost of care.[49] A system offering support and information resources for caretakers of Alzheimer's patients in Cleveland, Ohio, showed similar results.[50] Researchers from Case Western Reserve University who studied the ComputerLink system found that patients whose caretakers had access to it used fewer traditional health and social services than those without access. In fact, researchers reported that the cost of implementing ComputerLink was recovered in the first year of operation. The program cost $84,000—for placing computer terminals and modems in 47 homes, and to pay a nurse to answer caretaker questions. As more and more people buy personal computers, iPhones®, or Web TVs, the future cost efficiency of e-care programs such as ComputerLink might be even greater.

In addition to on-line computer bulletin boards, some organizations are building successful e-care patient support networks with the help of IVR technology. Phone bulletin boards consist of voice mailboxes that are shared by groups of patients. Say, for example, that a member of an expectant mothers' support group has a question about morning sickness. She can initiate a topic title and then share a recorded message with other members on that topic. When another member calls the system, she can choose "morning sickness" from a list of current topics and listen to the first member's question. If she has an answer or a comment, she can leave a message for the first caller and others to hear. The computer will then call the first caller and alert her of this new item, as well as new items on other topics to which she may have contributed. All interactions are confidential and no patient names or phone numbers are provided to the other patients.

Such telephone bulletin boards are viewed by some as a valid alternative for patients who cannot attend support group meetings and do not own a computer. Like computerized and face-to-face support groups, these networks may help reduce utilization. In a Cleveland State University study of 53 drug-abusing pregnant women, for example, those who used a telephone bulletin board reported significantly lower rates of outpatient clinic visits than members of a control group.[51] Lower utilization did not lead to poorer health status or more drug use. Additionally, those who were offered the telephone support group were eight times more likely to accept the invitation to participate than a similar group that was invited to attend face-to-face meetings.

The reach of the e-care support group concept can be extended even further through a concept being explored by The NewSof Group, a division of HealthOnLine and the American Cancer Society (ACS). In this case, participants can use a toll-free number 24 hours a day to access the Cancer Survivors' Network (www.cancersurvivorsnetwork.org; CSN) (Figure 6–11). This IVR and Web-based program includes 14 topical discussions categorized for long-term survivors, newly diagnosed cancer survivors, and caregivers. Listeners hear real cancer survivors telling their stories and providing supportive advice. All the programming is formatted to have the sound and feel (and look on the Web) of talk radio. This structure allows people to feel as though they are part of a conversation, even though they are not actually calling in themselves. Callers also can be connected to the ACS National Cancer Information Center for further information and support. In the ACS system, the overriding mantra is that all information for cancer survivors will come from other cancer survivors. All experts used in each recorded session are themselves cancer survivors.

Participants can access the ACS program via a Touch-Tone telephone or the Web, through the use of a computer audio card. This same content is provided on both channels. With the Web, however, participants can be hot-linked to experts who have participated in the service, as well as other organizations delivering care and support. This ACS e-service also offers the opportunity to be graphical,

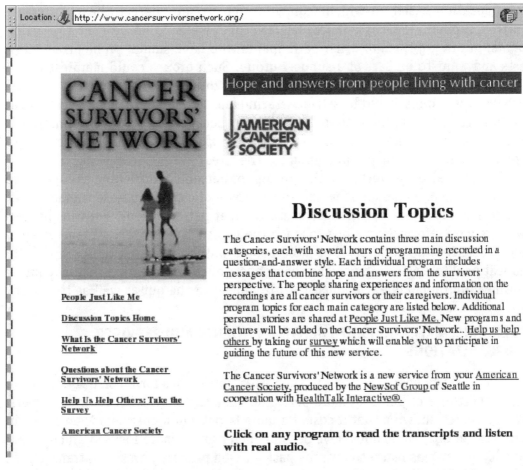

Figure 6–11 The Powerful World of Electronic Support Groups. *Source:* Reprinted by the permission of the American Cancer Society, Inc. All rights reserved.

allowing users to simply click on pictures of people who have a similar demographic or disease background to theirs and be directed specifically toward programming pertinent to them. Rather than surfing the Web site, they are provided with a totally tailored guided tour. In addition, when users choose the Internet version, the overall cost of delivering the program is lower.

It is possible for e-care systems such as the one described above to be integrated with other services. That is because the system not only tracks usage, but also creates a detailed accounting of which segments users found interesting. These IVR/Web data can then be used to generate tailored print materials with customization based on which segments each person chose to hear. To create further support, low-cost, tailored letters or e-mails could be sent to participants, informing them of other participants who have similar problems or interests and want to be part of a support group. Such groups could manifest themselves as computer or telephone-based chat groups or as in-person support groups. The groups would be self-generating and regulated by the participants at no cost to the delivery system. In addition, because all of the information is being carefully tracked, it provides a high level of data, enabling programmers to create fresh, pertinent programming for the site.

The CSN is also committed to the concept of personal storytelling as a means to communicate and change behavior. In the arena of chronic disease management, information is essential but insufficient to meet patient needs. Nor can the network rely on information alone to reach the health care delivery system's desired outcomes. It is no accident that more people watch and listen to Oprah than to educational television. To achieve the richness of communication that is required for meaningful change, we must learn to appeal to the gut as well as the brain.

9. ENHANCED RELATIONSHIPS BETWEEN PATIENTS AND PROVIDER ORGANIZATIONS

Across nearly every industry in the 1990s, businesses have come to recognize the importance of building more permanent relationships with their customers. With research showing that it costs far more to get a new customer than to retain an existing one, companies have become increasingly more focused on customer loyalty.[52] Whereas marketing in the past focused primarily on single transactions emphasizing product features, today it emphasizes real-time customer service, commitment, and contact.

Perhaps nowhere is "relationship marketing" more relevant than in the fields of disease management and health promotion. If one views healthy behavior change as the "product," patients as the "customers," and health care providers as the "sales force," it is clear that closing the sale requires a strong relationship between buyer and seller. Research shows that the effort is worthwhile, however. According to Dr. Dee Edington's research at the University of Michigan's Health Management Research Center, organizations reap significant financial benefits by helping high-risk individuals in their populations move into low-risk categories and by helping low-risk people stay low-risk.[53]

In the past, the ability to influence a patient's health behavior was highly dependent on the quality of the one-on-one relationship between provider and patient. To help a person tackle a difficult problem such as tobacco addiction, for instance, the provider needs to know a great deal about the patient's lifestyle, motivations for smoking, and barriers to quitting. Ideally, there is a strong sense of trust and intimacy between patient and physician, allowing them to get to the heart of the issue and plan a workable strategy for quitting. Because of today's resource constraints, however, physicians rarely have enough time for this kind of relationship building. That is where new e-care technologies can be useful. Organizations can use computers to "talk" to patients and to gather and store bits of information about their risks, lifestyles, and psychodemographic characteristics. They can then use this information to create personally tailored responses. Such "virtual e-care relationships" don't replace the patient–provider relationship; they enhance it. Providers can use these new e-technologies to assess problems and make treatment recommendations based on information that is gathered in a thorough, consistent manner. This allows them to better direct their patients' care and to provide interventions that are highly relevant to each patient's situation and lifestyle.

A familiar example of how this relationship building works in other industries is the Amazon.com on-line bookstore. When you buy books from Amazon, the company's computer keeps track of your purchases. Then it automatically compares your purchases to the purchases of others who have bought the same books you bought, and recommends books you might like to read next. In effect, it is like walking into your favorite bookstore, where the clerk knows you so well that he can intuit what you would like to read. In the case of Amazon, however, the recommendations are not based on intuition. They are based on concrete information about your buying behavior and the buying behavior of others like you.

Creating this type of individualized profile of each patient, based on information supplied by that patient, is the idea behind health-related IVR and Web-enabled e-care tools. One new system, for example, allows providers to communicate with patients via recorded, tailored messages that address common patient concerns.[54] And because it is possible for the program to gather information about the patient's stage of change, health beliefs, learning style, and so on, the provider's message can be automatically tailored to address the patient's problem in a personally relevant way.

To prevent the message from sounding too automated, a provider can provide a personalized introduction, and all the information is given in the voice of the provider that consumer has always dealt with in the past. For example, a health educator might begin, "Hi, Jane. This is Mary from Dr. Smith's office. I got the information you sent in over the phone yesterday. It sounds as though you're doing well, but you could be a bit more consistent about your medication." From this point on, the patient hears Mary offer helpful tips for remembering to take pills on time—tips Mary recorded earlier and stored in a voice bank for use by all her patients. After the tips, Mary may conclude with a patient-specific comment such as, "We'll see you at the clinic for your appointment on the 25th." In this way she is able to create a 5-to-10-minute personalized message for her patient, while actually spending only two minutes creating a new message and adding messages from her personal voice bank. This allows Mary to handle far more patients while still maintaining a personal connection and impact with each patient in her assigned population.

In the future, as more powerful artificial intelligence systems are developed, computers will be able to generate the appropriate responses for the vast majority of cases without Mary's spending any time on the "call." At the same time, the computers will flag specific cases that indicate the need for highly personalized real-time intervention, allowing Mary to focus on patients where her time will create the greatest value.

This is not to imply, however, that patients don't feel a sense of relationship with computerized tools. In fact, research from Stanford University's Center for the Study of Language and Information reveals that people relate to computers and new communication technologies in ways that are astonishingly similar to the way they interact with other human beings. For example, people are usually quite polite to computers, say Stanford professors Byron Reeves and Paul Edwards in their book *The Media Equation*.[55] The two describe an experiment in which subjects were asked to evaluate a computer's performance on a particular task. Half the participants responded to the evaluation on the same computer that performed the task; the other half were moved to a second computer and asked to evaluate the computer they had just left.

The result? Those who moved to the second computer were less positive than those who stuck with the computer they were evaluating. In other words, participants felt freer to criticize the computer they worked with when they could do so behind the computer's back. Sound familiar?

At the same time, Reeves and Nass point to research that shows people are often more willing to share sensitive information about themselves with computers than with human interviewers.[56] This is consistent with findings we refer to in Point #5—that patients using IVR-based interventions for alcoholism and mental disorders were often more willing to disclose sensitive information with an automated system than with a live provider. Such findings lead us to believe that new e-care technologies help patients share richer, more accurate information with their providers, which can result in better quality of care. All of this presumes, of course, that patients know how and why sensitive information will be used. They must also be assured that information will be kept confidential and secure.

10. INTERVENTIONS USE ENTERTAINMENT AND EMOTIONAL CONNECTION TO INSPIRE BEHAVIOR CHANGE

To understand how the media affect health behavior, watch a morning of children's network television shows or thumb through the pages of *People* magazine. The television ads bombard children with loud, colorful, exciting images of happy kids eating sugary cereals and high-fat snacks. The magazine ads show sexy, sophisticated, healthy-looking people smoking cigarettes and drinking alcohol. And although examples are rare, the mainstream media sometimes influence people to adopt healthy behaviors as well. Witness the cattle industry's claim that beef sales plunged after talk show host Oprah Winfrey expressed her fears about the safety of eating beef. If the cattlemen's claims were true, perhaps Oprah's one brief but widely televised comment did more to change America's eating habits than millions of dietitians' pamphlets ever could.

The difference between Oprah and traditional health education pamphlets is clear. Unlike most pamphlets, Oprah seems entertaining, trustworthy, and relevant to her viewers. She interacts with her audience. She is one of them. They do not have to read anything to get her message. And every afternoon, she is in their living rooms—the very environment where they eat, exercise (or not), pay their bills, and experience their lives. Oprah is part of their daily lives. The CSN is built on this same premise, creating a comfortable yet emotionally charged environment in which people can learn and share very personal information and stories.

Such are the promises of many of the new technologies available for disease management and prevention. With segmentation and tailored messaging, health organizations can make sure their messages are relevant. With real-time call centers, IVR, and the Internet, they can deliver interactive messages anywhere, anytime. And with the expansion and convergence of telephones, television, and the Web, they will be able to use the power of multimedia to entertain as well as inform.

The University of Michigan's Dr. Victor Strecher is using many of these concepts in an innovative pilot program to bring preventive health messages to underserved populations. The Michigan Interactive Health Kiosk Demonstration Program is setting up 100 sites in stores, shopping malls, and worksites located in highly populated, disadvantaged areas of the state.[57] With touch-screen monitors, users can choose from five health modules: smoking cessation, prostate cancer, breast cancer, immunizations, and bicycle helmets. Adolescent drinking, adult drinking, sexually transmitted diseases, cardiovascular risk reduction, and cancer risk reduction will be added in the next year.

The modules include audio, animated video, and text. The idea is to make interactive health programming easily available to people who do not normally have access to it. But the program will work only if it can capture and hold the attention of its target audiences. That is why a spot for children on skin cancer risk reduction, for example, features a cartoon character with his skin melting off into a disgusting blob. Though unappealing to most adults, the scene is highly entertaining to the average eight-year-old, the age group for which the spot is intended.

New e-care technologies are also useful in expanding beyond our traditional ideas of behavior–change intervention. User research from the NewSof Group, for example, has revealed that people typically approach behavior change in three different ways: planning, tracking, and storytelling.[58] Planners change by looking forward, setting goals, making plans, and following those plans until they achieve their goals. Trackers change by keeping records of their behavior and then looking back and analyzing patterns. They then adjust their behavior based on what they learn from that retrospective reflection. Storytellers neither plan nor track. Instead, they find the inspiration and strength to change after sharing anecdotes and testimonials with others.

The NewSof Group is developing an assessment to determine which of these three categories best describes individual patients. They believe that classic behavior-modification techniques—which include goal setting, tracking, and rewards for progress—can work well for the planners and trackers. But storytellers may benefit from new and different kinds of intervention that allow them to share their own stories and listen to the stories of others. Patients are encouraged to share their experiences on Internet bulletin boards. Phone counselors urge storytellers to see movies, watch television programs, or listen to tapes with narratives related to themes of behavior change. High-quality entertainment can arouse emotions, causing people to see their behaviors in new ways. Storytellers may also be able to participate in interactive health "talk shows" available via telephone IVR systems and Internet "real audio," much like the CSN, described earlier. They are encouraged to read about people just like themselves in tailored newsletters and Web pages. In this way, they can harness the emotional power that music, video, and personally relevant storytelling have to inspire and transform.

CONCLUSION—THE E-CARE FUTURE

The e-care future of the next generation of disease management and prevention is exciting, and new technologies can launch health care providers and organizations into a complete transformation of the way care is currently delivered.

As you lead your health care organization down this path, use the following action steps on the journey.

1. *Resist going after technology just for technology's sake.* As those in the field of disease management and prevention continue to develop and use new technologies, desired outcomes for patients and organizations must be kept in mind. Today's technologies allow the design and creation of amazing efficiencies. Instead of being dazzled by glitz and glamour, select systems and tools that strengthen your relationships with e-customers—and that are easy for providers and patients to use.

2. *Remember that one size does not fit all.* When you are creating supported self-care and disease management interventions, remember that no one modality of communication and intervention is the correct approach. Different people have different needs, and you must account for all of them.

3. *Look for ways to integrate e-care technologies.* With the continuing expansion of communication bandwidth into the home, there will be opportunities for patients to start an intervention on the Net and, in the course of the session, be connected to a live clinician, who can be reached for a two-way video meeting through the click of a button.

4. *Rally the physician troops.* If you want to change the entire care delivery system, you must show physicians the potential of new technologies and how they can enhance their status and practices.

5. *Develop a new mantra: "from knowledge to action."* Health information is insufficient to change consumer behavior. Focus all interventions on helping the consumer take action, whether that be changing a personal health behavior, purchasing appropriate care products, or scheduling appointments when they are needed.

6. *Start with the human, not the risk or the disease.* To effectively reach consumers and patients, and to fundamentally change their behavior, health care professionals must learn about them—beyond the traditional medical and risk information collected today. Frankly, knowing patients' hobbies may be more important in helping them manage their diabetes than knowing their most recent blood sugar levels.

7. *Invest in systems that capture information.* In order to build personal relationships with consumers and patients, specific information is needed. To prepare for future adaptation and innovation of products and e-services, collect data about consumers. Doing so will allow your organization to constantly learn from doctor–patient interactions, and to adapt its systems and e-tools accordingly.

Whether we accept it or not, we are in a new age of health care that is racing to keep up with the e-worlds of commerce, communities, and care. We have to open our minds to new approaches to disease management, be sensitive to the power of communication, and strive for new models of e-care support. This chapter has only touched on the great strides and advances that are transforming health care into a new era of customized care. These are truly exciting times for those who are ready to embrace new capabilities and new paradigms while making exponential improvements in how we support and empower better health and medical e-care.

REFERENCES

1. D. Van Brunt, "Internet-Based Patient Information Systems: What Are They, Why Are They Here, How Will They Be Used, and Will They Work?" *Managed Care Quarterly* 6, no. 1 (1998): 16–22.

2. R.W. Amler and D.L. Eddings, "Cross-Sectional Analysis: Precursors of Premature Death in the United States," in *Closing the Gap: The Burden of Unnecessary Illness,* eds. R.W. Amler and H.B. Dull (New York City: Oxford University Press, 1987), 181–187.

3. D. Edington and L. Tze-ching Yen, "The Financial Impact of Changes in Personal Health Practices," *Journal of Environmental Medicine* 39, no. 11 (1997): 1037–1046.

4. "Data Source Profile: The MEDSTAT Group Is a Market Leader in Health Care Databases," *Health Care Strategic Management* 14, no. 2 (1996): 14.

5. "Products and Services," The MEDSTAT Group Web site (www.medstat.com), accessed March 1998.

6. Interview with Virtual Integrated Health Management Systems officials at UniHealth, March 1998.

7. J.O. Prochaska and C. DiClemente, "Stages and Processes of Self-Change of Smoking: Toward an Integrative Model of Change," *Journal of Consulting and Clinical Psychology* 51 (1983): 390–395.

8. J.O. Prochaska et al., "Standardized, Individualized, Interactive, and Personalized Self-Help Programs for Smoking Cessation," *Health Psychology* 12 (1993): 399–405.

9. V.J. Strecher et al., "The Effects of Computer Tailored Smoking Cessation Messages in Family Practice Settings," *Journal of Family Practice* 39, no. 3 (1994): 262–270.

10. C. Skinner et al., "Physicians' Recommendations for Mammography: Do Tailored Messages Make a Difference?" *American Journal of Public Health* 84, no. 1 (1994): 43–49.

11. J. Brug et al., "The Impact of a Computer Tailored Nutrition Intervention," *Preventive Medicine* 25 (1996): 236–242.

12. A. King et al., "Increasing Exercise among Blue Collar Employees: The Tailoring of Worksite Programs To Meet Specific Needs," *Preventive Medicine* 17 (1988): 357–365.

13. Strecher et al., *Journal of Family Practice,* 262–270.

14. M. Kreuter et al., "Using Computer-Tailored Calendars To Promote Childhood Immunization," *Public Health Reports* 3 (1996): 176–178.

15. Strecher et al., *Journal of Family Practice,* 262–270.

16. B.H. Marcus et al., "Evaluation of Motivationally Tailored vs. Standard Self-Help Physical Activity Interventions at the Workplace," *American Journal of Health Promotion* 12, no. 4 (1998): 246–253.

17. Interview with David Bulger, Micromass, April 1998.

18. J. Schwartz, *Clinics in Chest Medicine* 12 (1991): 4.

19. J. Cromwell et al., "Cost-Effectiveness of the Clinical Practice Recommendations in the AHCPR Guideline for Smoking Cessation," *Journal of the American Medical Association* 278 (1997): 1759–1766.

20. S.J. Ceci et al., "Don't Forget To Take the Cupcakes out of the Oven: Strategic Time-Monitoring, Prospective Memory and Context," *Child Development* 56 (1985): 175–190.

21. S.J. Ceci, *On Intelligence...More or Less: A Bioecological Treatise on Intellectual Development* (Englewood Cliffs, NJ: Prentice Hall, 1990).

22. I. Lazarus, "Medical Call Centers: An Effective Demand Management Strategy for Providers and Plans," *Managed Health Care* 5, no. 10 (1995): 56–59.

23. J. Connolly, "More Managed Care Plans Add Nurse Phone Lines," *National Underwriter*, 29 April 1996.

24. C. Orleans et al., "Self-Help Quit Smoking Interventions: Effects of Self-Help Materials, Social Support Instructions, and Telephone Counseling," *Journal of Consulting and Clinical Psychology* 59, no. 3 (1991): 439–448.

25. N. McAfee and N. Sofian, "Smoking Cessation at GTE Northwest," *Wellness in the Workplace*, 1988.

26. HealthTalk Interactive Web site (www.htinet.com), accessed April 1998.

27. R.H. Friedman et al., "A Telecommunications System for Monitoring and Counseling Patients with Hypertension: Impact on Medication Adherence and Blood Pressure Control," *American Journal of Hypertension* 9 (1996): 285–292.

28. K.A. Kobak et al., "A Computer-Administered Telephone Interview To Identify Mental Disorders," *Journal of the American Medical Association* 278, no. 11 (1997): 905–910.

29. J.S. Searles et al., "Self-Report of Drinking Using Touch-Tone Telephone: Extending the Limits of Reliable Daily Contact," *Journal of Studies on Alcohol* 56, no. 4 (1995): 375–382.

30. Friedman et al., *American Journal of Hypertension,* 285–292.

31. Kobak et al., *Journal of the American Medical Association,* 905–910.

32. S. Krishna et al., "Clinical Trials of Interactive Computerized Patient Education: Implications for Family Practice, *Journal of Family Practice* 45, no. 1 (1997): 25–33.

33. M.A. Cross, "Disney's City of the Future," *Health Data Management*, October 1997.

34. R. Herzlinger, *Market-Driven Health Care: Who Wins, Who Loses in the Transformation of America's Largest Service Industry* (Reading, MA: Addison-Wesley Publishing Co., 1997).

35. L. Liao et al., "Impact of an Interactive Video on Decision Making of Patients with Ischemic Heart Disease," *Journal of General Internal Medicine* 11, no. 6 (1996): 373–376.

36. M.J. Barry et al., "Patient Reactions to a Program Designed To Facilitate Patient Participation in Treatment Decisions for Benign Prostatic Hyperplasia," *Medical Care* 33, no. 8 (1995): 771–782.

37. *Consumer Health Infomatics: Emerging Issues,* a report to the chairman, Subcommittee on Human Resources and Intergovernmental Relations, House Committee on Government Reform and Oversight, (United States General Accounting Office, 1996), 12.

38. Foundation for Informed Medical Decision Making Web site, www.dartmouth.edu/dms/cecs/fimdm/index.html, accessed April 1998.

39. Interview with Eric Boberg, Center for Health Systems Research and Analysis, University of Wisconsin, April 1, 1998.

40. J.O. Taylor et al., "The Comprehensive Health Enhancement Support System," *Quality Management in Health Care* 2, no. 4 (1994): 36–43.

41. F.M. McTavish et al., "CHESS: An Interactive Computer System for Women with Breast Cancer Piloted with an Under-Served Population," *Journal of Ambulatory Care Management* (1995): 35–41.

42. N. Krause, "Understanding the Stress Process: Linking Social Support with Locus of Control Beliefs," *Journal of Gerontology* 42, no. 6 (1987): 589–593.

43. S.E. Taylor et al., "Attributions, Beliefs about Control, and Adjustment to Breast Cancer," *Journal of Personality and Social Psychology* 46, no. 3 (1984): 489–502.

44. J.A. DiPasquale, "The Psychological Effects of Support Groups on Individuals Infected by the AIDS Virus," *Cancer Nursing* 13, no. 5 (1990): 278–285.

45. C.T. Orleans et al., *Journal of Consulting and Clinical Psychology*, 439–448.

46. F. Alemi and M. Mosavel, "Telephone Bulletin Boards Reduce Clinic Utilization," *Wellness and Prevention Sourcebook* (1998), 306–314.

47. J.O. Taylor et al., *Quality Management in Health Care*, 36–43.

48. S. Krishna et al., *Journal of Family Practice*, 25–33.

49. J.A. DiPasquale, *Cancer Nursing*, 278–85.

50. F.C. Payton et al., "Cost Justification of a Community Health Information Network: The Computer Link for Alzheimer's Disease Caregivers," Nineteenth Annual Symposium on Computer Applications in Medical Care, New Orleans, LA, November, 1995.

51. F. Alemi and M. Mosavel, *Wellness and Prevention Sourcebook,* 306–314.

52. M. Christopher et al., *Relationship Marketing: Bringing Quality, Customer Service and Marketing Together* (Oxford, England: Butterworth-Heinemann, 1991).

53. D. Edington et al., "The Financial Impact of Changes in Personal Health Practices," *Journal of Environmental Medicine* 39, no. 11 (1997): 1037–1046.

54. Lexant Corporation internal research, 1997.

55. B. Reeves and C. Nass, *The Media Equation: How People Treat Computers, Television, and New People Like Real People and Places* (Cambridge University Press, 1996), 23–25.

56. B. Reeves and C. Nass, *The Media Equation,* 21.

57. Interview with Amy Parlove, project lead, Michigan Interactive Health Kiosk Demonstration Project, University of Michigan, April 10, 1998.

58. Lexant Corporation internal research, 1997.

CHAPTER 7

Telemedicine Becomes a Reality with Web-Enabled Applications and Net Devices

Richard L. Nevins and Ronald J. Pion

FOR YEARS, patients and physicians have sought solutions for several dilemmas in the health care delivery system:

- How can patients in underserved areas, both rural and urban, access primary care and specialty physicians, as well as other health care professionals, when none are available in their immediate area?
- How can medication and treatment compliance be improved for reduction of disease, risk factors, and management of chronically ill patients?
- Are there ways other than a visit to the physician's office or the emergency department for patients to receive health information, education, and decision support regarding care?
- Can homebound patients—such as chronically ill, disabled, and hospice patients—be monitored and treated in ways that do not require as many visits to the physician's office, thereby improving convenience and reducing costs?

Until now, there have not been feasible and cost-effective solutions to these kinds of problems. But with the advent of the World Wide Web, Web-enabled applications, and advances in telecommunications technology, a solution now exists: telemedicine exists in the home or anywhere.

This chapter outlines some of the areas in which telemedicine can be effectively used to reduce the cost of health care and improve the quality of that care, while making care delivery more convenient for both the patient and the provider.

DEFINING TELEMEDICINE

Health care by telemedicine includes any interaction between a patient and a provider—or other source of advice, information, and treatment—that is not face-to-face and that can be delivered over the telephone, the Internet, or wireless technology. In its broadest sense, telemedicine incorporates audio, data, image, and video technologies to enhance health care–related activities. Telemedicine merges computers, teleconferencing equipment, interactive television, interactive telephones, pagers, and the Web for the delivery of e-care services.

The range of telemedicine services varies from on-line appointments to remote surgical procedures directed by a surgeon to a nonsurgeon via telecommunications technologies. Assessment of patient problems, establishing and confirming diagnoses, physician-to-physician consultation, patient-to-provider consultation, data transfer, transmission of X-rays, and interactive education and training are all examples of telemedicine applications in health care delivery.

Telemedicine began with the introduction of the telephone. For many years, health care providers have given advice, health education, and information to patients over the telephone. Then two pioneers emerged. Dr. Albert Jutras began teleradiology and Dr. Cecil Watson, a psychiatrist, began treating his patients through interactive video in the late 1950s.

It was in the late 1980s and early 1990s, however, when digital technologies were developed that could support image, data, and video telemedicine. The systems initially were used almost exclusively for physician-to-physician consultations, because the interfaces and screen displays were inadequate for clinical evaluation, which made them awkward for direct patient care delivery from the provider. Video-conferencing equipment was the most commonly used tool. This equipment was cumbersome, difficult to use, and extremely expensive. In the early stages of its development, the telemedicine consultation, as described above, involved upwards of $150,000 worth of equipment on each end of the link, and required physician availability on each end as well. The cost could be as much as $1,600 per consultation. Most of the telemedicine systems and programs were funded by research grants or sponsored through government programs.

But that was then, and this is now. It is important to understand that "doing telemedicine" today does not necessarily require expensive conferencing equipment. The equipment can be as simple as two personal computers (PCs), each with a particular Web application, software, and a video camera. And video-conferencing systems have become less expensive. In one Colorado rural health network, for instance, a system that cost $65,000 in 1995 was replaced in 1999 by a more compact system that performs the same functions for $11,000.[1]

Telemedicine has continued to expand, with a variety of applications, as better bandwidth technologies have developed. Added to that, the Internet has evolved as a common platform with many more functional tools and devices that can be used for patient care, all at a much lower cost than other telemedicine systems. And, as compression technology has improved, image transmission and storage capabilities have expanded, which has facilitated the development of teleradiology and picture archiving and communication systems.

For a number of reasons, telemedicine programs are increasing in number and functionality. A 1998 survey by the Association of Telemedicine Service Providers and *Telemedicine Today* magazine found 139 interactive telemedicine programs nationwide in 1998, up from only 9 in 1993. The number of estimated teleconsultations was 40,000 in 1998, an increase from only 1,715 in 1993.[2]

Increased access to broad bandwidth is making telemedicine and digital medical networks for the home and worksite realistic and viable options that did not exist just a few years ago. Physicians are seeing the benefits the Internet can bring to their practices. In 1999, 85 percent of physicians surveyed used the Internet—an 875 percent jump since 1997. More than 63 percent use e-mail daily and 33 percent have used e-mail to communicate with patients.[3]

Patient and physician acceptance of e-care technology as a reliable means of care delivery is a dynamic that is driving the expansion of telemedicine services. Certainly, the use of computers and the Internet is increasing exponentially, and many surveys have shown that patients are increasingly turning to the Internet for health care information and decision making support. It is completely conceivable that patients' first stop for solutions to health care needs may, in the not too distant future, become an e-care telemedicine application. We believe that widespread accessibility of broadband cable and the assimilation of Net devices—such as interactive television and iPhones® (www.MDtel.com), personal digital assistants, and other Web-enabled e-service applications—will be the catalyst for integrating telemedicine as a health care system and taking telemedicine into the home. Telemedicine will facilitate in-home monitoring, and cyber visits will become increasingly more common. It will not be only tertiary care centers that have telemedicine programs in place but also homes, long-term care facilities, physicians' offices, worksites, mall kiosks, and home health agencies. Imagine a video cell phone—technology that already exists—as a telemedicine application for e-care delivery.

The new generation of telemedicine also brings "space age" technology into the fold. At the high-tech end of telemedicine are products such as HANC (Home Assisted Nursing Care), a robot that acts as a live-in nurse. HANC collects blood pressure, electrocardiogram, pulse, and temperature information, then transmits it back over the telephone line to a central nursing station. Nurses there monitor the patient's condition and intervene when the data show that the patient needs to schedule an appointment or increase his or her medication.

And who says high tech cannot be high touch? The developer of HANC, HealthTech Services, Inc., uses a bit of humor to aid in patient compliance. HANC reminds patients when it is time to take their medicine by saying, "Excuse me, excuse me," louder and louder until the patient responds. A top-of-the-line HANC costs $12,000, but lower-end models that get good results cost less than $1,000.[4]

Will telemedicine replace physicians? Of course not. There will always be a need for appropriate physician office and emergency department visits, as well as inpatient admissions for intensive care, procedures, and surgery. But many physician–patient interactions—especially those for minor problems, injuries, and disease prevention—can be conducted more efficiently at a patient's home or worksite through e-care.

And these interactions can often result in better outcomes, for several reasons. On the practical side, few people enjoy a visit to a physician. The visit interrupts schedules and consumes time patients could be using for other activities, including work, child care, and other duties at home. People with chronic diseases and physical limitations can be further burdened by the mobility and transportation issues around going to see the physician. Also, going to physicians' offices or emergency departments can produce substantial anxiety in some patients.

On the outcomes and satisfaction side of the equation, patients who are more knowledgeable about their disease or more informed about acute problems have been shown to have better outcomes and satisfaction rates. And physicians treating these patients have higher satisfaction rates and decreased incidence of malpractice issues, because the patients are better informed.

Telemedicine is not limited to patients in rural areas. By eliminating the barriers of time and distance, telemedicine can radically transform health care delivery to busy Americans anywhere. Consumers at all socioeconomic levels can benefit from telemedicine through greater access to providers and specialists, more convenient treatment, and reduced travel time and time away from work. Telemedicine is the future of how physicians and other health care providers will manage care, educate patients, and transfer clinical data electronically—and the Web is the platform that is making telemedicine more easily accessible and cost-effective. Telemedicine will increase convenience, decrease cost, and improve quality of care.

TELEMEDICINE SAVES MONEY AS WELL AS LIVES

What if the cost to treat the patient population you manage—whether your organization is a health plan, employer, hospital, or clinic—could be reduced without sacrificing care or patient satisfaction? What if the volume of clinic visits, hospital admissions, and emergency department visits could be reduced while maintaining or even improving clinical and human outcomes? Each of these is possible using advanced telephonic and Web-enabled technology. Here are some examples of the financial impact of telemedicine on health care costs:

1. *Reduces days per thousand and physician visits for chronically ill patients.* Using telephony to remind patients to take their medication or using a Web-based application to monitor glucose readings are two ways telemedicine keeps chronically ill patients healthier.
2. *Decreases costs of managing patients with chronic disease.* Continuous monitoring and education—which can be automated with telemedicine—reduce costs. Patient Infosystems, a provider of integrated health care, disease management, and Internet services, for example, demonstrated an average savings of $7.83 per patient for every dollar spent on CareSense, the company's asthma management program. The program—which incorporates patient self-reports, medical records, and claims data—resulted in 52 percent fewer urgent physician visits, a 67 percent decrease in visits to the emergency department, and a 36 percent reduction in health care costs compared with patient data from before the study.[5]
3. *Expands service area for providers using telecommunications technologies.* Providers can efficiently and effectively manage more patients at lower cost per unit of care. This is important in fee-for-service, discounted fee-for-service, and capitated environments.
4. *Reduces travel costs to and from medical education seminars.* Physicians and nurses at Example Healthcare, a Denver-based health care organization, saved $18,000 in travel costs in the organization's hospitals around the state by broadcasting medical education seminars via telemedicine.[6]

Despite what payers would like employers and patients to believe, what is happening is managed cost, not managed care. Care is being managed by providers; however, financial constraints are affecting many of the care decisions they make. The only thing that is being measured and managed is cost. No one is carefully tracking what is done for each patient as it relates to patient needs or needs of the injury or disease affecting the patient at that time. What is being tracked is cost, and that is the driving force for care in the reimbursement system today.

Few providers use care guidelines to standardize care delivery and predict outcomes. Likewise, many disparate computer systems and software programs exist among providers. Therefore, it is difficult or impossible at this stage to really understand how a particular treatment or procedure affects the overall cost and quality of care. Simply put, many health plans, health systems, and clinics are not equipped to manage care and manage costs in an appropriate and measurable way.

A telemedicine cyber-revolution can and will provide solutions to these problems. Imagine an Internet server-based, thin client solution that provides both transactional and analytical functions for receiving, transmitting, and managing clinical as well as financial data for patients. Increasingly, health e-care executives and providers are realizing the need to expand information management—one of the core competencies for success in the emerging health care delivery system. The transition to managing disease and promoting wellness using e-care Web applications requires a fundamental shift in e-care delivery strategy and philosophy. It is clearly the wave of the future.

NET DEVICES BEGIN TO MAKE TELEMEDICINE EASIER

As your health care organization considers telemedicine e-care technology investments, it must look beyond just the use of PCs and consider new devices that enhance the marriage of clinical care and technology. A simple example: A diabetic who uses a home glucometer to determine blood glucose levels can now enter these data into a Web-enabled device, allowing a provider on the other end to monitor the patient's condition and contact the patient to give acute care advice or recommendations regarding subacute or chronic follow-up.

There are a variety of new devices that allow easy connectivity to the Internet and, therefore, an improved way for physicians and patients to communicate electronically. These "Net devices" (which are also referred to as information appliances) connect consumers and patients to the Net, but they are not PCs or laptops. Net devices have proliferated into a number of forms and include hand-held computers, two-way pagers, set-top boxes and interactive televisions, interactive smart iPhones®, smart houses and appliances, and car PCs. They are paving the way for the Internet to become an integral part of the way we live—in our work, our play, and our health. How? Net devices can make it possible to access the Internet even when you are mobile. There is no requirement to sit down at a computer and log on for several types of Net devices.

The Net device industry is exploding. Intelliquest found that 3.7 million Internet users access the Net with a hand-held computer, and television set-top boxes (such as WebTV) are used by 3.1 million people. Intelliquest forecasts that the market for Net devices will exceed $2 billion in the year 2000.[7] Companies such as America Online (AOL), Microsoft, and Excite have pursued initiatives to make content universally accessible, regardless of the device or network being used. In 1999, Yahoo! inked a deal with Online Anywhere, a company with technology that allows Internet service providers to rapidly reformat and deliver content to televisions, personal digital assistants, and wireless devices.

Anyone with a Net device will be able to access data from anywhere. For the health care industry, this fact will be a boon to productivity and improved care delivery. But health care's data transmission capabilities will not be maximized until all Net devices can access data. Standardized protocols are necessary. Like the exponential effect of Hypertext Markup Language on the World Wide Web, the widespread acceptance of new standards is essential to fuel the utility and adoption of Net devices. Initiatives such as the Wireless Access Protocol Forum for wireless access device space and the Advanced Television Enhancement Forum for the enhanced television marketplace are developing the future standards for Net devices.[8]

Net devices make it possible for the Internet to be accessed in the car, the kitchen, and the living room. Interactive television such as WebTV allows consumers to access the Web on a television screen. Interactive telephones, such as the iPhone® by InfoGear,® give consumers Internet access via the telephone, from any telephone jack (www.infogear.com®). And just imagine your refrigerator reminding you when the milk hits its due date. Swedish appliance manufacturer Electrolux premiered its Screenfridge at tradeshows in 1999. The device is equipped with a Web camera, touchscreen, bar-code scanner, and Integrated Services Digital Network access. The major Net devices are described in general terms below.

1. *Hand-helds.* Palm-sized devices get high marks for their small size and are excellent choices for users who need notebook-sized keyboards and screens with minimal weight and expense. Because physicians and other health care providers are mobile—going from office to hospital to nursing home—hand-held devices make data access fairly simple.

2. *Web pads.* The legal pad-sized devices are lightweight and wireless and, because of their comparatively large color screen, more usable than hand-helds and smart phones for heavy Web and e-mail activity. Currently, these devices are wireless analog modems, but when they connect to the larger digital wireless infrastructure, they could be the true notebook replacements.

3. *Interactive smart phones.* These are the mobile Net devices with flash—the ones used by James Bond—where you can see data and images. iPhone® by InfoGear® (Figure 7–1) and the WebTouch One Internet screen phone by French manufacturer Alcatel are two popular products. AOL has also released a number of devices that allow consumers to jump on the Net without the use of a PC. AOL partnered with Alcatel for the use of its Le Minitel, which includes a screen and small keyboard.

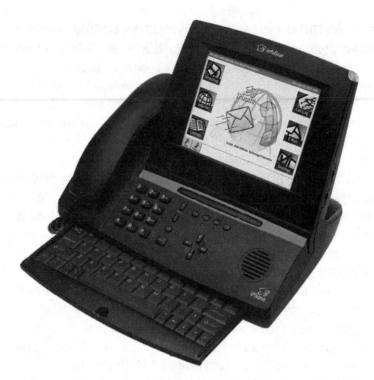

Figure 7–1 The iPhone® Offers On-Line Access Using a Touch-Screen and Small Keyboard. *Source:* Reprinted with permission from InfoGear® Technologies, © 1999.

Analysts believe that smart phones will occupy a significant niche in the Net device market, and this fact offers a huge new advantage to managing care. First, the use of smart phones would utilize a piece of technology equipment that most Americans are completely comfortable with and nearly every American already has. Smart phones are not without their limitations, however. The screen size is limited, which makes them marginal for extended e-mail and Web use, no matter how good the underlying microbrowsers are. And standards must emerge to allow near-universal roaming. Still, smart phones are a nonthreatening way to easily introduce telemedicine technology into the average American home.

4. Net TVs. These come in a variety of forms, but the most well-known is Microsoft's WebTV, which had about 800,000 subscribers as of June 1999.[9] Consumers using WebTV can browse the Web, send e-mail, and chat. The other major Net TV category is set-top boxes. These are not sold in retail outlets; they are installed by cable operators. As 40 million American homes had cable access in 1999, it is assumed that this will be the fastest-growing segment of Net TV in the coming years.[10] An instant hit with TV-focused Americans, interactive television could be the solution to home-based cybervisits, as the physician or other health care provider and the patient can interact while the patient is in the comfort of his or her own home, using a familiar system—the television and the remote control.

5. *Two-way pagers.* These may not be popular as stand-alone devices because paging capabilities will be built into other types of devices. However, the telecommunications connectivity of two-way pagers can be an important component of mobile health care, providing patients with automatic medication and appointment reminders, as well as relaying important clinical information.

The widespread use of Net devices will facilitate implementation of telemedicine by making it easier for both patients and physicians to use Web-enabled e-care technology. Like cellular phone service companies before them, Web-enabled health care device vendors are giving away end-user Net devices to encourage the user into a long-term service relationship. For example, the health care e-commerce site ePhysician plans to give away 10,000 PalmPilots to physicians and other health care professionals to generate future business.[11]

ePhysician has positioned itself to be a fully Web-enabled practice management system for the future (Figure 7–2). Providers connect to the ePhysician site to order lab tests and prescriptions or check their appointments. With the ePhysician software loaded on a PalmPilot, the health provider can make the request, dock the PalmPilot to a PC, and place the order. This process sends the order to ePhysician, which then sends it to laboratories and pharmacies either electronically or via fax. Initially, the ePhysician software worked only with the PalmOS, but subsequent versions work with the wireless Palm VII and Windows CE devices.[12]

Accessing the Internet by means of Net devices is changing the way physicians and health systems deliver services. Allowing patients to be cared for in their own homes, using a device such as a smart phone or interactive television two-way video connection, is the wave of the future. When Net devices are fully embraced by e-consumers, e-patients, and e-physicians, the Web will be an accepted way of delivering health education, information, and care. Cybervisits will become as commonplace as office visits. Elderly patients will be treated in the security and comfort of their own homes, and those with chronic disease can perform their own daily e-checkups—such as testing their blood sugar level or performing a pulmonary function test—and log them in so physicians, nurses, and other providers can monitor and direct care on line.

Helping patients evolve into e-patients includes its own set of issues, however. Understanding the culture, habits, attitudes, and behavior of individuals is the

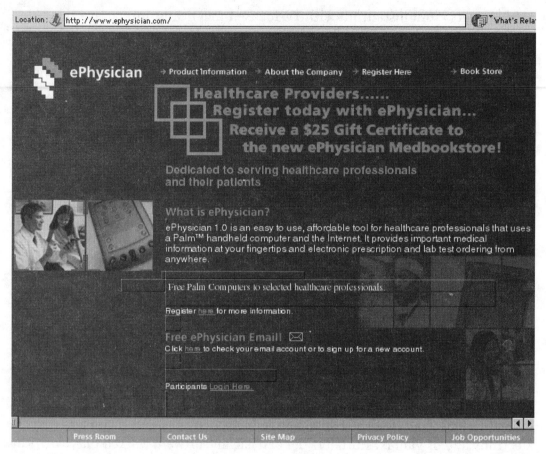

Figure 7–2 ePhysician: A Web-enabled Practice Management System. *Source:* Reprinted with permission from www.ephysician.com, © 1999, e-physician.

key to building a successful e-patient practice. Comfort and familiarity are crucial to ensuring effective use of any new technology. True implementation of telemedicine—especially for the home—involves training patients to communicate through technologies. It is unrealistic to assume that this can happen overnight. Telepartnering between health care providers and patients is perhaps the greatest challenge for telemedicine in the home.

The power of the Internet as a vehicle for building health and medical e-communities and e-care delivery around Net devices cannot be underestimated. In the past, the Web has spawned incredible applications, such as LinkExchange and HotMail, that have become legendary. Services like these captured the imagination of e-consumers, and it is believed that Net devices will too.

E-CARE APPLICATIONS OF SMART PHONES AND NET TV

The two primary Net devices that are most likely to drive the proliferation of telemedicine in the home are smart phones and Net TVs. Described below are the health care applications of each.

Smart Phones

Who would have thought that Alexander Graham Bell's invention in the 1800s would be a primary tool for carrying digital information and delivering e-care? Because of its ease of use and ubiquitousness, the Touch-Tone telephone is a widely used tool for delivering care at home. With modifications of existing equipment, data, images, and video can be transmitted directly over home telephone lines.

The telephone can be used in simple ways with patients. For example, telephone reminders are effective for improving patients' immunization and medication compliance, appointment keeping, and preventive care procedures. Twenty-four-hour access to emergency telephone consultations from home health care providers has reduced emergency department visits and hospitalizations. Ongoing support by telephone has proven valuable in improving patients' emotional status and satisfaction with their care.

Interactive voice response (IVR) systems, a more sophisticated use of the telephone, enable users to receive prerecorded messages, mini-lectures, and reminders; make and change medical appointments; and access answers to questions about common symptoms and specific diseases. IVR systems are just as effective as printed questionnaires in obtaining health information and screening, and are used in telemedicine and by medical call centers to disseminate information and gather data.

The "new" telephone—the smart phone—facilitates telemedicine at new levels. Smart phones use standard telephone lines, plain old telephone system, to transmit voice and data to and from the patient's home. They have touchscreens that allow patients to access the Web, manage their own schedules, and send e-mail. In the telemedicine e-care world, the smart phone is connected to a monitoring site (physician's office, home health agency, etc.), where health care professionals monitor data to facilitate symptom and disease management. Exhibit 7–1 shows some of the many uses for telephone e-care delivery using smart phone technology. Health care providers can monitor patients with chronic diseases, manage utilization of services, and educate consumers using interactive tools and frequently asked questions (FAQs).

Exhibit 7–1 Smart Phones Can Be Used for a Variety of Home Health Telemedicine Functions

Coronary heart disease	Cardiac monitoring Rehabilitation Information support
Diabetes	Glucose monitoring Nutrition and exercise Other self-help services
Cancer	Home infusion therapy Support services
Health promotion, emergencies	Information support
Osteoarthritis, Alzheimer's disease	Patient education
Smoking cessation	Reminders
Medical compliance	Monitoring
Appointment scheduling	Counseling

Sources: Data from E. Balas et al., Electronic Communication with Patients, Evaluation of Distance Medicine Technology, *Journal of the American Medical Association*, Vol. 278, No. 2, pp. 152–159; and R. Pion et al., Trends in Home Health Care: Past, Present, and Future Interviews with the Experts, *Home Care Consultant*, Pilot Issue, p. 21, © 1994.

The smart phone also makes patient education much more effective. For example, a patient educator could call a smart phone meeting with newly diagnosed diabetics to discuss nutrition. In the comfort of their own homes, patients would call in at a specified time, to a specified telephone number. And because technology now allows users to communicate on the telephone and surf the Web simultaneously, the patient educator could help meeting attendees maneuver through a Web site and download recipes and planned menus as part of the learning experience.[13]

Net TV

Net TVs are devices that make being on the Web nearly as easy as turning on the television. Literally, Net TV is a television set that is connected to a broadband, high-speed data line and can bring the wonders of the Web into the American living room.

As increased bandwidth becomes commonplace across the country, the use of Net TVs continues to increase. And advances in WebTV technology are far-reaching. First-generation WebTV did not allow users to watch television and surf the Web simultaneously. Now technology allows both signals to be merged into one medium so they can be accessed together. A news program can download links, pictures, Shockwave movies, and additional video in the background. When the information is displayed on the screen, an information icon appears. A click on this icon shrinks the video screen into a picture-in-a-picture screen and allows users to surf through the additional content that has been downloaded without interrupting their television viewing.

The biggest player in the Net TV marketplace is Microsoft's WebTV. But on-line multimedia giant AOL has also joined the scene. In 1999, AOL announced AOL-TV, a joint venture among the on-line service, Hughes Network Systems, Phillips Electronics, and Network Computer Inc. AOL-TV combines broadcast content and interactive content delivered through Hughes' DirecTV unit. Phillips will build the set-top box, and NCI's operating system and server will provide Internet services.

When this technology is available to large numbers of the population, Net TV will facilitate many cybervisits. If your child has what appears to be a cold, surf over to the local pediatrician's Web channel and check in. Interacting with a physician or nurse on Net TV allows for simple diagnoses such as colds and flu— as well as management of more complicated, chronic medical problems.

TELEMEDICINE FACILITATES SHARED DECISION MAKING

When patients access health information and obtain health education, they become informed participants in their own health care decisions. The supported self-service tools of telemedicine empower patients with knowledge for the decision-making process. This sharing of accountability between providers and patients is a departure from the traditional system, in which accountability has resided primarily with the provider. When patients become more accountable, compliance often increases and outcomes are improved. Patient Care Technologies, for example, is an on-line company that Web-enables homebound patients to participate in their own care (Figure 7–3).

Patient Care Technologies (www.ptct.com) is an example of a point-of-care system (POCS). POCSs are Web applications that enable e-patient recordkeeping from a central e-provider base. A POCS is a digital interface between patients and

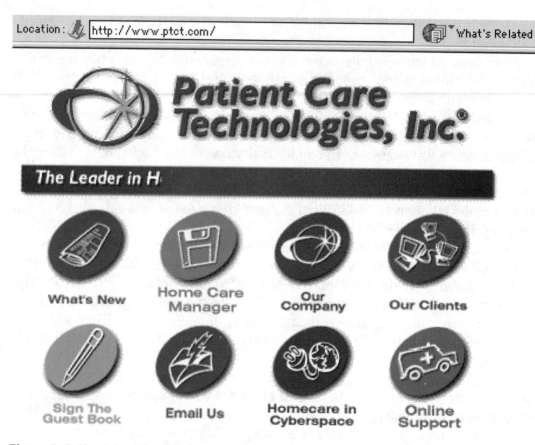

Figure 7–3 Home Care Manager Improves Outcomes and Overall Health of Homebound Patients. *Source:* Reprinted with permission from www.ptct.com, © 1999, Patient Care Technologies.

providers that offers 24-hour access to care. The technology is pushed into the home via the patient's computer or telephone, and is instrumental in monitoring and managing the e-patient's treatment plan, drug therapies, and status. POCSs have been shown to result in a significant decrease in office visits and admissions.

POCSs are rapidly becoming the common denominator of home telemedicine, quality assurance, and cost accounting. They empower providers to partner with patients in cyberspace to deliver and adjust treatments, provide counseling and education, and evaluate care. And because the data are cumulatively tracked— via e-patient input and e-provider monitoring and input—POCSs actually offer an opportunity to analyze the costs and benefits of treating disease. HeartCard is one POCS product that offers this service to patients.

Coronary heart disease is America's number one killer, despite major advances in both prevention and management.[14] The incidence of heart disease death rates reflects an aging population and the need for Americans to make drastic changes in their sedentary lifestyles and high-fat diets. Taking care of these patients is one area where home telemedicine can help.

At the very least, home telemedicine applications for heart patients include condition monitoring, nutrition education, and meal planning. Using HeartCard, patients are monitored on a 24-hour basis from their homes.[14] A device worn by the patient detects potential cardiac events by tracking irregular heartbeats. The patient uses the telephone to transmit these data to a physician for evaluation and recommendations. The payoffs for monitoring cardiac patients this way are obvious: more accurate and expeditious diagnoses, fewer visits to the emergency department or the intensive care unit, and decreased costs.

In addition to interacting with a physician, HeartCard patients can interact with others by participating in a home-based, on-line cardiac recovery program. Having to leave home can be highly problematic for many cardiac patients in rehabilitation. Sharing experiences in an on-line support group results in re-duced anxiety and increased confidence, and often promotes physical activity. The program has resulted in an added benefit: many of these patients become friends.

MANAGING THE WORRIED WELL

According to a General Accounting Office study released in 1996, approxi-mately 55 percent of patients who visit an emergency department do not need to see a physician in an emergency situation. Their questions or problems could be managed on a more elective outpatient basis, either through a traditional office visit or through education. Other studies have shown that over 60 percent of office visits are for health information that could be obtained in a less costly and more convenient venue.

Real-time call centers—a strategy that many health systems put in place in the early and mid-1990s—have evolved to be one of the best tools for handling patient requests for health information, education, and triage. (See Chapter 8 for more information.) Consumers and patients talk with nurses stationed at the central call center (which is usually staffed 24 hours a day, seven days a week) and are asked a series of questions based on clinical protocols that are housed in a demand-management application program. This information moves consumers or patients to some type of decision that typically eliminates the worry they had when they called.

Web-enabled technology and telemedicine can take the concept of a call center one step further by offering customized information to the worried well. Answers to FAQs, audio streaming, video streaming, and ultimately an interactive video window for the e-consumer or e-patient to speak with a nurse are all improvements on the traditional call center model. And, as Exhibit 7–2 shows, the use of telemedicine in this way offers the significant advantage of collecting data for improved outcomes and future decision support.

Home- and worksite-based telemedicine applications can provide the patient with information, education, and decision-support tools, and thus reduce the number of provider visits, which incur both time and dollar cost. Using Net devices or kiosks at worksites will significantly reduce long-term costs: the low cost of implementing technology that will keep consumers healthier outweighs the cost of emergency department visits, hospital admissions, and procedures.

IS THERE A CODE FOR A CYBERVISIT?

Despite the incredible technology advances and the long-term cost savings, there is unfortunately little incentive for physicians or health systems to adopt

---

Exhibit 7–2 Using Telemedicine To Capture Data and Improve Decision Support

Collect data	Using a Health Risk Assessment (HRA), consumers or patients are asked to complete information about their condition.
Provide information	As HRA questions are answered by the consumer or patient, unique, customized data are pushed to the consumer based on his or her responses.
Impart knowledge	Based on the information received, consumers can understand their risk of having a certain condition. Logically, they can ascertain, "I only have 2 of 10 risk factors, therefore my chances of having this condition are slim. I don't have to worry."
Enable wisdom	Electronically captured data from consumers and patients are compiled universally and used in decision support applications. This collection of outcomes data uses the world's wisest information and can create an expert system. In 1999, this database did not exist. With telemedicine, it can.

Courtesy of Ronald J. Pion, MD, 1999, Los Angeles, California.

telemedicine technologies. Reimbursement for teleconsultations has been a key stumbling block for telemedicine. Few, if any, private insurance companies reimburse physicians for telemedicine services. And although home telemedicine has the potential of saving millions of dollars, existing health care benefits, reimbursement, and medical licensure requirements are disincentives to providers of these services.

The Center for Telemedicine Law, a nonprofit foundation in Washington, D.C., was instrumental in educating Congress for the passage of reimbursement for some telemedicine services. Although the reimbursement is limited to select Medicare-approved situations and is only for live video consultations, it is significant for the future of telemedicine. Clearly, store-and-forward functionality needs to be included soon in reimbursement strategies. Although the Health Care Financing Administration (HCFA) does have some progressive leaders, the organization needs support and input from physicians and health care executives regarding the next steps for telemedicine reimbursement.

Medicare still uses a payment mechanism that reimburses when elderly people get sick. The equation needs to change, and that will require out-of-the-box thinking. For example, why not provide beneficiaries with a smart phone or a PC and with Web-enabled software that holds them responsible for managing preventive care? The purchasing power of HCFA could most certainly result in a significant discount from any manufacturer who would like the opportunity to sell millions of units. Connecting Medicare beneficiaries offers the chance to enhance the quality of life through access to knowledge bases, and someday to wisdom bases. Imagine the robust and useful electronic database that could be created.

Instead of struggling to cut costs, HCFA and other payers should adopt a different method of cost reduction: initiating strategies for improved return on investment. HELP Innovations is one company that is creating opportunities such as these. Its Web site (www.helpinnovations.com) offers data that can help providers and plans determine the return on investment for employee home health techniques. What is your organization doing when it comes to e-commerce and e-care?

CHALLENGES TO TELEMEDICINE AND E-CARE IMPLEMENTATION

Although implementation of telemedicine is inevitable, it will most likely occur at a slower pace than other technology initiatives. Several issues that exist in various stages of evolution and resolution have and will negatively affect telemedicine's growth. The American Medical Informatics Association has brought many of these issues to the fore[15]; some of them are described below, along with some potential solutions.

1. *Confidentiality*. Security of medical records and maintenance of confidentiality are prime considerations for health care providers. The instantaneous access from multiple locations, while extremely beneficial to health care delivery networks and to telemedicine applications, increases the risk of breaches of confidentiality and security.

Clearly, the issue of confidentiality has lessened over the past several years. Americans have become much more accustomed to entering their credit card numbers for making purchases, banking, and buying stocks on line. For those who remain concerned, encryption, authorization, keystroke tracking, and auditing can all be used to ensure confidentiality.

Or why not consider paying people for their willingness to provide medical information? Doing so will send the message to consumers that their data are valuable—and may encourage them to supply the basis for a rich and robust database that can go a long way to managing outcomes information.

2. *Responsibility*. It is possible that a number of providers could have input, via telemedicine technologies, to the care of a patient. If physicians and other providers are connected electronically, e-mailing information and attaching critical records, data, images, and video and documents is not only possible, but simple. Within this electronic communications network, the primary care physician can still maintain overall care management, and he or she will have greater access to data than ever before to delegate or manage care decisions.

3. *Licensure and accreditation*. Although electronic data transfer knows no geographical boundaries, licensure, credentialing, and accreditation do. Medical licenses and nursing licenses are issued by each state, monitored and disciplined by the state, and maintained by the state if the licensee meets certain requirements. Those licenses permit the practice of medicine or nursing in a given state. Only a handful of states honor the licenses of other states.

Historically, American physicians have been held to the standards of the average physician in the same geographic area. This "locality rule" has been significantly eroded in the past 20 years by the nationalization of medical education, residency training, and continuing medical education. Telemedicine is poised to eliminate it entirely. Sometime in the next few years, we will probably see litigation arise over whether a telemedicine consultant met national standards of accuracy in diagnosis, informed consent, and treatment.[16]

There is a debate among a growing number of organizations—such as the American Association of Ambulatory Care Nurses, the American Medical Association, the Center for Telemedicine Law, the Council of State Boards of Nursing, and others—about whether licensure in one state should convey privileges to practice medicine or nursing in other states. This model would follow that of drivers' licenses, which are issued by the state but allow the licensee to drive in other states. Telemedicine in all of its forms—audio, data, image, and video—will survive or flourish depending on decisions about licensure, accreditation, and credentialing.

4. *Fraud.* How can a patient verify the accuracy and relevance of information received during e-care? The source of the information, and its currency and application, are more difficult to determine in distant patient–physician relationships than in a traditional face-to-face relationship.

A reputable pre-Internet source of advice, information, and education is still reputable on line. We do not see fraud as a big barrier to telemedicine implementation as long as the best-of-breed telemedicine applications—those that are trusted in the industry by physicians and consumers—are used. Information filters can also be created.

5. *Ethics.* How will remote diagnosis and treatment compare in accuracy and relevance to diagnosis and treatment delivered in the traditional face-to-face model? Is the physician–patient relationship measured by the same legal standards in the telemedicine model as it is in the traditional model? How will informed consent, release of information, durable power of health care attorney, and living wills be managed in the cyber-environment?

These questions are relevant to the historical system. Up until now, patients have not played on a level field. Access to information was closely held by physicians and other medical professionals. With the advent of the Internet, however, e-patients have access to information, decision support, and, ultimately, wisdom. Wisdom-based consent, not informed consent, should be the operative term for the future.

6. *Reimbursement.* HCFA has just begun to reimburse for teleconsultations—but only "live," not store-and-forward. Physicians are like other professionals: they are paid for the service they perform, which includes their expertise and advice. Not paying physicians for telemedicine is not an option. The challenge is how to modify the entire reimbursement system to meet the needs of telemedicine services. Creative solutions must be sought.

7. *Access to technology.* A modification of the "access to care" problem is "access to telemedicine technology," which has so far been a major hurdle. Whether it is a solo practitioner who cannot afford the hardware, software, and staff to manage telemedicine in the practice or the inner-city family who cannot afford the electric bill—let alone a PC—cost has been a significant barrier to widespread use of telemedicine.

Thankfully, that is changing—and fast. With the advent of low-cost Net devices, the e-care model we will probably see is that of companies providing the device free and charging a service fee, or simply "paying" for the device via the lowered cost of overall care. Like ePhysician's plan to give away 10,000 Palm Pilots, smart health care organizations and plans could consider giving away smart phones. Give them out to chronically ill and elderly people so they can monitor their own care, have access to on-line support groups, and be empowered to manage their own outcomes.

What is your organization doing to further the implementation of e-care telemedicine initiatives? In what way can empowering your patient population lower overall health care costs and improve outcomes and quality of life? Health care executives and physicians must join together to address these challenges and substantiate the overriding number of positives that result from telemedicine initiatives.

CONCLUSION

We are clearly at the threshold of redefining the way health care is delivered. The marriage of telecommunication technologies with health care can provide many improvements in the cost, quality, and convenience of care delivery. What an opportunity for providers, payers, patients, consumers, and health educators to design and implement significant changes that will benefit all participants in the health care equation!

Today the primary care setting is the physician's office; tomorrow the primary care setting will be the home. With the help of e-care technology, patients will manage much of their own care. The number of times they visit the physician will decrease—and the quality of clinical outcomes will most likely increase, as will patient satisfaction. Consider how connectedness could liberate hospice and nursing home patients from care facilities and return them to their homes. Isolation would no longer be a problem. Touch a screen, see a nurse, talk with a nurse. Request medication refills, interact with other homebound Americans—all of these activities produce an added level of comfort and security, and reduce worry and anxiety.

Not surprisingly, the biggest e-care hurdle is resistance to change. Truly embracing telemedicine requires significant changes in the way physicians practice, the way patients access care, and the way providers are reimbursed. Technology is not perceived positively by everyone. Whether it is an aversion to using an "inhuman" piece of equipment or an aversion to investing in that piece of new equipment, many people are concerned about modifying the "old way" to a way that is as yet uncharted. What will it cost? How much money will it really save? What do patients and physicians have to change about their lifestyles in order to use telemedicine? These are some of the many questions that will be asked in the next several years as Net devices and telemedicine converge.

Here is a set of steps you can take in your health care organization to move the telemedicine ball down the field:

Action Steps for Providers

1. Recommend to your patients a Web site that you approve, one that will provide them with high-quality health information, education, or advice.
2. Create a Web service for your practice or join a channel provided by your hospital or integrated delivery network.
3. Offer an interactive telemedicine option, such as a Net device or WebTV, for patients to communicate with your office.
4. Consider the use of a Net device that enables e-patients to be dismissed from the hospital early; for example, newborns with jaundice or patients whose surgical wounds need to be monitored.
5. Encourage payers and legislators to establish reimbursement for telemedicine and e-care services.

Action Steps for Payers

1. Define populations that have mobility and transportation issues, such as homebound or long-term care facility patients.
2. Install Net devices in one or two locations, and monitor patient and provider satisfaction levels while tracking changes in office and emergency department use resulting from the availability of simple audio/visual technology.
3. Begin to develop reimbursement methodologies for telemedicine services.

Action Step for Health Educators

1. Incorporate the use of telecommunications and Web applications into the clinical curriculum for medical students, interns, and residents.

Action Steps for e-Patients

1. Ask your provider, employer, or health plan to recommend Web services and other telecommunications solutions to make care more convenient and less costly.
2. Encourage payers and legislators to establish reimbursement for telemedicine services.

The future is now. The telemedicine technologies are here and there are only a few barriers in the way of our e-care future.

REFERENCES

1. R. Fillion, "Technology Expands Long-Distance Care," http://www.denverpost.com/enduser/ telemed0405.htm (5 April 1999), accessed 24 May 1999.
2. Fillion, "Technology Expands Long-Distance Care."
3. "Research Shows 42% Growth in Physician Use of the Internet in Last Three Months" (from Healtheon Corporation's Internet Survey of Medicine), *AOLNews@aol.com*, 6 May 1999.
4. E. Nagourney, "Visiting the Doctor, Via the Dining Room," http://www.nytimes.com/library/national/ science/ (6 April 1999), accessed 24 May 1999.
5. "Patient Infosystems Demonstrates Significant Cost Savings and Improved Health Outcomes with CareSense Asthma Disease Management Programs," Patient Infosystems press release, Rochester, New York, 19 November 1998.
6. Fillion, "Technology Expands Long-Distance Care."
7. "More People Online without PCs," http://www.cyberatlas.internet.com/big_picture/demographics/ quest.html (20 April 1999), accessed 22 April 1999.
8. D. Rimer and P. Noglows, "Internet Appliances and Universal Access," http://www.iword.com/iword41/ iword41.html (March 1999), accessed 14 June 1999.
9. "WebTV Networks Launches Next-Generation WebTV Classic and Plus Products; Provides Free Service Upgrade," http://www.webtv.com/company/news/nextgen.html (2 June 1999), accessed 14 June 1999.
10. D. Rimer and P. Noglows, "Internet Appliances and Universal Access."
11. D. Haskin, "Write a Prescription, Get a PalmPilot," http://www.allnetdevices.com (13 May 1999), accessed 14 May 1999.
12. "Products," http://www.ephysician.com (June 1998), accessed 14 June 1999.
13. R. Pion et al., adapted from information in *Home Health Telecommunications* (New York: McGraw-Hill, April 1999).
14. "Warning Signs," http://www.americanheart.org/warning.html (1998), accessed 14 June 1999.
15. M. Gardiner Jones, adapted from information in "Electronic House Calls: 21st Century Options," *Consumer Interest Research Institute* (Washington, DC, June 1995), 21–22.
16. L. Fentiman, "Opinion: Internet Medicine Holds Promise," http://www.newspage.com/cgi-bin/ pnp.GetStory?story=t0611006.5kr&topic=171&date=19990614&inIssue=TRUE&mode=topics (10 June 1999), accessed 14 June 1999.

CHAPTER 8

Real-Time Customer Information and Health Management Centers

Loree Jurgens and Douglas E. Goldstein

Is YOUR HEALTH AND MEDICAL CALL CENTER READY for expansion or ready to discover new ways to manage higher-volume, lower-agent, or higher-touch interaction? Do you need to develop focused and profitable products for your call center? Are you developing an Internet on and off ramp for your organization's Intranet, or building Extranet relationships with business partners? Is your organization or call center considering the use of Web technology to drive self-serve transactions, deliver e-commerce, provide e-care, and develop e-communities?

If you answered "yes" to any of these questions, a real-time customer information and health management center—one that reduces health care costs, enhances revenues, and offers consumers meaningful choice—may be the solution for your health care organization.

Through high-level customer service delivered in a call center and over a monitored and supported Web channel or portal, you can reach a high volume of customers at the lowest possible cost. A health care organization cannot only keep pace with the ongoing demand, it can stay connected to patients and customers. Instead of developing services and then finding customers for them, you can develop your customers and find the service capability to meet their needs.

It is important that you understand what market forces are demanding that you reevaluate—and re-engineer—your health care call center to keep pace with electronic digital technologies. This transformation of health care service delivery is being driven by the need to:

- Consolidate care management business units as new technologies arrive with real-time transaction capabilities.
- Integrate and offer meaningful consumer medical management care delivery.
- Respond to consumer demand for meaningful choice at the moment of a health care need.
- Use the infrastructure to sustain consumer loyalty and brand equity.

This chapter provides information, describes leading-edge health care call center experiences, and takes a look at the call center future as an integrated real-time customer service center—today. The action plan that is proposed will affect your health care organization and providers by:

1. Offering greater ability to combat negative pricing trends for services by lowering high fixed costs by means of lower-cost products and services, and by taking advantage of the declining costs of technology.
2. Re-engineering call center services and resources and using technology that alters the cost efficiencies of mass production via one media channel (the telephone), to delivering mass customization via multiple media channels, including the Web.

In response to the demand for change, many integrated health care delivery networks are rushing to get truly e-connected. Here are some e-facts:

- The digital integration of regional delivery networks was up from 30 percent in 1997 to 46 percent in 1998.[1]
- Technology capital spending was up 6 percent in 1998,[2] which is a significant jump for an industry that is known for spending only 1 percent to 3 percent of revenues on technology.[3]
- And regional delivery networks are getting on line too—the Voluntary Hospital Association reported that 52 percent of hospitals have Web-based platforms, and 30 percent operate Intranet systems.[4]

WHAT EXACTLY IS A REAL-TIME CENTER?

A real-time customer information and health management center—which we will refer to in this chapter as a real-time center—is a sophisticated health care call center that uses Web-enabled technology to bring together high tech and high touch to serve e-patients and e-consumers (Figure 8–1). Other terms for this next generation call centers include multimedia customer relationship management center and integrated customer service center. Real-time centers can improve e-communications, e-communities, and e-care delivery to e-consumers in your markets. By capitalizing on the e-consumer's desire for self-service and your organization's existing call center staff, you can create a real-time center that offers simultaneous cost savings and increased e-patient satisfaction. Real-time centers:

1. Provide needed brand value experiences through highly individualized and transparent consumer or patient call center and on-line interactions. The

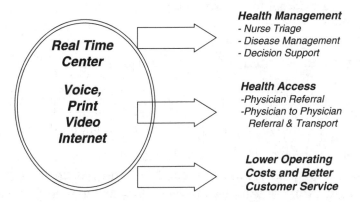

"Real-Time" Customer Service and Health Management Centers

Figure 8–1 A Real-Time Customer Service and Health Management Center. *Source:* Copoyright © 1999, Douglas Goldstein.

interactions typically result in a transfer of information and clinical decision support.

2. Offer e-consumers and e-patients on-line choices of products and services that are endorsed by a health care provider or partner.

3. Increase access to channels of information and service delivery using various media. Your health care organization can keep pace with e-consumer and e-patient demand and active use of other media channels, such as the Web and interactive television.

4. Reduce health care costs and enhance revenues by offering consumers a meaningful choice any place, any time they need health care products or services.

BETTER HEALTH MANAGEMENT THAT FOCUSES ON POPULATION HEALTH

Few people would argue that today's health care delivery system needs improvement. To control costs, the current managed care system restricts access, requires procedure authorizations, and mandates case management. Failings of this system include insufficient chronic care programs, inappropriate uses of health care services, and poor health prevention programs.

In addition to e-consumer demands, the push toward digital integration and the transformation of health care services is being driven by the need to consolidate the care management business using real-time transaction capabilities. Imagine that your system could offer meaningful e-consumer medical management and e-care delivery, and respond to the demand for meaningful choice at the moment a consumer has a health care need. The development of such an integrated system could maintain your organization's brand equity and e-consumer loyalty in a whole new way.

Real-time center technology using Internet tools and multimedia will revolutionize medical management as we know it today. It will also significantly lower the cost of moving data, voice, and images. A real-time center can also offer real-time, longitudinal tracking of health and disease status for organizations that are at financial risk to deliver and care for the total health of a population. Management of utilization, morbidity, perceived consumer needs, patient/enrollee preference, and nonhealth motives (for example, qualifying for sick leave, disability, or workers' compensation benefits) are all possible with a fully integrated real-time center.

The new e-consumer is an e-care participant and partner! These consumers are demanding *choice* and a role in their own care management. Web and telephone technologies are poised to enable this e-consumer; and they will essentially collapse medical management as we know it today.

Forced to be real-time by knowledgeable e-consumers and e-patients, health care organizations that wish to keep the administrative management portion of the premium dollar will see their call center business evolve into real-time centers, where state-of-the-art technology can deliver the health care transactions demanded by e-customers. Demand, disease, and case management will be digitally integrated to achieve population health management. It will also be unbundled for targeted risk intervention products. *Technology is the e-tool that will make this e-care delivery method possible.*

UNDERSTANDING "REAL TIME"

Real time is the space that is created when time, distance, action, and response collapse simultaneously, aided by technology (Figure 8–2). In other words, real time is *right now, where I am, in a way that lets me take action with a click, call, or touch, and responds to me on the basis of additional actions and information that I have provided.* The real-time phenomenon is also known as a *transference* or *virtual* experience. It can occur in an integrated customer information and health management center when technology collapses time, dis-

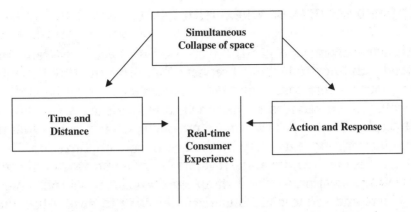

Figure 8–2 Real-Time Consumer Experience. *Source:* Copyright © 1999, Loree Jurgens.

tance, action, and response through the use of calls, videos, kiosks, streaming audio, and Web transactions. This process is described as real-time because users click, call, or touch a screen or button, and receive an immediate response.

One example is the experience of taking a Web-enabled health quiz in which audio and text responses determine the next question the e-consumer receives. The quiz experience is customized based on the answers the e-consumer provides, and additional learning content is pushed to the on-line screen.

Another example is that of the patient who is told by his physician that he needs to undergo open-heart surgery. After he leaves the physician's office, he realizes that in his shock he forgot to ask some important questions, so he calls a cardiac nurse at the real-time center. The nurse answers his questions using a customized set of responses, along with her expertise in the field and her intuitive judgment. Additional custom information is delivered at the pace that is right for this particular patient.

Clinicians call these "teaching moments." They are real-time moments that give clinicians the power to teach when the patient is the most willing to learn. The *time* is the moment you have a question, the *distance* is eliminated by the immediacy of the diagnosis, *action* is needed, and the patient must *respond* to make a difference in the outcome. In an integrated real-time customer information and health management center, these moments happen by the hundreds and thousands through calls, audiotapes, videos, and Web encounters. They can be extremely effective when technology is used to facilitate a real-time response from the patient.

PRODUCTS AND SERVICES OF A REAL-TIME CENTER

Health management and health access services have large categories of customer need fulfilling products and services that drive the three financial models in a real-time center: cost reduction, cost savings, and revenue production. Health management services are designed to reduce the cost of care by controlling utilization by the e-patient and to provide cost savings by lowering the cost of the product or service delivery by the health care organization. Health access services are designed to generate revenue by bringing in new business to the health care organization in the form of service utilization and patient acquisition. Products and services are organized this way to ensure the alignment of product goals and the emphasis of service delivery and staff training.

• HEALTH MANAGEMENT

A twenty-first century integrated real-time information center can provide the tools to ensure the integration of management for both longitudinal care and acute episodic care. The business tools include a combination of clinical decision support tools for the professional and the patient: telephony, telephones, personal computers, faxes, Web technology, e-mail, and an on-line digital medical record. Real-time centers can improve patient satisfaction and lower costs. Some of the primary product lines and an overview of services follow.

Health management services can include health risk identification, primary prevention, self-care support, nurse triage for immediate care (self, physician, emergency department), major medical decision support, disease or condition management, secondary prevention, and communication with patients/enrollees about health management programs.

• RISK ASSESSMENTS

Risk assessments take a given database of a population and its clinical information and, usually by using a Boolean logic, stratify the population into risk groups and assign interventions to manage health status prospectively. The outcome is the intervention before treatment is needed, avoiding unnecessary cost. Adjustments to the clinical management of a given patient can lower overall costs and improve individual outcomes. The following are elements and services of the health status evaluation, risk assessment, and prevention promotion:

1. Health Risk Identification and Planning

- Annual health appraisals
- Health risk assessments and clinical screenings
- On-line referral authorizations
- Personal action plans to support better health and appropriate health care utilization

2. Primary Prevention

- Group health education classes
- One-on-one nurse counseling meetings
- Outbound telephone health information
- Outbound telephone behavior modification support
- Health information materials
- Provider profiling and referral

e-Fact: The market demand for risk identification technology solutions is expected to increase from $20 million to $210 million, an excess of 60 percent over typical annual sales by 2002.[5]

• DEMAND MANAGEMENT

Demand management results in more efficient health care service utilization and improved patient satisfaction and outcomes. Call centers that deploy integrated Web technologies can reduce call center staff by 2.5 nurses or non-nurses for every computer telephony integration (CTI) Internet terminal in the call center.

1. Nurse Triage for Immediate Care (NurseHelp Line)

- 24-hour telephone nurse triage
- After-hours telephone nurse triage
- Provider locator and appointment setting
- Follow-up calls to high-risk patients/enrollees
- Specialty referral

2. Self-Care Support/e-Care Support

- Self-care books
- On-line self-care information

- Video and audio library on health topics
- On-line catalog services

e-Fact: The market for demand management technology solutions is expected to grow 35 percent annually for the next three years, from $200 million today to $900 million by 2002.[6]

- **SECONDARY PREVENTION AND DISEASE MANAGEMENT PROGRAMS**

  Secondary multimedia prevention and disease management programs optimize care for chronic health conditions that integrates health care delivery across all points of access to truly manage the specific disease for a group in a given population over time. Call centers that deploy Web technology to aid in the care management of this population can increase the patient caseload for discrete types of patients from 40 cases to 400 uncomplicated cases.

  ### 1. Secondary Prevention

  - Lifestyle change assessments
  - Outbound telephone behavior modification support
  - On-line registration to programs and classes

  ### 2. Major Medical Decision Support

  - Third-party counseling about medical treatment alternatives
  - Collateral materials to support decisions
  - Associations with nationally recognized centers of excellence

  ### 3. Disease or Condition Management

  - On-line and telephonic disease management products
  - On-line and telephonic prenatal care management programs
  - On-line and telephonic chronic disease management programs (asthma, diabetes, and congestive heart failure)
  - On-line, telephonic, and elder day care programs

  ### 4. Communication with Care Support Patient/Enrollee Populations

  - Collateral pieces to introduce program to target populations
  - Identification card to demonstrate eligibility

e-Fact: **It is expected that the demand for technology solutions that support disease management and case management combined will collectively grow 40 percent annually, to over $800 million by the year 2002 from less than $150 million today.**[7]

• HEALTH ACCESS

Health access means that e-consumers can choose efficiently. Design health access marketing services intentionally with a blend of multimedia channel technologies (Exhibit 8–1). Include physician-to-physician teleconferencing or on-line consultations and referrals, telephone and Web health information, on-line class registration, hospital registration, physician referral and appointment where the consumer can self-serve, and call centers staffed with specialty nurse experts. These nurse experts consult and facilitate a direct referral to a specialty program, physician, transport, and if needed, family hotel accommodations. Automate some of these interventions in the form of push promotions, messaging, literature, health surveys, appointment reminders, and monitoring reminders using real-time consumer and patient data about interests, conditions, survey results, and on-line self-care logs, all with digital media solutions.

Initiating multimedia self-serve technologies allows nursing staff expertise to be directed to clients who represent high economic and long-term-relationship value (such as those in need of a physician referral) and yet leaves "light shoppers" feeling that the real-time center has value. What will leap forward as technology is available is a whole new set of specialty products and services that attract the cost-conscious e-consumer to improve and sustain his or her health status. High-volume, high-self-satisfaction services such as physician referral

---

Exhibit 8–1 Health Access Revenue Services

- Physician referrals
- Emergency department visits
- Classes, seminars
- Urgent care clinic referrals
- Patient retention programs
- Physician-to-physician referral programs
- Specialty programs

Source: Copyright © 1999, Douglas Goldstein.

and appointment, health information, and class registration can be shifted in part to the automated telephone and cyberspace. The following are some additional tips for the successful implementation of health access services.

1. *Offer widespread health access.* Widespread health access means that consumers can choose the information they want and have it delivered when they want, where they want, in the form they want, and by the media channel they want. The real-time space of the call center 24 hours by 7 days, along with the Web, has widened the applicability of information, exceeding the boundaries of paper and direct mail, to the delivery of products and services.

Health care has entered the era of retail, where location, location, and location are the foundation of the consumer-oriented service and marketplace (Exhibit 8–2). Be as strategic about the positioning of your uniform resource locator (URL) as you have been with the organization's 1-800 numbers. Include it in specialty services, senior programs, school-based programs, and even hospital rooms and clinics.

2. *Design opportunities for one-on-one dialogue.* With the proliferation of products and the media vehicles to promote them, the consumer is headed for broadcast message overload. Broadcast messages disseminate the same information to the masses in a "monologue" form. In one-on-one marketing, the monologue approach is replaced with a dialogue-based approach, where the needs of the individual can be a factor in customization. A real-time call center with Web-enabled applications can cultivate a dialogue with consumers by:

- Offering products and services that consumers can test at low risk, providing an experience of health care at your organization.

Exhibit 8–2 Market Opportunities

Market Opportunities...

- Meet consumer needs for access to health information, services, and decision support 24 hours a day
- Reduce inappropriate and unnecessary health care expenditures
- Deliver outstanding customer service
- Differentiate your organization from the competition
- Build brand loyalty with consumers

Source: Copyright © 1999, Douglas Goldstein.

- Connecting them with people who have the same problems via support groups, on-line discussion groups, and monitored chat rooms.
- Taking real-time surveys to cultivate, and capture data about, e-consumer interests.
- Providing high-touch service by individualizing the health information, referrals, and resources at each encounter.
- Offering an option to escalate the call or Web contact to the attention of a "live" professional who will manage the encounter at a higher level, promote access to providers, and provide valuable expertise.
- Providing product and service features that tell the client that you value his or her time.

3. *Provide true high-touch human contact points.* If there is anything to be learned from the banking and telephone industries, it is not to pull all your customer service people overnight. People need time to adjust to the fast-paced Web environment and, frankly, some of them never will. Buying health care is not like buying a soft drink. You give greater consideration to who does your open-heart surgery than to selecting a cola. Removing access to a professional because it is less costly is no excuse for compromising the time given to consumers who need assistance making significant health decisions.

The consumer recognizes that you value his or her time in two ways: (1) when an actual human takes the time to listen and individualize the information or resources and (2) when you do not keep customers on hold forever—allowing them the ability to self-serve if they do not really need to talk with an expert.

4. *Follow through on promises.* Do not make the promotion promise that "all calls are answered on the third ring" if your real-time center cannot deliver. Consumers do not have time to complain, nor do they want to risk the anger of the person who is telling them about the best cardiac surgeon. What the consumer wants is the experience of talking to a person after the third ring. They will not count rings, try to figure out how to complain, or take the time to complain. They just will not call back.

WHY DEVELOP A REAL-TIME CENTER?

There are two primary reasons to develop a real-time center: e-consumers want it, and real-time centers save money in the short and long run. The transformation in the way information and care are e-delivered will have an incredibly "healing" effect on health care organizations. The cost of providing this in a Web-enabled environment is very low. Fewer telephonic and in-person transactions lower costs even further. Using real-time health information and service centers, your system can outperform large vendors and competitors with better, cheaper, faster services and still maintain a personal, consumer-focused feel.

Real-time centers can reduce health care costs, enhance revenues, and offer e-consumers meaningful choice. Through high-level customer service, delivered in a call center and over a monitored and secure Web channel, your health organization can reach volumes of customers at the lowest possible cost. A real-time center allows the health organization to not only keep pace with ongoing consumer demand but also to stay connected to e-patients. If your health care organization would like to accomplish the following goals, a real-time center can be an effective strategy:

• Bring the cost of health care down to the lowest unit cost of care.
• Provide on-line, phone, and multimedia self-serve options to the 60 percent "worried well" who use services in response to their perception of illness.
• Offer access to prevention and health care service options that optimize health.
• Keep the front door open to the community so consumers can experience low-risk products and services at retail prices.
• Offer access to qualified health care professionals by making the expert available at the critical time in the decision-making process.
• Enhance the quality of a consumer's health care experience and his or her actual health status.

WELCOME TO TWENTY-FIRST CENTURY E-CARE DELIVERY!

It is time for health care organizations to catch up with e-consumers' high expectations for access, information, choice, and health status, by initiating self-serve, multimedia channels. For instance, health organizations must have access to information, data, and communication systems enterprise-wide that include physician-specific information, medical records, clinical pathways, insurance plan information, facility information, and more. To accomplish such a huge task, communications tools such as the telephone, PC, e-mail, video, television, and the World Wide Web must be integrated. All are part of the electronic digital integration of health care services. These mega-highways of communication can be organized around internal business transaction services and partners, self-service, and multimedia channels in the following ways:

• The telephone and Intranet connect resources within the health care organization and offer security behind a firewall.

- The telephone and Extranet link the health care organization with suppliers, distributors, retailers, and strategic partners.
- The telephone and the Web link the health care organization with regional and local communities, one e-patient or e-consumer at a time.

REVITALIZE MARKETING AND BUILD MULTIMEDIA BRAND VALUE

Brand is a virtual experience derived from the consumer's experiences with the product, service, or company—not from the messages of broadcast media. The development of brand requires that an infrastructure of distribution, support, and service be in place when and where the consumer wants it. Real-time technology delivers the brand experience anytime, anyplace.[8]

Essential to putting "care" back into health care is the ability to complete a watershed transformation that allows the e-consumer to experience brand value through various traditional and new media channels. Begin with an evaluation of the relationship between your marketing endeavors and the organization's overall information technology strategy and the streams of information that are necessary for this shift. In most cases, the terms "marketing" and "technology" have historically not been used in the same sentence. The executives in these departments rarely attend the same meetings and probably do not know each other's core strategies or competencies.

The prime strategy is to be able to access real-time information vital to early product testing with consumers, to ensure that appropriate and profitable products reach the marketplace. The fast paced-environment of telephone and Web transactions allows new product testing at no risk because "time and cost to market" are no longer factors. Real-time information flow ensures a quick, low-cost decision by product managers, as eager e-consumers test new products in real time. You can cut your losses quickly on a product that is a lemon (Figure 8–3).

This shift is critical for real-time center success. E-consumers must be able to identify your brand with their telephone and Web real-time experiences, which results in a new brand value for your organization. This brand value can be achieved only if your organization's current marketing strategy is enhanced by, and functions in tandem with, your technology strategy. The revitalized brand should include e-communications and e-care delivery.

Health care marketing is being transformed from the ground up. Marketing budgets must be reallocated based on the market size of each multimedia chan-

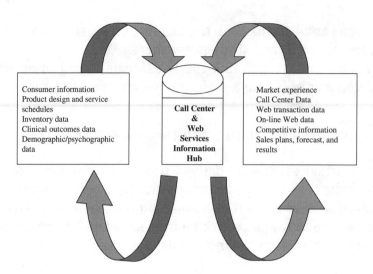

Consumer information
Product design and service
schedules
Inventory data
Clinical outcomes data
Demographic/psychographic
data

**Call Center
&
Web
Services
Information
Hub**

Market experience
Call Center Data
Web transaction data
On-line Web data
Competitive information
Sales plans, forecast, and
results

Figure 8–3 Real-Time Information Flow. Courtesy of Loree Jurgens.

nel. Your new marketing strategy is about much more than glossy printed materials, health fairs, and radio commercials. The marketing team's tool kit should be repacked to include on-line e-connections, interactive television, computer kiosks, self-service terminals, and customer real-time call centers. Marketing must catch up with e-consumers and the many ways in which these consumers communicate their needs. *This shift is about transforming marketing to the "level of one;"* mass marketing campaigns no longer cut it (Figure 8–4).

Patients do not want to be treated equally; they want to be treated individually. E-consumers are already used to being treated in an e-personalized way. Look at Amazon's (www.amazon.com) OneClick service, which recognizes the visitor each time he or she logs on. Or CDNow (www.cdnow.com), where e-customers set up their own on-line pick lists for friends and relatives who want to purchase just the right CD for a special occasion. To e-consumers or e-patients, the experience with your brand is not a statistical event. It is an e-care delivery experience that creates an environment of privacy, information, assurance, and comfort—*just for them.*

Ask the physicians and other health professionals in your organization for help when you are creating this "level of one" marketing strategy—they have been creating patient relationships this way for years. For example, all male patients over the age of 45 with chest pain receive a cardiac protocol and workup. But the physician tailors his or her discussion and the next steps of the

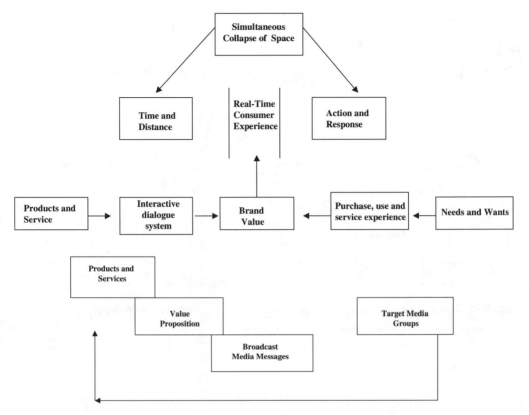

Figure 8–4 Real-Time Space and New Brand Value Chain. Courtesy of Loree Jurgens.

treatment plan to the test results and the patient's individual history. Customizing the treatment plan to the individual patient in this case is an example of "marketing" to the level of one.

Let us take this example into cyberspace. When health care information and products become available on line, the e-consumer can browse and compare the health care treatment options for coronary artery disease. Within this real-time space, a purchase decision between heart surgery or medication and diet management is a complex, information-intensive, and high-risk decision (Figure 8–5). In real time, the health care e-consumer will not only make the decision, but will be responsible for managing a variety of lifestyle changes and a number of on-line clinical monitoring support tools (which in this example could be a blood pressure cuff and a daily weight log).

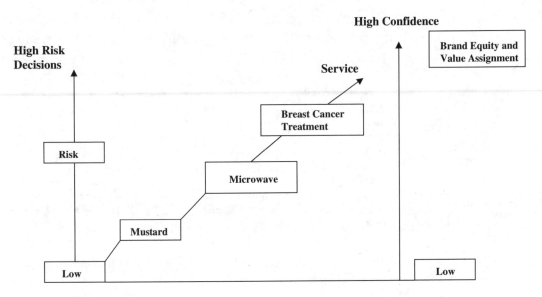

Figure 8–5 Building Brand Equity and Assigning Value. Courtesy of Loree Jurgens.

REAL-TIME CALL CENTERS ARE HERE TO STAY

While health care executives debated the success or failure of the national managed care strategy, the public quietly decided that call centers are a market expectation for choice and health care assistance. Consumers want the low premiums of managed care *and* choice of providers and services. They expect multimedia real-time call centers to be available at *their* convenience. And since disease and demand management are critical services that reduce health care expenditures, and call centers deliver this service to consumers, there are both financial and consumer satisfaction reasons to further integrate your organization's call center strategy. *E-care or real-time call centers will continue to expand despite the reverse of capitation in many markets.*

Most health care organizations already offer a physician referral program, either through their own call center or a vendor call center. At least half of these offer access to health information and symptom triage as value-added services to their physicians, health plan members, and the community. Within the past three years, a lot of attention has been paid to this type of demand and disease management and the cost reductions it can provide—so much so that 20 percent of health maintenance organizations (HMOs) have implemented disease management initiatives in the areas of asthma, congestive heart failure, and diabetes. HMOs are also investing in call centers, to manage the risk of patients in markets where the provider network is capitated by the health plan, or where the HMO encourages member use of plan products and services, and open enrollment modifications.

Health systems, beware! Several of the top health insurers—such as Kaiser, Blue Cross Blue Shield, CIGNA, and United HealthCare—are taking a very significant position in the demand and disease management industry through the investment in and expansion of such real-time services. For example,

- CIGNA is aggressively recruiting demand management executives and setting up national call centers to support its insurance operations.
- United HealthCare is a leader in the field of demand management and has developed an affiliated company called OPTUM, which is marketing nurse triage and other on-line demand management services.
- Kaiser Permanente has traditionally offered extensive nurse triage, on-line appointments, and mails print versions of various self-care support newsletters and books to members. Kaiser has moved to integrate and improve its nurse triage services with its members only www.kponline.com real-time service.

Watch this trend carefully. Managed health plans and health systems will compete for control over medical management through advanced demand and disease management strategies and real-time systems, which will evolve into real-time centers. If you do not offer these e-services to your e-patients, a competitor will.

These trends and market challenges offer an opportunity to become the premier e-consumer information and health management real-time center in your markets, offering access to health information and resources 24 hours a day, seven days a week. This strategy can reduce inappropriate and unnecessary health care expenditures, deliver outstanding e-customer service, source new business, and differentiate your organization from the competition—while you build brand loyalty among e-consumers and e-patients.

Expect new technologies to entice e-consumers and e-patients to try multimedia technologies such as the Web, e-fax, e-mail, and video-conferencing for self-care and disease management. The response to Web-enabled physician referral and appointment programs has been overwhelming, and mandates for patient choice in managed care are prevalent. If your organization wants to influence loyalty and offer wide-area access to services, developing your call center into a real-time center that uses Web-enabled technology is a necessity that your e-patients will love.

REAL-TIME ACTION PLANS FOR ADVANCED CALL CENTER AND WEB SERVICES

Call centers are one of the lowest unit cost services provided in health care today. Savvy business leaders of health care organizations are now turning to the Web for even lower-cost ways to deliver high-volume transactions with low-cost solutions.

The evolution from a single-product call center to an integrated real-time centers continues to be a dynamic process. E-services are redefined as quickly as technology provides a new innovation, and clinicians identify new care strategies that improve or manage health better. Call centers have begun to move from a simple, single-product, single-agent telephone transaction environment to a complex network of multimedia transactions. These complex transactions are handled by multiple agents or technology solutions, such as television video-conferencing and in-home observation, interactive Web self-care products, computer-telephony-driven messaging systems, telephony-and-Web-monitored disease management, and low-cost automated intervention delivery via personal computer. Numerous high-profile health care organizations have laid out plans to move in this direction.

Allina Health System

Allina Health System of Minneapolis is a 30-hospital system with multiple medical groups and a million member health plan (Medica). Allina consolidated all calls from its hospital community programs, outpatient clinics, physician practices, and health plan into a call center called Medformation, which handles more than 500,000 calls each year. Allina has launched an evolving Web-enabled extension of its call center—a real-time center—called Medformation.com to shift a large number of these calls to a new set of Web-based products and services, with www.medformation.com, www.allina.com, and www.medica.com.

Catholic Healthcare Partners

Catholic Healthcare Partners (CHP) is a health system with 16 hospitals, 6,000 physicians, and locations in three states. The corporate offices are in Cincinnati, Ohio. CHP consolidated its three call centers into a single high-functioning call center and added Web-enabled supported self-serve features to the set of call-based services. In re-thinking the mission of the call center, CHP chose to define its functions with the new term "patient contact center." The new entity, e-

HealthConnection, your community health resource (www.healthonline.com/clients/chp), operates under two separate strategic divisions: health management and hospital services. Products and services are being repackaged and sold directly to physicians and other strategic third parties, such as employer groups. In addition, a consumer on-line channel e-HealthConnection.com is offered throughout their regions.

Both of these systems are on their way to creating a twenty-first century integrated customer information and health management center. Such a real-time center can successfully integrate clinical concepts, technology, new products, and medical management services by weaving the e-consumer or e-patient right into the fabric of the organization—in *real time*—as a partner in e-care. Equipped with a telephone that has computer telephony, video integration, on-line access to physicians' offices, appointment scheduling functions, a list of participating insurance companies, hospitals, strategic partners and physicians, and some level of electronic medical record, the clinical desktop can be transformed into an autonomous e-tool for real-time center nurses. E-consumers and e-patients will receive a high quality of care through on-line, video, and audio services.

10 STEPS TO BUILDING A REAL-TIME E-CUSTOMER INFORMATION AND HEALTH MANAGEMENT CENTER

The following e-action plan was initially designed to re-engineer traditional call center operations for more advanced practices. It has been adapted as a model for building a real-time center. Before you begin, remember that although call centers and Web technology may already be a part of your organization's infrastructure, it is likely that to continue to expand services and make improvements, your organization will require justification in the form of return on investment (ROI). The business model not only addresses the ROI but positions the business as a predictive model that estimates the reduction in utilization. The model is based on health information, e-care support services such as the next generation of demand and disease management, and revenue projections from health access programs such as physician appointments, health information, and other marketing efforts.

Step 1. Align Strategies and Principals—Organize the Project Team

Assemble the right team for this strategic exercise, one that can project the future path for your real-time center. Expected outcomes from this session include the selection of the project team, positions to be held by senior management, degree of support available, identification of key stakeholders, financial performance expectations, and a laundry list of the issues you face.

Step 2. Perform a Market Evaluation—Assess Strategic Market Opportunities and Target Markets

While call centers are operated in many health care organizations, they reflect their markets in the services and products they provide. Each health care market has its own economic, social, and health care issues. That is why a market evaluation is the first step for organizations that are developing on-line, multimedia products and services (Exhibit 8–3). Many research-based health systems use a call center to promote clinical trials and recruitment efforts. Markets in which capitation exceeds 30 percent use call centers that offer 24-hour triage services and charge physicians a fee when patients use them. Other call centers offer special contracts for workers' compensation follow-up calls, employer health screenings, or 24-hour health information and triage services.

As you evaluate your own market, consider the following factors:

- Size of the market—be sure to project call volumes, cost, and profit structures.
- Capital need to Web-enable existing call center services or use automated computer telephony.
- The organization's management imperatives—cost reduction, revenues, or cost savings related to the evolution of the call center.
- Size and interest level of your organization's internal and external markets. Do not just build it and expect them to come; ask your internal customers—

Exhibit 8–3 Market Evaluation

Market Evaluation
• Determine Market Opportunities and Priorities
– #1. Employer Services
– #2. Physician Services
– #3. Revenue Producing Services
– #4. Reduce Health Expenditures

Source: Copyright © 1999, Douglas Goldstein.

as well as e-consumers and e-patients—which products and services would serve their needs.

Distribute a survey to a cross-section of your internal constituents—call center nurses, physicians, operations managers, front-line staff, marketing and technology teams. Collect external market data by surveying patients by paper, telephone, or focus groups. Bring key partners such as employer groups into the fold as well. Once the data are in hand, you must further evaluate each project based on a cost-benefit analysis. Segment the target markets and calculate the cost of each service. Each service will require a complete set of financial cost assumptions, worksheets, and benefit assumptions based on a standard market formula for the type of service you evaluate. These are discussed in more detail later in this chapter.

Step 3. Perform an Extensive Evaluation of Current Call Center Operations

The call center assessment should include the infrastructure, staffing, product performance, product portfolio, and future product management capabilities. At the same time, a project team member can meet with the chief information officer and marketing representatives to determine the technology strategic plans and timelines and assess current and future real-time information, data, and communication flow within the organization.

Step 4. Define and Package Products and Services Using Market Evaluation and Survey Data

Depending on the outcome of the market evaluation in step 2, you might determine that the organization can take advantage of existing products and services:

- Partner with independent physician associations (IPAs) and physician organizations to provide a nurse help line and e-care support service suite. Sell either a nurse help line or a complete suite of e-care support services to IPAs with Medicare, Medicaid, and commercial risk capitation agreements. The single-service, lower-cost nurse help line would be the easier sell; after six months to a year, an expanded e-care support suite of services could be added to provide further savings for allied physicians.
- Partner with employers, using health information and empowerment services. Deliver valuable cost-containment and consumer services to keep consumers healthy and reduce overall medical costs. Demonstrate that providers

are the employer's best friend when it comes to improving health care quality and cost-effectiveness.

- Support providers in the quest to contain unnecessary medical expenses for at-risk populations and improve access and self-care support. Provide critical demand management and medical management services that manage at-risk commercial and Medicare populations. Reduce unnecessary utilization at the appropriate location, cost, and service level. Retain and save millions of dollars in unnecessary expenditures as a result of various care support programs and services.

- Retain control of medical management as a core capability of health care organization. Retain control by using advanced e-care support and disease management services. This can support the health care organization's contracting efforts and preempt the strategic and operational initiatives of major competitors efforts by helping the health system retain a high percentage of the premium dollar and deliver a value-added benefit to employers.

Because of multiple product lines and the complexity of services, packaging your real-time center's products and services is critical to success. The breadth of e-care support services in a real-time center ranges across communication platforms—from telephone, print, and audio health libraries to Web-enabled video, Intranet, and one-on-one counseling. The services include telephone-based inbound and outbound services, nurse triage, primary and specialty care referral, emergent/urgent or specialty care preauthorization, health care decision support, chronic disease management, and other health promotion services. The goal of each service is to offer safe, clinically effective, convenient, user-friendly screening and guidance services that route consumers and patients to the most effective care delivery—whether that be emergency department, urgent care, physician office visits, or self-care alternatives. The value of these services should not be underestimated.

One approach to the design of real-time center products and service packages is to bundle them based on your marketing or care management goals, need for results, and the product cost-benefit.

The financial assumptions for specific product and service packages typically fall within two broad categories: utilization projections and cost savings. Defining financial assumptions is an attempt to identify costs and revenues associated with these services and to quantify medical utilization savings for managed care populations under management for the client. For example, one of the focuses of the nurse triage service is to demonstrate cost reductions—this potential cost reduction should be factored in when you price the service package. Services can be marketed on a per member per month pricing system, with some element of risk sharing built into the program as a discrete product, alone or bundled with additional services, such as a total care support package (Exhibit 8–4). After starting with a service like inbound nurse triage, expand multimedia services that can leverage revenue. Also, substantial cost reduction can be achieved by additional targeted e-care support programs.

Services can also be packaged to meet the need of a clinical initiative. For example, if the hospital wants to reduce the number of readmissions for congestive heart failure patients, deploy a disease management program. Try out an on-line pilot project in which each congestive heart failure patient is monitored on line and via a telephone health tool that collects vital sign data. The e-patient enters data elements each day for heart rate, weight, and medication, and receives automatic real-time feedback and recommendations for action if guideline thresholds are over or under baseline. In this scenario, the patient could also be given access to an on-line health library and a Heart Team that fields patient questions, assists in meal planning, and provides instructions about medication dosages. Deploying multimedia disease management programs can reduce readmission rates for congestive heart failure patients. See Chapters 6 and 9 for an indepth discussion of these approaches.

Step 5. Devise Pricing Strategies and Address Financial Issues

Developing a product and service pricing strategy requires two things: (1) knowing the unit cost per product, transaction, or service in your call center

---

Exhibit 8–4 Packaging Products and Services

Real-Time Services Packaging

"e-Care Support" Suite of Services
1. Population Assessment and Tracking
   – Health/Cost Risk Assessment Profile and Plan
2. e-Care Support (Print, Video, and Online)
3. Symptom Assessment and Triage for Appropriate Care with Major Medical Decision Support
4. Next Generation Disease Management Programs
   – Internet Diabetes Trial
5. Multimedia Communication with Patients

Source: Copyright © 1999, Douglas Goldstein

and (2) applying the cost to a distribution channel. For example, a health screening includes the unit cost to mail, follow-up, enter data, and perform results reporting, and may cost $10 per survey. If you package the survey as part of a health screening program with a clinic visit, you can predict your cost for the survey and add the cost of the clinic visit for your total package price. However, if a customer only wants to survey its employees, you could price the menu item to be cost ($10) plus a profit (Exhibit 8–5).

By developing a menu of product, program, and service costs, you can mix and match your service offerings as packages. Your product and service fee structure will need to consider the organization's position as a not-for-profit, sensitive to physician inurement issues. Pricing and fees can be arranged in a variety of ways:

- Fee-for-service—cost plus 10 percent markup for "fair market rate."
- Family discounted rate—direct and fixed costs subsidized by the organization.
- Per member per month—price based on number of covered lives.
- Cost per call, per survey, or per Web transaction.
- Per physician rate—rate charged to physicians aligned in an affiliated IPA or medical group.
- Joint risk sharing—cost allocated through intercompany transfer, with cost savings split quarterly and used to cover the cost of the service.

Step 6. Develop Innovative Advertising, Promotion, and Sponsorship Strategies

Create advertising that promotes your real-time center. In 1996, the American Hospital Association completed a report that outlined Americans' perception of

---

Exhibit 8–5 Pricing Options and Issues

Pricing Options and Issues

- Real-Time e-Service Pricing Options:
  1. Below cost (subsidized)
  2. Cost
  3. Wholesale—Cost plus
  4. Market Competitive
  5. Retail

Source: Copyright © 1999, Douglas Goldstein.

health care advertising. An important finding of this study is that *consumers respond only to advertising that provides them with immediate and useful information or services that maintain their own health status.* Health care call centers and real-time centers do just that.

Real-time centers can improve the overall competitiveness of a health care delivery system because, as multimedia centers offering immediate and personal information access, they invite entry into the system through a number of different doors. But consumers need to be told about each door! Develop promotional and advertising messages that communicate the accessibility of information and the ability of consumers to receive assistance in various ways—from self-serve automation on the Web to one-on-one, patient-based interactions with highly trained staff at the 1-800 number. Position the center as a systemwide initiative, and focus on local services by adding a targeted look and feel to the ad design or adding a local telephone number and organization's name. The direction you choose will be unique to your organization, market, and customers. While one market may focus on physician satisfaction with its referral program, another might encourage use of mental health facilities during a crisis. Still others may want to enhance clinical integration and promote their on-line cardiac risk screening tool.

Remember your marketing basics: be sure to track each activity back to the media channel used, to validate the impact of the promotional campaign. Whether you plan a large advertising blitz or just a Web push campaign to targeted patients, the cost benefit can be derived from the response data collected, and from quickly adjusting promotional plans that are not working.

One way to approach the launch of a new service is to recruit sponsors. Approach pharmaceutical companies, local pharmacies, agencies such as Planned Parenthood, and donors for selective sponsorships. Conduct fundraisers, establish membership programs, create local sponsor banner ads for Web pages, and consider the development of a coalition of providers for a healthier community.

Step 7. Develop the e-Business Plan for the Real-Time Center

In writing the business plan for the new real-time center, the most complicated aspect is the financial model. First, you build the model, pulling all assumptions together for services, volume, promotion, and so on. Next, you project the benefits for cost reductions and incremental revenue. Finally, you run the model with current data and refine and adjust your tables by comparing them with actual performance data (Exhibit 8–6). For presentations to executives, it is important to focus your financial analysis on a topline summary of the return on investment. If an organization invests $1.00, how much benefit will there be in

Exhibit 8–6 Cost-Benefit Assumption Table

Cost/Benefit Analysis Summary: Key Findings

- Year 1
  - Incremental Revenue Benefit Ratio = $1/$1.75
  - Cost Reduction Benefit Ratio = $1/$2.20
- Year 3
  - Incremental Revenue Benefit Ratio = $1/$4.90
  - Cost Reduction Benefit Ratio = $1/$3.50

Source: Copyright © 1999, Douglas Goldstein.

---

year one, two, and three? The real-time call center is an investment, not an expense. An effective financial model will be able to project the ROI over time.

Consider presenting the cost of the new business development along with the projected revenues and benefits to ensure organizational understanding of what to expect. The cost assumption tables that define the total unit cost of every call type, survey done, and Web transaction completed are critical to the accuracy of the cost-benefit projections for targeted populations and program performance. Employ a business analyst to assist with this aspect of the real-time business plan development. Overall benefit projections should include the qualitative as well as the quantitative, as shown in Exhibit 8–7. Qualitative measures need to be con-

---

Exhibit 8–7 Benefit Elements

Real-Time Benefit Projection—Elements

- Quantitative-Financial:
  - Cost Reductions for capitated populations based "Health Management" supported by Real-Time e-services
  - Incremental Revenue from all other customers from "Health Access" e-services
- Qualitative with Measures:
  - Enhance customer retention
  - Improved medical management infrastructure
  - Enhanced access and patient satisfactions
  - Improved market share

Source: Copyright © 1999, Douglas Goldstein.

sidered too, including benefits such as enhanced patient satisfaction, which often leads to higher retention.

Step 8. Re-engineer the Call Center into a Real-Time Center

In a call center environment, where product lines are complex and clinical data are vital, initiating process redesign may seem a daunting task. Actually, re-engineering any business process is no easy task, and we will not attempt to provide an in-depth process here. You should anticipate, however, that this process can take up to nine months with a dedicated team that coordinates not only the re-engineering process, but the technical innovations, e-service flowcharts and planning, program and product development, and staff training. One of the first tasks is to determine the services you will offer in the real-time center and the customer-focused strategies you want to adhere to, as we have discussed in this chapter (Figure 8–6). Traditional medical management is giv-

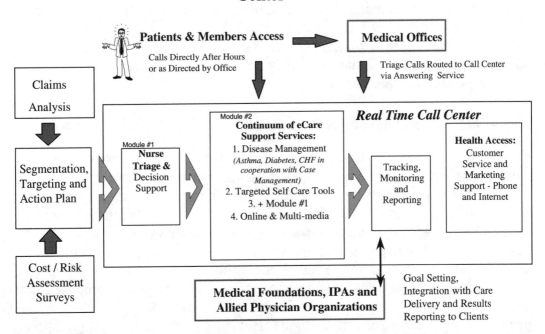

Figure 8–6 Real-Time Customer Information and Health Management Center. Source: Copyright © 1999, Douglas Goldstein.

ing way to a more prospective prevention and disease management role and involvement with the patient delivered through a suite of call center services that integrate the care from getting a doctor to registering for a class, to seeking advice for chest pain.

For some organizations, re-engineering will involve the development and implementation of health management services. Others may want to leapfrog the local competition and offer e-commerce, e-communications, and care delivery by Web-enabling many existing call center services. Products and services that are high volume and self-serve are perfect for Web applications. Move health information, surveys, class registration, physician referral, streaming voice audio-health topics, and specific disease programs to the Web. Promote your URL and your call center telephone number together on all marketing and communications materials designed to drive business to the real-time center.

Regardless of your re-engineering need, there are a number of call center and Web software products available to make the work go more easily. Call centers use the software application "Erhlang C" to develop appropriate customer service levels, call response times, and appropriate staffing. Web software tools that aid in planning, forecasting, and management include e-mail software. The software supports two-way communication between the patient and the agent; central help desk software to manage technical difficulty response time; contact management tools for CTI call transfers from the Web; and Java software that will allow a corporate browser to download to Web browsers. In addition, high-quality telephone and Web performance standards and certifications, endorsed by national organizations, are available.

Step 9. Act and Implement e-Service Now!

The key to a successful implementation is the ability to develop a detailed implementation plan and manage all the parallel efforts and timelines. A significant amount of time must be set aside for negotiations with external vendors for call center and Web products. This is often an underestimated task in terms of time and knowledge, so you may want to employ an external content expert to help you. Other key implementation tasks include technical preparation, personnel preparation, internal and external marketing and communication plans, account management and contracting preparation, equipment and product installation, database development for clinical and marketing data tracking, and population downloads for initial clients. Moving quickly after appropriate planning is essential for success in real-time e-services and center development.

Step 10. Evaluate Real-Time Center and Program Performance

Concurrent evaluation of the real-time center should be based on functional performance criteria. Once performance standards are established, the real-time center is tracked and monitored to manage performance to meet best-of-breed real-time center practice. These criteria might include telephone occupancy and service levels, average talk time, speed of answer, abandonment rates, hit rates, page views, page load times, page audit trails, and bugs and glitches.

Evaluation of core products, programs, and e-services requires the establishment of baseline data and information and the development of process objectives and outcome objectives that represent best practices. *Process objectives* that would affect performance include compliance, dropout rates, participation levels, program awareness, adherence to the process, and instructional materials. *Outcome objectives* might include screening measures, mortality/morbidity risk, general well-being, medical measures, utilization patterns, productivity, and efficacy. These objectives form the basis for reports and evaluation through specific statistical analysis, high-cost/high-risk patients, risk-cost association, identification of major risks, medical care cost indexes, delta values between time one and time two, trend analysis, and recommended interventions.

CONCLUSION—DELIVER E-SERVICES THROUGH REAL-TIME

Here are some real-time thoughts. The expansion of your call center is really a set of strategic questions. You have to answer the question, Are the call center and the Web-enabled extension of the services that can be provided—such as e-commerce, e-communities, and e-care—a part of our corporate communication, data, and information system strategy? Are we open to the possibility that by implementing real-time systems and changing working relationships between doctors and patients we may actually gain customer loyalty and discover new ways of taking care of e-patients? When you pose these questions, it begins to make sense to refine your primary patient relationships with e-consumers, who demand greater personalization, higher touch, and continued high tech.

The reversal of capitation and the push of point-of-service plans indicate that consumers are not satisfied with the "one-size-fits-all" commodity business of managed care. You are in business to serve the customer. If a mega-highway infrastructure of computer, telephony, Intranet, and Extranet is being built at your organization, create a series of missions that capitalize on it. Serve your e-customers and e-patients. Keep them satisfied using self-service e-communications, e-services, and e-care, and they will be loyal to your brand.

REFERENCES

1. Punk, Ziegel & Company, *Closing the Loop—The Digital Integration of the Health Care Industry* (New York City, June 1998).
2. Punk, Ziegel & Company.
3. C. Clark, "Healthcare Information Systems," *Value Line* report (7 April 1995), 679, quoted from M.L. Millenson, *Demanding Medical Excellence* (Chicago: University of Chicago Press, 1997), 91.
4. Punk, Ziegel & Company.
5. Punk, Ziegel & Company.
6. Punk, Ziegel & Company.
7. Punk, Ziegel & Company.
8. R. McKenna, *Real Time—Preparing for the Age of the Never Satisfied Customer* (Cambridge, MA: Harvard Business School Press, 1997).

CHAPTER 9

Technology and On-Line Care Management

Sandra J. Feaster, David J. Howell, and LuAnn Joy

INTRODUCTION

As managed care programs proliferate and costs continue to rise, the challenge of managing finite budgets while meeting the infinite cost demands of chronic disease looms ever larger.[1] In the past, health care administrators have met this challenge simply by reducing resource allocation.[2] They need not do so any longer: The repositories of medical knowledge are not confined behind medical school walls. Documented works are now readily available on line. The volume of information and data is daunting. Good search engine capability and keyword knowledge, however, enable anyone to search efficiently for medical and pharmaceutical information. Web pages, portals, and channels designed specifically for the layperson are increasingly available. They provide instant access to information across the medical and disease spectra.

In addition to information resources, one can also reach e-services that will "follow" an individual and provide ongoing teaching, monitoring, and coaching to meet specific health or disease management goals. A pager can be used to remind a person of certain activities; for example, medication schedules and exercise regimens. Physicians can access their patients' information on protected Web sites specifically designed for computerized patient records. They can also provide patients with new information electronically, information that may assist in disease prevention as well as in the management of an active condition. Physicians must, however, lead their patients to become actively involved in their own personal disease management.

And this responsibility is not only on the physicians' shoulders. Health care administrators must also be accountable in the area of electronic care. For health care executives to achieve maximum benefits for chronically ill patients, they must inculcate self-care skills in patients within their managed care environments. These patients must become de facto case managers of their own health.[3]

The arrival of electronic care has been both a tool of empowerment and a clarion call to physicians and health care administrators. The challenges of electronic care are now being met by well-designed electronic programs for on-line consumers. On-line disease management, health improvement, and information portals have significantly increased the knowledge of the consumer and have in turn increased the consumer's demand for up-to-date services and care techniques.

HARNESSING TECHNOLOGY TO MANAGE CHRONICALLY ILL PATIENTS

People with chronic diseases such as congestive heart failure (CHF), diabetes, chronic obstructive pulmonary disease (COPD), and asthma are ideal patients for electronic monitoring because their health status indicators are quantifiable.[4] Electronic monitoring allows the patient, physician, and caregivers the chance to see all factual information that is collected by both individual data points and trend records. With routine data entry, the electronic record remains updated. The electronic record can also be set to "alarm" when certain specific parameters have been violated. Fortunately, software programs that provide trend data also provide a measure of security. For example, a single blood pressure reading may engender an alert within the system. This single alert is not nearly as valuable as a trend of many daily data points.

Trained medical professionals who look at both short-term and long-term data collection are integral to wise electronic health care monitoring and disease management. The professionals provide a margin of safety coupled with a healthy medical skepticism to keep inappropriate data from disabling the monitoring system. Continuous analysis, evaluation, and trending of data—such as blood pressure, heart rate, blood glucose levels, weight gain or loss, peak flow, and disease-associated symptoms—can be efficiently executed via sophisticated software programs that link to home-based computers.[5] These programs constantly scan accumulated data to detect aberrations or parameter-exceeding information preset by the physician. When parameter-exceeding events occur, registered nurses (or other health care professionals) can follow up with the patient to determine the nature of the problem. The patient's physician now has an early warning system for early intervention.[6] The result of the early intervention is reduced patient morbidity and fewer emergency department visits and hospital admissions.[7]

COMBINING HIGH TECH WITH HIGH TOUCH: THE CHALLENGE OF E-CARE

The cost of touch-based, or traditional, nursing care in the home is becoming prohibitive.[8] At the same time, improvements in overall care and the management of disease can reduce health care costs. The answer lies somewhere in between continuous touch-based care and the use of technology in the management of disease. From the technology perspective, there are five key elements of chronic disease management, all of which can be managed using e-care technology: (1) patient selection (opt-in versus opt-out enrollment), (2) timely data gathering, (3) ongoing monitoring, (4) early intervention, and (5) behavior reinforcement. But although these five technological elements are crucial to the success of a comprehensive disease management program, health care professionals must recognize that they are not the only building blocks of success. Using only technology misses a big element—the human element. Disease management programs that are technology based must not be driven only by technology. Rather, these programs must combine technology ("tech") and human interaction ("touch") for optimal health care delivery, improved quality of life, and effective cost containment.[9]

As more people with chronic health conditions become e-patients who use the Internet for information about their conditions, the cybercommunity of people with chronic diseases will increase exponentially.[10] What will happen, then, to "traditional patients" who are enrolled in disease management programs? Will these programs remain sufficient for efficient and reliable disease management? The answer to that question depends on the particulars of the disease management program under consideration. Regardless of whether the program uses e-care technology, patients need personal coaching by medical professionals who understand how to deal with expected relapses.

We believe the most effective way to manage care for persons living with chronic disease is to combine the use of e-care technology with patient self-advocacy and professional vigilance. Doing so creates a partnership referred to as "supported self-care." Supported self-care allows all patients to participate in disease management programs, regardless of their level of technical expertise. All of us have friends and family with varying degrees of computer literacy levels. The use of a variety of technologies—such as interactive voice response, or Web-enabled applications—allows direct data and symptom information to be captured into the disease management system and appropriately managed by health care professionals.

E-PATIENTS AND ON-LINE CARE

Living with a chronic disease can be difficult and disheartening. For patients with chronic disease, communication with family and friends helps maintain a semblance of normality. The value of the familial support system cannot be overestimated. However, the Internet offers opportunities for another kind of support: support from other people who are living with the same chronic illnesses.[11]

Talking with others who have the same disease provides psychological support to e-patients. On-line chat groups allow opportunities for sharing information and the creation of a community of individuals who have been diagnosed with a chronic condition. Reviewing national standards, learning about alternative medicine, and sharing experiences with others most definitely make e-patients better informed. This community of e-patients needs access to the most efficient health care search engines for assistance in locating timely information. The opportunities for shared information, however, are a liability when the information shared is incorrect or misleading. Health care providers must help e-patients distinguish between evidence-based information and hearsay.

"Indeed, for every dollar Americans spent on books last year, they spent four on prescription and over-the-counter medications, industry executives estimate. The drugstore totals: $90 billion on prescriptions, $20 billion on over-the-counter health goods, $20 billion on personal care items, $20 billion on vitamins and other 'wellness' products, and $15 billion on beauty aids and cosmetics."

EMPOWERING PATIENTS TO MANAGE THEIR OWN ILLNESSES

Empowering patients to manage their chronic illnesses is one element of efficient case management in today's marketplace. Another element is wise use of technology. Indeed, the fact that this book has been published is proof that e-care of patients is rapidly becoming an accepted component in a disease management delivery system.

Second-generation disease management systems can now deliver quantifiable data about physiologic parameters and symptom changes to health care providers.[13] These systems include easily accessible technology—Touch-Tone telephones, interactive video players, computers, and, of course, human interaction.[14] For health care executives and providers, these second-generation disease management systems offer cost- and time-efficient interventions. Moreover, the best of these systems are easily customized and individualized to each patient living with a chronic disease or with disease comorbidities.[15]

SUPPORTED SELF-CARE: THREE CASE STUDIES*

LifeMasters® Supported SelfCare[SM] (www.lifemasters.net) is a company that is pioneering cost-efficient e-care programs to monitor patients in the home set-

---

Source: Case studies reprinted with permission from LifeMasters® Supported SelfCare[SM], Case Studies 1, 2, and 3, © 1998.

ting. These programs provide easy-to-use technology in the home environment and a staff of clinical professionals to reinforce healthy behavioral changes and to watch out for potentially harmful changes in patients' physiological status. Three case studies about managing patients with CHF and attendant disease comorbidities have been selected from the Supported SelfCare annals. These case studies illustrate the benefits of using well-designed technology and human interaction to improve both the physiologic and emotional health of patients, and preserve the economic health of payers. Case Study 1 relates improvements in clinical indicators. Case Study 2 discusses important quality-of-life issues. And Case Study 3 provides quantifiable data about the economic benefits of monitoring patients on an ongoing basis to avert costly hospitalizations.

Case Study 1: Clinical Indicator Improvement in a Patient with Congestive Heart Failure

Rationale

Patients who receive continuous monitoring and access to early intervention can successfully keep clinical indicators in a healthy range. Daily monitoring, scheduled telephone nursing appointments, and well-designed patient education materials help patients make wiser and healthier lifestyle decisions. The following case study illustrates the value of LifeMasters Supported SelfCare specific to access to early intervention by primary care providers.

Patient Profile

74-year-old married white male with a history of CHF and frequent short-term emergency department and hospital admissions for the past three years.

Before Enrollment in the LifeMasters Program

This patient, with documented Class IV CHF, had an ejection fraction of 17 percent and a prescription for at-home oxygen. Over the past several years, the patient's presence in the hospital emergency department and intensive care unit (ICU) had increased. In the most recent calendar year, he had already had four visits.

With his worsening CHF symptoms, the patient and his spouse had learned the importance of monitoring daily weight and blood pressure (Figure 9–1). Because of his daily monitoring, he was aware that his symptoms were worsening, but he did not inform his physician of the decline. Over a period of several weeks, the patient's dyspnea became quite pronounced. At night he required oxygen and had to sleep upright in an armchair. In an attempt to make him feel better one

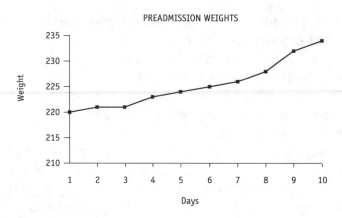

Figure 9–1 Preadmission Weights

afternoon, his wife fed him canned chicken noodle soup for lunch. Six hours later, the patient had visibly deteriorated. His spouse called 911.

The patient was admitted directly to the ICU, where he remained for four days before being transferred to the floor for six more days. During that period, a pulmonary artery catheter and intravenous line were inserted. He received titrated dobumatine (Dobutrex) and furosemide (Lasix). The cost of his hospitalization was approximately $20,000.

Results of Participation in the LifeMasters Program

After discharge, the patient enrolled in the LifeMasters program. He and his spouse learned how to control fluid intake and sodium consumption. They also learned how to use an automatic blood pressure device and electronic digital scale to send daily vital signs and weight to LifeMasters Supported SelfCare over the telephone. The patient succeeded in bringing his vital signs within acceptable limits, even in the face of advanced CHF disease (Figure 9–2). Understanding the importance of physician notification, the patient and his wife kept the physician informed of any worsening symptoms. For a period of nearly a year, the patient continued his participation in the LifeMasters program without any additional hospital admissions.

Comments

Most people genuinely desire to manage their health as wisely as possible. The difficulty for them is knowing how to do it and getting started. The LifeMasters program provides skill training, personal coaching, and data management for people to make savvy lifestyle decisions.

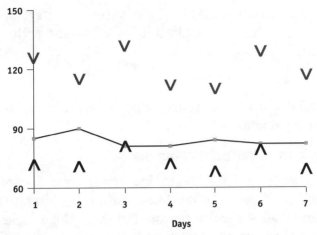

Figure 9–2 7-Day Sample of Vital Signs during Participation

For this patient, the cycle of deterioration followed by exacerbation and hospitalization stopped when he began active participation in his own care. The results speak for themselves: a sustained period of acceptable quality of life at home, without hospitalization and costly medical admissions.

Case Study 2: Quality of Life Improvement in a Patient with Congestive Heart Failure and Coexisting Chronic Conditions

Rationale

The National Committee for Quality Assurance (NCQA) is a significant force influencing the trend toward informed patient populations and the development of quality care programs. As the importance of NCQA accreditation continues to increase, the need for quantifiable measurements of patient health becomes ever more pressing. Quantifiable success of a disease management program can be shown by parameters such as decreased hospitalizations and improvements in functional status of patients.

Patients equipped with knowledge and self-care techniques are empowered to take an active role in modifying their behavior, improving their outcomes, and improving overall quality of life. Condition-specific education materials and personalized patient training forms the foundation of the LifeMasters Supported SelfCare program. Patients also benefit from daily vital sign and medications monitoring, proactive nursing intervention techniques, and scheduled telephonic nurse support and interaction.

The following case study illustrates the value of LifeMasters Supported SelfCare specific to the physical functioning of a patient with several chronic health conditions.

Patient Profile

70-year-old married white male, retired chef, with a history of CHF, diabetes, COPD, and multiple myeloma.

Before Enrollment in the LifeMasters Program

This patient has multiple life-threatening conditions: documented Class II CHF, diabetes, COPD, and multiple myeloma. Before beginning the LifeMasters program, the patient had difficulty performing even the simplest activities of daily living. He felt that his physical health was worsening and also that his lifestyle was increasingly limited by his morbidities. This perception of failing health was not unwarranted: the patient had experienced multiple hospitalizations and emergency department visits over a fairly short period of time.

Results of Participation in the LifeMasters Program

The patient was referred by his physician and enrolled in the LifeMasters program. Vital signs and quality-of-life assessments (in this case, the SF-36 survey) were conducted at program entry and at 24 weeks (Figures 9–3 and 9–4). Al-

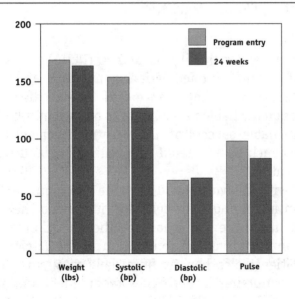

Figure 9–3 Vital signs

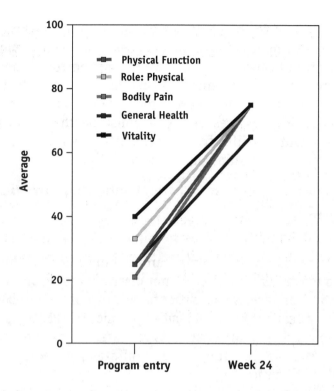

Figure 9–4 Quality of Life

though this patient experienced additional health problems—fractured ribs, chemotherapy, phlebitis, and poor wound healing—his program participation did not falter. He remained committed to changing his behaviors.

The patient learned about lifestyle choices to improve his health and has begun to alter his daily regimens. His diet, initially loaded with high-sodium foods, has been replaced with healthier food entries. His activity level, hampered because of pain and hospitalizations, has not halted his commitment to increasing his physical stamina. In addition, the patient has stopped drinking alcohol with his dinner. He has become more knowledgeable about his medications and their effects on his body. He feels that his overall health is improving.

Comments

LifeMasters Supported SelfCare focuses its resources to customize and tailor services to the specific condition or comorbidity of the individual patient. The program supports both the physician's treatment plan and the need for reliable patient data that pertain to the intervention and decision-making process. Patients make both large and small lifestyle changes that result in improvement in even the most complex health situations. By taking control of their own health management, even the most chronically ill patients begin to feel better when faced with other health problems that diminish their physical condition.

This patient's behavioral choices clearly demonstrate that changes in attitude affect changes in quality of life: five months after beginning the LifeMasters program, he boarded a cruise ship bound for Hawaii.

Case Study 3: Financial Benefits for a Patient with Congestive Heart Failure and Other Cardiac Illnesses

Rationale

The costs of managing patients with cardiac illness in the United States is significant. Although cardiac illnesses do not discriminate according to socioeconomic class, gender, or race, some patients within population-based memberships (also known as capitated, per member per month [PMPM] payment reimbursement) may incur disproportional costs for care. For example, patients with chronic conditions such as CHF often exceed capitated payments, even with well-controlled resource utilization.

This case study dramatically illustrates the value of LifeMasters Supported SelfCare in reducing costs of care for a patient suffering from CHF and other cardiac illnesses.

Patient Profile

72-year-old white male who lives alone in a retirement complex and has a history of Class II CHF, coronary artery disease, angina, multiple myocardial infarctions, angioplasties, and coronary artery bypass surgery.

Before Enrollment in the LifeMasters Program

Before enrollment, the patient had undergone numerous expensive procedures. In the previous year, his costs of care for cardiac illnesses alone exceeded $58,000. This figure includes costs of angioplasties, bypass surgery, emergency department admissions, and hospital stays.

Results of Participation in the LifeMasters Program

As a result of Supported SelfCare and behavior modification training, the patient began to make lifestyle choices that contributed to improved health. By 12 months after enrollment, his weight had dropped 16 pounds. During the second year, his weight dropped another 8 pounds for a total weight loss of 24 pounds. As part of his program participation, the patient has taken up daily walking. He attributes his weight loss to his increased daily activity. The patient's systolic and diastolic blood pressures have also decreased over the two-year period.

At the end of his first year of participation in the LifeMasters program, this patient's total cost of care for cardiac illnesses was slightly more than $11,000. This reduction represents a savings of $47,396 for the managed care organization. His PMPM cost for cardiac care fell from $4,895 to $945.

In addition, the patient's average number of bed-days was reduced by 60 percent (Figures 9–5, 9–6, and 9–7).

Comments

Participation in the LifeMasters Supported SelfCare program results in quantifiable savings for providers. For this patient, cost reductions for cardiac illnesses were more than 80 percent at the end of the first year of program enrollment. The patient's behavioral changes are equally impressive. Over a two-year period, he has reduced his weight by 24 pounds and lowered his blood pressure to levels well outside the range of concern.

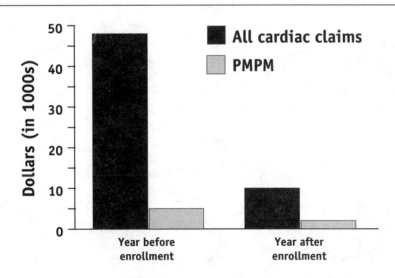

Note: Preintervention costs for multiple angioplasties and bypass surgery = $17,648; postintervention cost for single angioplasty = $1,132.

Figure 9–5 Annual and per Patient per Month Cost Reductions for Cardiac Claims.

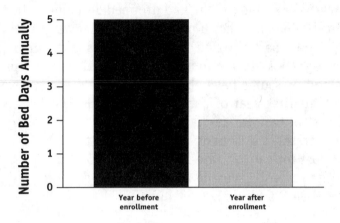

Figure 9-6 Reductions for Bed-Days

CONCLUSION—OUR MULTIMEDIA E-CARE FUTURE

Health care providers and managed care organizations must invest in e-care technology that meets the needs of people living with chronic conditions—as well as those who are at risk for chronic disease in the future. As consumers

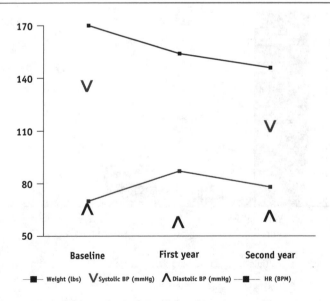

Figure 9-7 Weights and Vital Signs during Participation

increase their knowledge, they are better able to make the lifestyle changes and commitments necessary to improve or maintain their health. With improvements in health should come decreases in cost of health care. If a patient with a chronic disease becomes aware of choices that will improve his or her well-being, that patient is likely to make at least one choice to increase quality of life. Just by becoming more informed, the patient increases the amount of control over his or her chronic disease. Family members and friends can also help a loved one by becoming more informed.

In this age of information overload, it is necessary to help patients and their loved ones find quality, trustworthy knowledge and support quickly and easily. The e-care providers have already designed systems that work toward those goals. Customization to meet the individual's needs must always be the first consideration. With a variety of well-integrated e-care technology tools and human interaction, people with chronic health conditions now have access to better information, camaraderie, and monitoring to promote better health. The results are attractive on every count: efficient economies of scale for health care providers, demonstrable improvements in health and well-being of patients, and happier physicians in managed care groups.

Consumers, electronic and otherwise, are demanding information in the current environment of rapid communications. Proven disease management services and e-care software are available for purchase. These services and software programs can be customized for any health care services group. Developing systems and programs de novo is a luxury in which few, if any, health care organizations can indulge. Consequently, health service organizations that explore purchase or partnership opportunities with competent and efficient multimedia e-care tool developers are those that will emerge victorious in the e-commerce and e-care world of today!

REFERENCES

1. C. Marietti, "Seize the Disease," http://www.healthcare-informatics.com/issues/1999/03_99/disease.htm (March 1999).
2. R.H. Friedman et al., "The Virtual Visit: Using Telecommunications Technology To Take Care of Patients," *Journal of the American Medical Informatics Association* 4, no. 6 (1997): 413–425.
3. S.J. Feaster, "Nursing, Technology, and Patient Care: A Home-Based Model," *Nursing Case Management* 3, no. 1 (1998): 7–10.
4. L.C. Meyer, "Telecommunications and Disease Management in the Home Environment: New Strategies To Improve Outcomes," *Medical Interface* (June 1997): 78–83.
5. S. Moran, "Making House Calls Via Home Computers," *Internet World,* 3 May 1999, 44.
6. C.R. Hughes et al., LifeMasters Supported SelfCare Provides a Framework To Deliver Care to Patients with

Congestive Heart Failure (poster presentation at Cardiovascular Health: Coming Together for the 21st Century, San Francisco, CA, February 19–21 1998).

7. N.B. Shah et al., "Prevention of Hospitalizations for Heart Failure with an Interactive Home Monitoring Program," *American Heart Journal* 135, no. 3 (1998): 373–378.

8. R. Wootton et al., "A Joint US-UK Study of Home Telenursing," *Journal of Telemedicine and Telecare* 4, suppl. 1 (1998): 83–85.

9. C. Carrington, "Successful Disease Management Demands Human Touch," *Telehealth Magazine*, April 1999, 19–21.

10. M. Menduno, "Net Profits," *Health & Hospital Network* (1999): 44–50.

11. J. Hageland and A.G. Armstrong, *Net Gain* (Boston: Harvard Business School Press, 1997), 19–20.

12. B. Tedeschi, "Want To Be an Online Drugstore? Take a Number," *e-commerce report*, http://www.nytimes.com/library/tech/99/02/cyber/commerce/ (2 February 1999), accessed 23 August 1999.

13. S. Kellaher, "Take Two Units of Insulin and Call Me in the Morning," *Diabetes Interview*, May 1999, 1, 20–24.

14. I. Warner, "Telemedicine Applications for Home Health Care," *Journal of Telemedicine and Telecare* 3, suppl. 1 (1997): 65–66.

15. D.A. Perednia and J.Grigsby, "Telephone, Telemedicine, and a Technologically Neutral Coverage Policy," *Telemedicine Journal* 4, no. 2 (1998): 145–152.

CHAPTER 10

Beyond Web Portals to On-Line Health and Medical Channels

Douglas E. Goldstein and Margaret Fisher

AMERICA IS a consumer-driven society. Every U.S. business—whether it be a department store, drug manufacturer, private university, medical practice, or hospital system—is competing for consumer dollars. Because of this consumer-driven marketplace, consumers are bombarded with a myriad of choices, and often it is the recognized brand or the most familiar name that captures their loyalty and business.

Nonprofit organizations and businesses find themselves plunged into this world of capturing market share, advertising, and retaining existing customers. No longer is being the largest or lead business in a community or market enough to guarantee primary market share. Consumers are free to choose not only from a purchasing perspective, but from a geographic perspective as well. In an e-driven society, where the e-consumer is king and the Web offers access to information, services, and products, an organization's e-customers now have any number of choices to pick from—and the numbers increase daily.

How does this e-commerce shift affect the health care industry? Like businesses in other industries, medical product manufacturers, hospital systems and physician organizations compete for new customers and constantly scramble to retain and satisfy current ones. In an e-consumer-driven society that is powered by the Internet, health care organizations must also aggressively compete for consumers as other industries do—in cyberspace. Employing a strategy that embraces e-communications, e-commerce, and e-care is paramount to a health care organization's future success.

YOUR E-PATIENTS ALREADY LOVE DOING THINGS ON LINE

According to a recent study by IntelliQuest Research, more than 79.4 million adults—38 percent of the U.S. population age 16 years and older—are on line.

And with 18.8 million people planning to go on line in the next year, IntelliQuest predicts that nearly 100 million adults will be accessing the Internet in the year 2000.[1]

Who are these Internet users? The IntelliQuest study showed that the number of "mainstream" Internet users is growing: the Internet is no longer a medium for the elite or highly educated. According to the survey, only 36 percent of people on line have a bachelor's degree or more, and only 55 percent of people on line earn $50,000 or more.[2] These figures mean that in the twenty-first century a health system's average patient is likely to be on line right now and customers of other health care organizations are doing more and more on line.

Cyber-shopping and -purchasing have grown into common and acceptable ways for Americans to spend their dollars and for businesses to save time and money. Sixty percent of Internet users shop on line, and nearly 20 percent purchase on line. So far, books, music, and computer hardware and software are the most popular items to buy on line,[3] but that is rapidly changing. When e-consumers and businesses spend billions buying stuff on the Web, why not allow them to buy some of it from your health care organization?

According to a recent Harris Interactive poll,[4] in 1998, more than 60 million Americans went on line in search of health and medical information. Of people who used more than two types of health information sites, 36 percent said a page sponsored by a medical society was most useful; 32 percent cited patient-advocacy pages; 15 percent preferred pages run by pharmaceutical companies; and 11 percent favored hospital pages. It is no wonder that the business of e-healthcare is growing by leaps and bounds, and everyone wants a piece of the action.

As your organization struggles to remain competitive in this evolving marketplace and stake its claim to e-market share, are you making the best use of the far-reaching Web medium? How can passive marketing Web sites be transformed into dynamic e-services that grow market share? How can an e-healthcare organization build on-line services that effectively and efficiently meet the needs of these e-customers?

By describing how a leading health system used the e-healthcare revolution to achieve success in its own region, this chapter delivers insights for other health systems and physician organizations seeking answers. It also provides valuable lessons for other health care organizations seeking to leapfrog the competition. The challenge for the example health system was to stop the erosion of the doctor-patient-hospital relationship by various health Web portals. The opportunity seized was to build a regional on-line health and medical channel that capitalizes on a health system brand and delivers e-communications, e-commerce, and e-care to e-consumers and e-patients in the target market.

MEET ALLINA HEALTH SYSTEM

Minnesota-based Allina Health System has long been a national leader when it comes to innovative thinking and implementing effective ways to meet customer needs. Within the Allina system are a million-member health plan, Medica, 19 hospitals, 5,000 affiliated providers, and a continuum of health and medical services. As an innovator in structuring a consumer's experience, Allina documented that its employees had 14 million human contacts, handled more than 5 million telephone calls, and treated 89,000 inpatients and more than 2.5 million outpatients per year.

Strategic imperatives dictated that Allina and Medica develop new ways to leverage patient contacts and drive new business to their doctors, hospitals, and health services. Allina's goals for their "e" initiatives involved:

- supporting healthier communities
- cross-selling existing services and products
- generating offsetting revenue

Allina market trends research showed that consumers and women in particular were more involved than ever in their health care choices and decisions and the Web was a preferred medium. Allina identified an on-line consumer health care revolution and recognized the importance of leveraging the vast resources and expertise of the Allina delivery system to bring value to its customers, meet their expanding health and medical needs, and build brand loyalty. In addition, Allina research also showed that the ongoing "e-revolution" was resulting in a proliferation of new on-line consumer-focused competitors. Geographic delivery and financing boundaries were becoming less relevant with the creation of virtual services at the national level. Allina needed to clearly and *quickly* define and pursue second generation on-line strategy to differentiate itself within its market and retain patient relationships.

Allina Health Systems' first generation on-line effort, which was supported by IBM, led to two noncommercial Web sites. Allina's Health Village (www.allina.com; Figure 10–1) offered e-information about the system's hospitals, clinics, and services, as well as information on Allina-sponsored classes, events, community initiatives, and general health information. The second first generation Web site, Medica.com, was the on-line vehicle for e-communicating and servicing to Medica health plan members. The member-only area of this Web site offered physician search capability, class schedules, and a complete health information, symptom, and disease database. The public area of the site offered

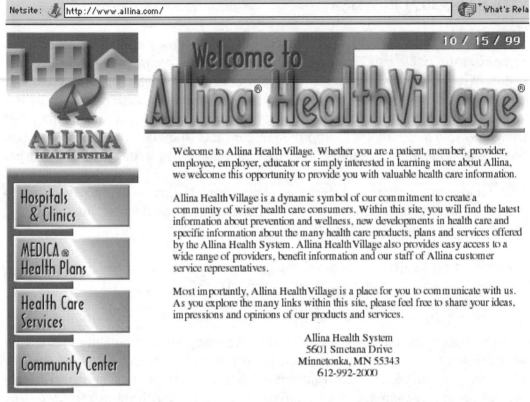

Figure 10–1 Allina Health System's HealthVillage Web Site. *Source:* Reprinted with permission from www.medformation.com, © 1999, Medformation.com. Medformation is a registered trademark of Allina Health Systems.

general Medica information. In 1998, both sites were successful and well utilized within the Allina region, generating more than 300,000 site visits annually.

But more could be done. In June 1998, Allina partnered with Medical Alliances, Inc., a nationally recognized health care e-commerce consulting firm to develop a dynamic Internet strategy for 1999 through 2002. Allina recognized the need for a more robust Web strategy that provided better e-health and medical e-information and supported traffic to its outpatient services, hospitals, and aligned physicians. Allina's other imperative was to support healthier communities by helping consumers connect directly with care resources. Allina health village governing council also recognized the wisdom of expanding its existing Web strategy with a third consumer focus Web service, one that capitalized on sponsorship and transactions, but they did not want to diminish the unbiased consumer focus of their two Web sites and the overall community mission of Allina.

Allina realized early on that when it came to delivering health and medical information on the Web, there were plenty of options on a national and world-wide basis, but these were not effective for local consumers to actually have their health and medical needs *fulfilled*. Allina leaders contemplated the need for a robust regional Web service that met e-consumer and e-patient needs and that would become integrated with their consumer health care call center, Medformation, over time. Medformation was a widely known brand in the market and handled 500,000 consumer information and nurse triage phone calls per year.

WEB SITE, WEB PORTAL, OR WEB CHANNEL?

As Allina moved its e-strategy forward, it had to make some fundamental decisions. A Web site seemed "last year," and besides, Allina and Medica already had two Web sites. As technology evolved and e-consumer confidence and use of Internet increased, the concept of a mere Web site seemed obsolete. In the e-planning effort Allina and Medical Alliances developed a methodology that segmented Web efforts in health care into four levels:

1. *Web site*: Sometimes referred to as *brochureware*, a basic Web site merely presents e-information to the site visitor. In the case of a hospital, for instance, this might include a picture of the hospital, information about the services performed there, contact information, and possibly directions or other miscellaneous content. This is a "flat" site that does not offer much user interactivity. The major focus of a Web site is marketing.

2. *Web portal*: These are highly promoted health Web brands seeking to be the health information gateway to the larger Internet. For consumers, the basic goal of a health Web portal is to deliver health information, sell products, and deliver consumer page view to advertisers.

3. *Web service*: This is the next level up from a Web site. A Web service typically offers interactivity for users and compelling reasons to return—e-communities based on disease states, on-line support groups, purchase of products, and other services. This is certainly a more useful Web destination than a simple Web site. The goal of a Web service is to move beyond information to facilitating access to care resource quickly and effectively through on-line technology.

4. *Web channel*: This delivers a series of robust Web services, along with information and much more. As Exhibit 10-1 illustrates, a Web channel offers unique Web programming that excites users, offers information plus real services and

Exhibit 10–1 Web Channel

An on-line regional health and medical channel offers

- A consumer focus that supports healthier communities off line and on line
- A regional focus and cross-sell of medical care services at appropriate opportunities
- Premium regional positioning on the homepages of local newspapers, television stations, cable companies, and Internet service providers
- Immediate access to medical call centers and health care services
- Web-enabled medical e-communities using advanced disease-focused Web and interactive voice response (IVR) applications
- Fulfillment of users' daily health and medical care e-commerce and e-care delivery needs

Source: Copyright © 1999, Douglas Goldstein.

transactions, and meets consumer needs for access to health services. A Web channel is more than a Web portal; a portal is often a high-volume gateway that Web surfers pass through on their way to the "great beyond" of the Internet, while a channel usually offers many unique and interactive applications and services that generate e-consumer loyalty and drive repeat business. Some examples of successful Web channels in the financial services industry are e*Trade (www.etrade.com) and Quicken (www.quicken.com) (Figure 10–2). Each of these channels and others like them offer the latest Web technologies that serve up robust on-line services and activities that keep e-consumers interested and coming back. One of the primary goals of a health and medical channel is to streamline access to health care services. It also seeks to move a cost center into a revenue center by obtaining revenue from advertisers, sponsors, and transactions. In Allina's case it always stays focused on being the leading regional health and medical destination.

The premise behind an on-line medical channel is that health care is a service business, not simply an information business. Medical services are primarily regional businesses and certainly more complex than selling tickets on line. As a hospital or health system, how do you decide which e-presence is the best for your organization? If your goal is to deliver quality patient care, foster customer loyalty, build market share, generate revenue, and leapfrog your competition, a simple Web site will not meet your needs. Even a Web service may not offer the comprehensive range of services you need to accomplish your goals in today's fast-paced and ever-changing marketplace. If you want to emerge as a market

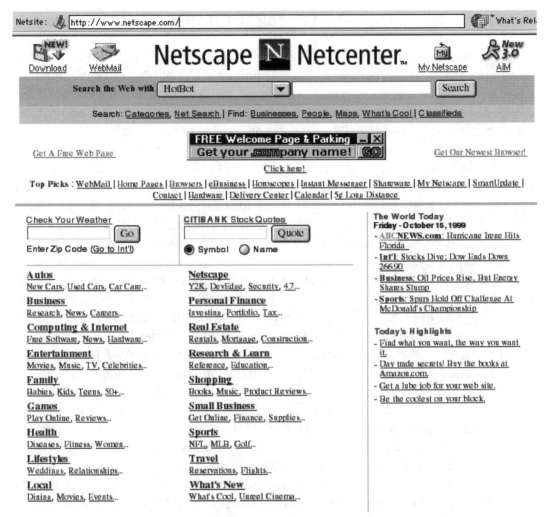

Figure 10–2 Netscape Web Channel Offers News, Shopping, and Search Capabilities. *Source:* Reprinted with permission from www.netcenter.com, © 1999, Netscape Navigator, America Online, Inc.

leader in e-care, your health system must position itself as an e-media channel, integrating call center activities, health and medical information, medical products, and site-of-care services. Don't just use the medium—*be* the medium! Be the leading regional on-line health and medical channel!

ALLINA BUILDS A ROBUST ON-LINE MEDICAL CHANNEL

Allina leaders decided that their best approach was to integrate their air space, telephone space, and cyberspace contacts on one medium—a fully developed on-line health and medical channel that offered much more than just information. Allina knew that it had significant on-line competition in the market and nationally, and moving ahead of its competition was a serious goal of its strategic marketing plan. Its visionary and innovative leaders understood the importance of capitalizing on the 14 million annual contacts they already had through the Medformation call center, Medica health plan, hospital admissions, and physician appointments. That reasoning supplied the foundation for Allina's on-line health and medical Web channel, Medformation.com (www.medformation.com), a community resource, which would also serve as an extension of the Medformation brand within a dynamic business model.

Allina selected Medformation.com as the name for its channel, taking the opportunity to build on its already well-known brand—the Medformation call center, which had been extensively advertised in billboard, radio, and print media. Allina's goal was to grow Medformation.com into the premier health and medical service center and on-line resource for the communities served by the Allina Health System in the upper Midwest. Medformation.com would leapfrog the competition by offering a *local* connection to health care services, resources, and transactions through the delivery of multiple applications, content services, interactivity, purchasing, and, over time, integration with legacy systems involved in care delivery. Medformation.com would also build on Allina's strong reputation as the leading regional health system and position the channel for placement on other on-line media outposts and distribution centers with leading regional Web portal operated by regional television stations and newspapers.

DEVELOPING AN E-STRATEGY

It is one thing to build a fully developed, integrated on-line health and medical Web channel; it is another thing to make it successful. In the good old e-days of "content is king," it was enough to have great content from reliable sources. But Allina realized that today's e-consumers expect more than that. On line health content is everywhere—now it is *service* and *function* that count. Allina decided to go beyond health and medical information and shoot for the future of health and medical service on the Web, as shown in Figure 10–3.

The left side of Figure 10–4 illustrates the professional process in handling a symptomatic consumer that could be seeking information and decision support

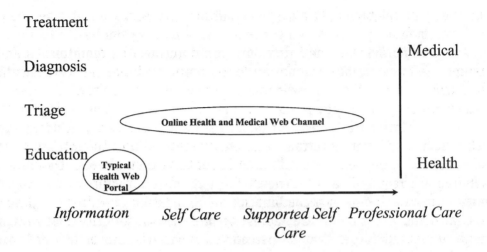

Figure 10–3 Online Channels Beyond Web Portals. *Source:* Copyright © 1999, Douglas Goldstein.

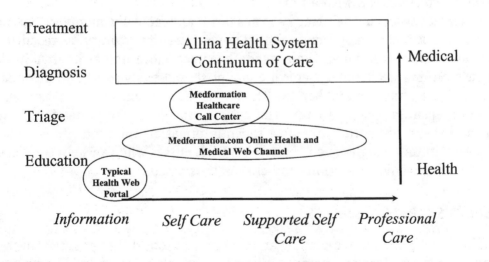

Figure 10–4 Medformation.com Integration with the Customer Care Call Center. *Source:* Copyright © 1999, Douglas Goldstein.

on line or by telephone. The gradient outlines the education, triage, diagnosis, and treatment steps taken as a consumer issue moves from health to medical for treatment by providers. The bottom gradient indicates the symptomatic patient's experience of accessing information, determining whether self-care is sufficient or do they need supported self-care, such as is given by a nurse in a health care call center or do they need professional attention. Most of the 15,000 health and medical Web sites are forced, for legal reason and the lack of a doctor–patient relationship, to be an entertainment/education medium. The symptomatic consumer of the twenty-first century is seeking answers and frequently professional services are required. An on-line medical channel integrates information and entertainment to deliver a combination of information, decision support, product sales and, most important, access to professional services within a community. Let us not forget that 85 percent of all health care dollars are spent on services, not pure information.

For a local health and medical Web channel to be successful, it must meet and exceed consumer needs and guide patients to the site of care in fewer stops. If e-consumers already log on to their local health and medical channel for information on juvenile diabetes, why not also offer them direct access to your health system's physicians, support groups, products, and other services over a Web channel over the telephone or in person? Does that e-consumer or e-patient have an immediate question? Open a telephonic link to a knowledgeable call center professional who can guide the patient to the answers he or she seeks through a telephone conversation with a nurse.

As Internet access in the home becomes faster and more commonplace through personal computers, televisions, and i-Phones, the opportunity to reach your customers and *really* meet their needs becomes more achievable. A health system's on-line health and medical channel should evolve its support of consumers with technology and bandwidth and move from text-based chat or rapid-response e-mail to real-time interaction with customer service professionals. The Web is a great medium to deliver low-touch information and products, but there is no substitute for high-touch connection with nurses who can help consumers with complex medical questions and cross self-services.

ALLINA'S E-STRATEGY EVOLVES

Allina had the vision to e-magine and e-plan for a robust Web channel that will bring patient care into the home. Allina's channel planning included a progressive version of what its information systems and patient support systems could realistically evolve on an annual basis within the context of a multiyear plan. But

Allina did not stop there. Company leaders envisioned an on-line channel of the future that offered immediate responses to the e-consumer and e-patient, integrated with physician offices and the health system services, and that served the health and medical needs of the entire community.

Allina recognized that this on-line channel effort was an ongoing development process that would grow and evolve along with the technology and consumer willingness to replace telephone calls with on-line communication, as Figure 10–4 illustrates. The phase one of the channel focused on positioning and building brand recognition. The important element of phase one was becoming known as the leading source of on-line health and medical information, e-products, and e-services for the Twin Cities region and the entire state of Minnesota. As phase one was being launched, the groundwork was laid for phase two, which offered even more robust services and increased functionality across a broader geographic area.

Figure 10–5 is a refined version of Figure 10–4 customized for Allina. It shows the integration of the on-line medical channel with a comprehensive 24-hour, seven-day per week health care call center (phone space), staffed by nurses and referral specialists who, in turn, are connected to site of care—both prevention and treatment.

POSITIONING AN ON-LINE HEALTH AND MEDICAL CHANNEL IN YOUR REGION

An element of a successful on-line health and medical channel is the assumption of certain levels of Web site volume, measured as "traffic," "page views," or "unique visitors." Viewership is key, not only because high viewership means that you are reaching motivated e-consumers and e-patients, but because it helps sell advertising and sponsorship—an integral factor for the channel's financial success. An integrated health care system has a built-in opportunity to generate traffic to its channel via patient contact promotions and call center referrals. But there are even more ways to build viewership and cultivate loyal patient-consumers who return to a Web site on a weekly or even daily basis. The keys to creating an on-line destination involve practical, useful, time and money saving "sticky" applications. In health care, this means helping consumers with their everyday health needs, whether it is purchasing diapers, refilling a prescription, or just helping with a symptom or condition. It also means understanding and addressing the needs of women who are the primary health care decision makers.

Repeat users and page view volume are key success factors for an on-line health and medical channel, because each drives direct revenue-generating ap-

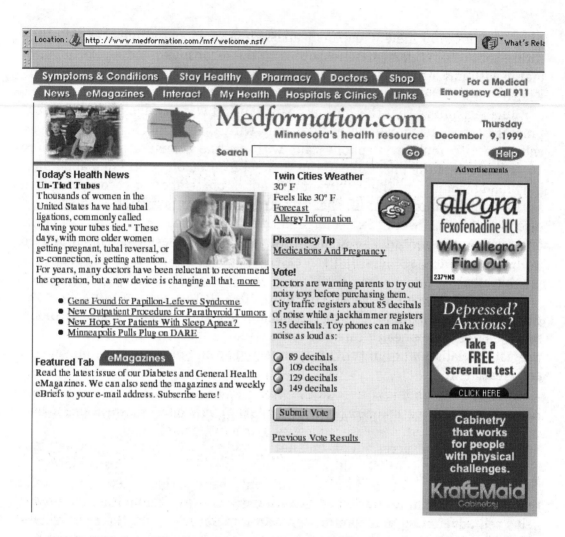

Figure 10–5 Meformation.com eMagazines Alert Users to News Items, Updates, and New Features. *Source:* Reprinted with permission from www.medformation.com/emagazines, © 1999, Allina Health Systems.

plications—such as increasing appropriate traffic to a hospital's outpatient services or scheduled appointments in doctors' offices, for example—and helps establish higher advertising and sponsorship rates. Also, high page view volume can ultimately result in an increase in hospital admissions, physician appointments, and health plan membership. Other benefits include value to the community, pull-through to existing system services, cross-sell and promotion of these services, and overall brand building.

The following are four major strategies with subtactics a health care organization can employ to increase traffic and usage of a Web channel:

1. Be the icon! Achieve wide exposure through cyber-outposts by taking a dominant position on high traffic regional Web portals, such as:

- Regional television and radio station Web sites
- Local telephone company home pages of their Internet services
- Local cable company home pages for high-speed cable modems
- Leading Internet service provider home pages

Today's typical on-line consumer enters the Web via the home page of his or her Internet service provider (ISP), cable modem, etc. Often, these consumers do not change their home page, so they see the ISP page first every time they log onto the Net. Through strategic positioning, a health care organization can be the meat behind the "Health" services or products Web buttons on these pages, driving additional viewers to your pages.

You can capture additional viewers and further build brand recognition for a robust Web channel through alliances with other high-traffic Web sites, such as newspaper, television, and radio station Web portals. Being the Health button on these pages reinforces your position as the leading provider of health and medical information, products, and services in a specific market.

2. Distribute Internet connect devices! Help consumers without access get on the Net through an interface you design.

- Distribute Internet-enabled information appliances. Through a large-scale sponsorship program, tens of thousands of Internet-enabled telephones, WebTV-type devices, or computers could be given away at point of care (discharge) to patients who otherwise would not have access. These devices would have a default icon or screen interface to your channel that would guide the majority of the health and medical e-communications, e-commerce, and e-care delivery needs of the patients.

3. Reach out to consumers the "e" way! Develop extensive channel webcasting (pushing information out to motivated viewers via the Web).

- Implement e-alerts—frequent e-mail messages to registered e-consumers who ask to be kept up-to-date on health topics that are important to them. As shown in Figure 10–5, the e-mail drives people back to sections of the channel for the story, product, or service.

- Deliver disease and condition focused e-magazines—consumers register to receive these periodic "magazines" via e-mail. The magazines can be centered around the clinical priorities of your health care organization and provide content as well as links to e-services.
- Generate special events notices—take advantage of additional traffic-building opportunities with notices and invitations to special events such as video/audio chats with experts, on-line seminars, and live surgeries.

4. Apply integrated marketing communication tactics.

Take advantage of every customer that your organization touches each year. Through its 14 million annual human contacts, Allina reaches over 50 percent of Minnesota's population multiple times. Allina is committed to integrating the Medformation.com Web channel with its off-line and on-line marketing communication efforts. Some key tactics include:

- Doing extensive piggyback marketing. Take advantage of the print collateral a health system produces every day. Display your channel uniform resource locator (URL) on billboards, radio ads, television ads, banners, flyers, and so on. These ads are being run by your system anyway—get your URL on there, too.
- Cross-selling through medical call centers and other promotions. Take advantage of your existing call center communications. Callers who are put on hold can hear about the latest offerings on your Web channel. Users who receive mailings can see your URL printed on the correspondence and know they can log onto the Web to receive information as well. Cross-sell through:
  —On hold messages
  —Voice reminders during calls
  —URL on mailed information
- Harnessing the power of existing customers. Your organization has customer databases with telephone numbers, but have you collected customers' e-mail addresses at work and at home? Get the word out and build e-databases via:
  —Patient registration e-mail capture with affiliated physicians
  —Hospital registration e-mail capture
  —Human contacts at all your facilities
  —System events, classes, health fairs
  —In-office and in-hospital promotions

Success in building Web traffic depends on an assertive and comprehensive database development and marketing plan. This means building a valuable customer database that you can use to promote your services. It also means limiting what you pay someone else for eyeballs when you can use your existing customer database through enhanced e-mail capture. Naturally, these strategies and tactics will vary whether you are a health system or medical products manufacturers, but principles and ideas can serve as foundations for your e-marketing plan.

PROMOTING MEDFORMATION.COM

Allina's Medformation.com channel e-team was made up of a cross-disciplinary group of information services, clinical (call center staff, physician medical officer), marketing decision makers, and key consultants from Medical Alliances, Inc. From the very first day, this team worked closely to coordinate channel development stages with other system initiatives.

Allina knew that its advertising and sponsorship sales depended on the ability to demonstrate e-consumer volume on the channel. Allina needed to do more than register its on-line channel in the well-known search engines; it needed to get the word out by every means possible that Medformation.com was Minnesota's most valuable source for on-line health and medical resource.

Allina took a multipronged approach to strategically position its channel. E-media outposts were identified: local television stations, radio stations, and newspapers with high-volume regional Web portals. Allina approached these outposts with the opportunity to make Medformation.com the Health button on their home pages and the rationale that this community resource would better serve customers. A reciprocal link strategy was effective because Allina would already generate a significant volume of direct traffic to its channel via its piggyback marketing strategy, so it was a win-win situation for the e-media outposts.

Next came Allina's actual piggyback or print marketing strategy. Representatives from the channel team coordinated with Allina's marketing and promotion department. A significant budget was established for revising existing marketing communications to reflect the URL for the Medformation.com channel. Most communications that went out from Allina—whether it was from the call center, the hospitals and clinics, billing, or affiliated Allina medical groups—would display the channel's URL: www.medformation.com, just as it would list key telephone numbers to call. In addition, the marketing department developed a takeaway card that featured five things a person could do at Medformation.com. This card, which was distributed through physicians' offices, was small enough to fit into a person's wallet and listed such things as "sign up for an aerobics class," "join an on-line support group," "renew a prescription," and "make a doctor's appointment."

Allina's strategy was to reach e-consumers and e-patients in every way possible and to promote Medformation.com as the leading source of on-line health and medical resources and services in their markets.

BE THE E-MEDIUM: USE YOUR OWN EYEBALLS

The secret behind the strategy for building page-view volume on an on-line health and medical channel is to make the decision to leverage your own patient and consumer relationships. Why pay a national Web portal or site for a link to your site? Rather than being just another advertiser buying eyeballs back from a third party, your health care organization is in the unique and enviable position of being able to *be* the e-medium that reaches out to e-consumers and e-patients in your area.

For example, Mary Smith lives in Minneapolis, Minnesota. Mary is looking for information on the chickenpox vaccine and a doctor who can administer it. She logs on to her computer through her telephone company's Internet service or America Online and clicks on the *Health* button and searches for information on chickenpox. She finds out about the vaccination, possible side effects, and recent recommendations regarding the diagnosis. But Mary wants to know more. Should she get her child vaccinated? What is the best age to receive the shot? Should she just let her child experience the chickenpox virus naturally? As it is now, Mary can receive most of the information she needs on line from national health Web portals. But where does Mary go for more? In this scenario, nowhere; perhaps a referral, but in the beginning of the twenty-first century, she does not get an appointment from most health Web portals.

Consider this better alternative.

Mary sits down at her computer and logs on via a local ISP. The browser window opens to the ISP's default home page, where Mary sees a *Health* button. She clicks on this button and is immediately transported to her local hospital system's regional health and medical Web channel. Mary searches for and finds most of the information she needs on the chickenpox vaccine—but she still has questions. Mary sees on her screen a message that prompts her to click for more information. She clicks and a window opens on her screen and she hears a voice through her computer speakers that welcomes her and says something like, "I see you're searching for information on the chickenpox vaccine. How can I help you?"

Mary asks her questions. The medical call center professional (nurse or referral specialist) on the other end gives her some of the additional answers and suggests that if Mary still has questions she should make an appointment with her family physician. When Mary indicates that she does not have a family physician, the call center person offers to find one for her who has convenient hours and is also on Mary's health plan. The call center person finds a physician and even schedules Mary's first appointment.

This entire transaction takes place on line via the on-line health and medical channel. An e-consumer searches for information, finds what she wants, and interacts with a professional from a health care organization. Through advanced Web technology, the e-consumer's needs are met and satisfied. Mary gets everything she needs in the course of a few minutes. When Mary visits her new family physician, she will go in more informed and comfortable—thereby starting off the new relationship positively for Mary, her family, and her new physician.

Best of all, through the efforts of Mary's regional hospital system, she is guided toward reliable information from a trusted source and effortlessly linked to care on a local level. If Mary had stayed with the national Web portal in 1999, she could have been stranded in a sea of information, but little service. The national portal could only give her what she needed to a point, and then she was on her own. Mary's local system, however, took advantage of its position and brand in the marketplace, employed an effective outpost strategy, and captured Mary's business.

It is up to you as a health care provider to capitalize on your own position within a region and aggressively launch e-services in cyberspace. Research shows that high numbers of people are searching for health and medical information on line with the majority of these consumers being symptomatic. If you do not provide the information and services they seek in that space, they will turn to other sources. Today's on-line consumers are becoming more and more sophisticated, and they expect more than simple information. They want products and they want fast access to care and experts. This is the age of e-commerce—easy e-transactions and personalized service using personal computers, interactive television, and interactive telephones (Exhibit 10–2).

During e-Christmas 1998, the Gap retail stores had huge banners in their Christmas windows displaying the phrase "Surf, Shop, Ship" along with their Web address, www.gap.com. The Gap figured if consumers were going to spend billions on line that, rather than ignore the e-trend, they would promote and capture on-line sales. The analogy to health care and the positioning for Medformation.com is

- Click (Web)
- Call (telephone)
- Contact (visit)

- e-Care

Exhibit 10–2 Comparison of Web Channel e-Positioning versus Gap.com.

Medformation.com e-Positioning	
www.Gap.com	www.Medformation.com
– Surf	– Click (Web)
– Shop	– Call (Phone)
– Ship	– Contact (Visit)
= Spend	= Care

Source: Copyright © 1999, Douglas Goldstein.

through the integration of key customer marketing and support systems. The bottom line goal for Medformation.com is care—better, faster, and more direct than competitive health Web sites and portals.

As a health system, it is in your best interest to position yourself now as the leading source of on-line health and medical information and services in your region. Take advantage of your contacts—merge phone space, air space, and cyberspace to reach e-consumers and e-patients in every possible way. If you do not act now to position yourself in this rapidly evolving medium, a competing organization will. And when someone else claims that space, you will find yourself scrambling to recapture the e-consumers and e-patients who were yours to begin with but whom you lost to the competitor across town.

Allina knew its competition and knew that if it wanted to maintain a leadership position in the community, it had to respond to the quickly growing population of local on-line consumers and patients. Its philosophy of proactive relationship building and offering the best possible care to its communities led Allina to pursue this novel and sensible approach to offering another level of care to its patients. Allina's multimedia approach was just one more way that this trailblazing system could reach its population. Use Allina as a benchmark as you outline key initiates for your health health care organization's Web initiatives (Exhibit 10–3).

Exhibit 10-3 Key Initiatives for Your Channel

Be the leading source of on-line health and medical e-care in your region:

- Create a recognized brand or extend one of your health organization's existing brands.
- Deliver multiple services and functions to meet your e-customers' health and medical needs and encourage repeated use.
- Provide a high-traffic, multiservice gateway and medical destination.
- Offer extensive search capabilities, health resources, service providers, self-care products, and other transactions for daily health care needs.

Source: Copyright © 1999, Douglas Goldstein.

CONCLUSION—ACT NOW!

Do not delay in staking your claim in the expanding frontier of Web space with an aggressive e-strategy! Every day, the face of the Internet universe is changing. More and more people are coming on line doing more and more things, and their needs and wants are becoming more sophisticated. The time to establish your e-services, build brand presence, and capture your market is *now*. As more and more organizations, from drugstore.com to on-line Amazon.com, move into the space of providing health and medical information and products, it is imperative that you guarantee your spot as the leading source not only for health and medical information and products, but for e-care as well. You owe it to e-consumers and e-patients to provide reliable e-information, e-products, and e-services that meet their needs as they surf for health care information and services for themselves and their families.

REFERENCES

1. IntelliQuest press release, http://www.intelliquest.com/press/release (3 March 1999).
2. IntelliQuest press release (3 March 1999).
3. "Online Shopping Growing Steadily, Lack of Connectivity a Barrier," http://www.cyberatlas.com/market/retailing/young.html.
4. Harris Poll #11, "Explosive Growth of a New Breed of 'Cyberchondriacs,'" http://www.louisharris.com/poll_fr.htm.1.

CHAPTER 11

Meet the Empowered, Interactive SuperNet Woman

Cheryl L. Toth and Kathi Marshall

WHO ARE THE HOTTEST e-consumers on the Internet? The short answer is women.

By now it is no surprise that the number of women using the Internet has grown significantly since 1995, when the Internet was primarily surfed by men. Cyber Dialogue reported that in 1998, 42 percent of Internet users were female—up from 20 percent in 1995. America Online claims that 51 percent of its 13 million members are female—up from only 16 percent four years ago.[1] Exhibit 11–1 gives a profile of the typical on-line woman: an empowered decision maker and purchaser of goods and services on the Net.

The Internet has empowered these "interactive" women—64 percent of whom work full time and 54 percent of whom are moms[2]—to make a variety of important decisions for themselves and their families. Trade stocks and manage the family's portfolio? She does it. Purchase vitamins, over-the-counter drugs, and gifts on line? Yes. Hunt for and download information about cancer prevention, her child's attention deficit hyperactivity disorder (ADHD), or her husband's intimacy issues? You bet.

Exhibit 11–1 Profile of SuperNet Woman

- The average female Internet user is 41 years old and has a household income of $63,000.
- 64 percent of women on the Internet work full time, and 54 percent are moms.
- Women Internet users spend an average of six hours on line per week.

Courtesy of NetSmart Research, 1998, New York, New York.

This chapter outlines some of the significant empowerment trends for women, as well as their increasing use of the Web as an interactive information-gathering tool. An understanding of this interactive consumer—we call her SuperNet Woman—is critical for physicians and health care executives who are targeting e-services and e-products to women on line. Use some of the examples from nonhealth care companies and commercial Web sites discussed in this chapter as your e-team targets women on line.

MOVE OVER WARD—JUNE'S IN CHARGE

June Cleaver she is not. Today's American woman makes many decisions on her own, without direction or oversight from the man in her life. She is an increasingly sought-after consumer and is seen as a major decision maker when it comes to household products, financial endeavors, and health care. There are several reasons for this, some of which are listed in Exhibit 11–2 and described below.

The first reason is a commonly cited statistic: America's 52 percent divorce rate. In 1998, 19.4 million American adults were divorced, according to the Census Bureau, which means that more than 9 million divorced adults were women.[3] Divorced women do not have a partner with whom they share decision making. Before divorcing in their 40s or 50s, some women may have had their household authority hampered or limited by husbands who insisted on being the head of the family. Many of these divorced women are able to make their own decisions for the first time in their lives—and they are taking advantage of their newfound freedom.

Single-parent households are another area where women have become—not always by choice—the primary caregiver, wage earner, and decision maker. The

---

Exhibit 11–2 Empowered Decision Makers

- 22.9 percent of married couples identify the woman as the "householder."
- 16.6 million children live in homes where the mother is the only parent.
- Nearly half of women over age 65 are widowed, and 70.1 percent of them live alone.
- Two-thirds of working women say they earn half or more of their family's income.
- A majority of married women say they earn half or more of their family's income.

Source: Data from The Official Statistics, October 29, 1998, Census Bureau and Working Woman Survey, AFL-CIO, 1997.

majority of the 19.8 million children under age 18 who live in single-parent households live with their mothers—84.1 percent.[4] And women are increasingly being identified as head of household even if they *are* married. The proportion of married couples that identified the woman as the householder tripled in eight years, from 7.4 percent in 1990 to 22.9 percent in 1998.[5]

Women also live longer than men. The average length of life for women is 79 years, versus 72 for men; thus, women often outlive their husbands. In fact, in 1998, nearly half of women 65 years and older were widows. Of these women, 70.1 percent lived alone in 1998 and made daily decisions autonomously.[6] Many of these empowered women have become so later in life; theirs was a generation in which women typically married early, became housewives and mothers, and had "breadwinner" husbands. Many widowed women over age 65 must overcome personal and generational culture issues to empower themselves—and many of them have done just that.

Finally, women are simply waiting longer to get married. In 1998, among people 25–34 years old, 13.6 million had never been married—that is 35 percent of the entire age group.[7] The women in this age group—some of them Generation X, some of them Baby Busters—were infants and toddlers during the 1960s civil rights movement and radical feminism days. These Brady Bunch generations were raised by women who worked and were not always home when they came home from school. They grew up to be more independent than previous generations. If they had to take care of their own dinner, safety, and recreation as youngsters, why wouldn't they do so as adults? Further, the girls in these generations were educated side-by-side with the boys, and got the message that they were just as capable of pursuing a career as a physician, lawyer, scientist, astronaut, or government official. Delaying or forgoing marriage is one way to pursue career opportunities.

EMPLOYED, WITH MONEY TO SPEND

Across the United States, women are altering the landscape of the American workplace. Women accounted for 46.2 percent of total labor force participants in 1997 and will make up 48 percent by the year 2005, according to the Bureau of Labor.[8] They have raised their families' standard of living by entering the work force and have increased their family's median income by 25 percent over the past three decades. Their efforts at the office have led to job sharing, flexible hours, and child care initiatives.

Women also lead the entrepreneurial boom—starting businesses at twice the national average. There are 8.5 million woman-owned companies in the United

States, with sales totaling $3.1 trillion in 1997.[9] These women entrepreneurs are changing the face of how America works, and they are making decisions about which benefits—including health care plans—to offer their employees. Although the wage gap still exists (in 1996 women earned 74 cents for every dollar earned by men), it is narrowing.[10] Empowered women earn and spend their own money.

Working Woman magazine (Figure 11–1), long an important reference for American women in the workforce, understands the power and influence of these women and has a successful, on-line version of its publication. WomenConnect service offers visitors information about their money, career, politics, and health. Surveys query women visitors about pressing business issues and salary information. The WomenConnect network also offers a search feature to help visitors locate articles in other women's publications (Figure 11–2).

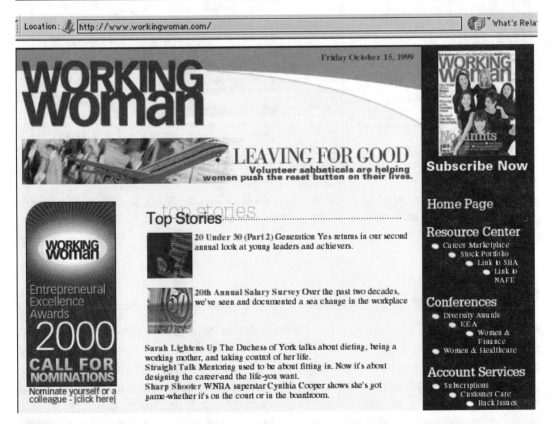

Figure 11–1 *Working Woman* Magazine Online. *Source:* Reprinted with permission from www.workingwoman.com, © 1999, Working Woman Magazine Online. For subscriptions call 1-800-234-9675.

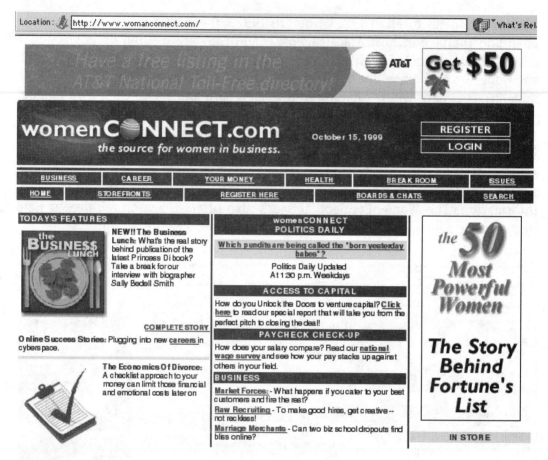

Figure 11–2 WomenConnect—A Useful Resource for Women in Business. *Source:* Reprinted with permission from www.womenconnect.com, © 1999, Women Connect.com.

IN CONTROL OF THE PURSE STRINGS

Women are fast becoming the chief financial officers of American families. About two-thirds of women surveyed in a 1998 *Working Mother* survey say they are in charge of managing the family's overall finances and spending. Sixty-three percent of working mothers say they are responsible for creating the household budget (when there is one), and 68 percent of working mothers say they are solely responsible for balancing the checkbook. A similar number pay the mortgage or rent and other household bills, and 55 percent prepare the household's tax returns.[11] By taking over these and other financial tasks, working mothers have acquired the power to set their families' monetary priorities—and part of this financial decision making includes health care expenditures.

Half of all working mothers say they are responsible for finding and analyzing promising new investments. Sixty-three percent of women in the *Working Mother* survey say they have faith in their ability to save and invest wisely or are becoming more active in managing their family's investments. In fact, PaineWebber reports that 42 percent of U.S. investors are women.[12] And, like the Beardstown Ladies, women are empowering their own investment decisions by initiating or joining local investment clubs. According to the National Association of Investors Corporation, women's clubs enjoyed an average return of 17.9 percent in 1997—beating the returns of both mixed and men-only clubs (17.3 percent and 15.6 percent, respectively).[13]

To attract financially savvy SuperNet women to its commercial site, Women's Wire (www.womenswire.com) dedicates an entire section to women and money management. This section includes tips about budgeting, financial planning, taxes, and retirement, alongside stock market indicators. It even includes Bloomberg's Women.com 30 Index—the first stock index ever to track top publicly traded companies headed by women.

IT HAS TO BE CONVENIENT

Ask just about any American woman about the way she likes to experience retail, health care, and any other service and she will tell you, "It has to be fast and convenient." With 42.7 percent of all families classified as dual-earners in 1996 (up from 20.4 percent in 1950), today's American woman does not have a lot of free time.[14] A full-time job, kids in tow, and a household to manage keep her plenty busy. The AFL-CIO's 1997 "Ask a Working Woman" survey concluded that time is in short supply for women. Survey respondents reported that they are working more hours than ever before. Most reported they are juggling work and family and have children at home or elderly relatives for whom they are caretakers.

In fact, 42 percent of women are concerned about work/life balance, compared with only 36 percent of men.[15] These women do not have time to stand in line, pore over reams of information, or wait for an hour in a physician's office. They have things to do, mouths to feed, and children to nurture. E-commerce offers these women a quick and convenient way to gather information and shop for products and services according to their own schedules. Health care companies must realize that the old days—when patients waited for extended periods of time to see the physician or took what the physician or health care provider said as the only explanation or care option—are over. Care delivery must evolve to meet the convenience and communication needs of America's new millennium woman. Success means rolling out health care e-commerce and e-care services.

EMPOWERED WOMEN ARE INTERACTIVE WOMEN

The empowerment trend marches on, as more and more women access the Web. If you thought authority over household decisions has come a long way for women, just watch as the Internet continues to explode. From a health care perspective, women are an important target market. Not only do they make up more than 50 percent of the American population, but they also make most of a family's medical decisions, use more health care services than men, and tend to maintain strong long-term relationships with their physicians. With the advent of the Web and women's increased access to information, women will become an even more powerful force as householder, mother, employee, and caregiver.

Health care executives and providers cannot afford not to target women consumers on the Net. If your health system, plan, or practice does not act quickly, commercial health care Web portals will continue to gobble up female on-line market share. What does that mean for your health care organization? It means that as the commercial Web sites focus more and more on women, and on health care, they stand to become the portals of choice for many women. Brands such as iVillage's allHealth (www.allhealth.com) and drkoop will become the first choice for women when they log on. What these brands will offer in the future is anyone's guess, but it is easy to see that they could offer health care services that will compete with local brands.

BUSTING OLD INTERNET PARADIGMS

If your organization already has a Web presence that offers information about your organization, an e-newsletter, and a physician finder, you have taken the first steps. But what does your health care company offer specifically for women? Have you targeted the SuperNet Woman niche, or is your Web site trying to provide information to everyone who clicks through it? If you do not specifically target the SuperNet Woman niche, it is time to explore this lucrative market. Following is information about how to do so successfully.

First, forget the theory that women use the Internet primarily for community—that theory is outdated. Women do more than simply surf around and post messages on bulletin boards. In fact, they spend as much time purchasing as their male counterparts, and spend more money overall. The fact that nearly 43 percent of American jobs are held by women, and that the wage gap continues to narrow, means that women have plenty of their own money to spend. Women have significant purchasing power and account for 70 percent of all retail sales; any smart consumer products executive is aggressively focused on how to attract the female buyer. An October 1998 survey of 1,016 adults, conducted for Clinique by Bruskin/Goldring Research, found these results for SuperNet Woman's on-line purchasing behavior:[16]

- *Women purchase at the same rate as men.* The percentage of men versus women with Internet access who have purchased on line is roughly the same—35 percent of women, 37 percent of men.
- *Women buy more.* Female buyers tend to purchase basic items such as books and music, but they tend to buy more than men do.
- *Women spend more.* The highest percentage of women shoppers (18 percent) report spending $100 to $200 per purchase, while the highest percentage of male shoppers (26 percent) spent $25 to $50.

The study also suggests that women want convenience when they shop on line. Among women, 52 percent who shop on line prefer to do it after 5 PM; 20 percent, after 8 PM. Similarly, 47 percent of men shop after 5 PM, while 19 percent shop after 8 PM. Your Web e-commerce service could offer a variety of health-related products—for example, supplements, books about prenatal care, or skin care protection products. The convenience of buying these products on line, at any hour women choose to shop, is appealing.

Create a Web service that also focuses on building relationships with women on line. Women like to customize information for their own needs and be remembered when they come back. Offering something similar to Amazon's OneClick service—whereby a customer establishes an account and subsequent purchases are made literally with one click—is a way of doing this. And since women like the opportunity to share ideas and hear opinions from other women, building message boards or interactive discussion groups can keep them coming back.

Similar to her desire in "real space," SuperNet Woman likes to contribute and be a part of something worthwhile. For example, women appreciate learning how to handle their teenager's rage from other moms who have had the same parenting experience. Women like to offer information about the breast cancer support group they found helpful when they were first diagnosed with the disease. They want to read practical information about how to provide nutritious meals for their families, and they are typically happy to complete a survey about women's issues. It is crucial to understand, however, that women do not like feeling as if they have been "sold." Boldly pushing a product will not excite female visitors; offering information and a sense of community is much more likely to bring them back.

SMART COMPANIES CASH IN

The secret is out: e-retailers know SuperNet Woman exists, she has money to spend, and she is making decisions that affect her and her family's daily life. Internet start-ups and brick and mortar companies alike are clamoring for a portion of SuperNet Woman's clicks.

Point your browser to an obvious women's site—www.women.com—and you will enter a network that has been around since 1992. The network offers interactive content in areas such as careers, relationships and sex, fashion, family, small business—as well as health and fitness.

Oxygen Media is another company that hopes to ride the wave of empowered on-line female consumers. It owns Moms Online, an interactive community for moms (www.momsonline.com); Electra, which describes itself as "women's survival guide to life" (www.electra.com); and Thrive (http://www.thriveonline.com), a site focused on women's health and well-being. Oxygen Media CEO Geraldine Laybourne, a former Disney and Nickelodeon programmer, envisions "a media revolution led by women and kids." She is betting that the Web will become a place where women communicate, shop, and look for information that has historically been found in women's health, beauty, and fashion magazines.

Online community iVillage.com (www.iVillage.com) is actually a network of Web sites that cater to women. One of the first national portals to recognize the complex needs of women, iVillage has assembled a community that offers women information about money management, travel, relationships, business and family issues, and much more. The service has deftly built, bought, or partnered with sites such as ParentSoup (www.parentsoup.com), instead of attempting to reinvent the wheel on content. In early 1999, iVillage became a publicly traded company and began running cutting-edge television commercials with images of interesting and varied women sharing their needs and desires with the camera. iVillage may end up being the Amazon.com of women's on-line communities; it should be bookmarked by anyone who markets products or services to women.

Companies that already have brand name awareness—L'eggs Pantyhose, for example—have begun to capture the unique interests of women too. The L'eggs Web site does more than just talk about pantyhose. Using (dare we say it?) "sheer energy" and a humorous writing style, the L'eggs Women's In.Sight Web service (www.leggs.com) offers content about how pantyhose are made, as well as how to recycle and reuse the perishable fashion items when they give way to nasty runs. To keep women coming back, the Web service lays out lively interviews and articles about politics, personal finance, fashion, health, and fitness. There is even a L'eggs Egg Game for those who think they are experts at the old Shell Game. Oh—and women can shop for products on line too. L'eggs has created an interactive environment where product purchases become almost secondary to the fun visitors have.

WOMEN'S HEALTH WEB SITES ARE FOLLOWING SUIT

Even a simple search of frequently visited women's on-line communities should send a strong message to health care executives and providers: women are searching for health care content and solutions on line. Cyberspace is the great new frontier that allows women to anonymously—and autonomously—surf for information about even "forbidden" health topics such as a low sex drive, lumpy breasts, or an eating disorder. Many women do not feel comfortable discussing certain serious health problems with their physicians, for fear these concerns may be dismissed as "overly emotional" or "all in their heads." Who can blame them? For years, medical research studies have not included women, and physicians have made light of women's symptoms. The Web empowers these women to seek information and answers—on their own, in the privacy of their own homes—that may help them or may lead to a physician who will respect them.

A plethora of women's health information already exists on the Web, and sites that carry it pull hundreds of thousands of eyeballs each month. According to Media Metrix, two such sites—allHealth and Mayo Health Oasis—scored 688,000 and 430,000 unique monthly visitors, respectively.[17] Both sites are filled with practical, printable information that is specific to women's health needs. allHealth (Figure 11-3), which is part of iVillage, contains reams of information on subjects from Alzheimer's to pets, relationships, and working from home. iVillage also encourages visitors to speak their minds on a variety of subjects— feminism and how to motivate yourself to exercise are just two examples. Women post their thoughts, which creates an on-line community where visitors can periodically review the latest postings.

The Mayo Clinic's Health Oasis (Figure 11-4) guarantees "Reliable Information for a Healthier Life," based on its world-renowned physicians and the Mayo brand. The site ties together information about pregnancy, diet and nutrition, and children's health, using headline news, articles written by Mayo providers, and a series of quizzes—the "Poop Quiz," for example, helps moms determine whether or not their child has serious bowel trouble. Mayo also opened a

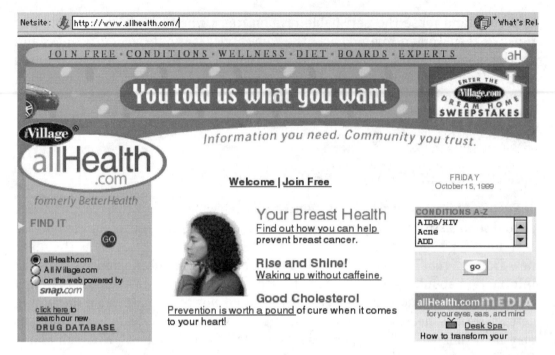

Figure 11–3 allHealth.com. *Source:* Reprinted with permission from www.allhealth.com, © 1999, iVillage.com.

Women's Health Center in Scottsdale, Arizona, in 1997 to further its quest of meeting women's health needs—in "real space."

Even traditional publishers have gotten into the act by offering women's health content. The *New York Times* Women's Health service (www.nytimes.com/specials/women/home/index.html) features medical news and information with little transactional quality but some decent content.

Late in 1998, yet another national health care community launched an on-line service. Dr. Koop Online, and specifically drkoop's Women's Health Resource page (www.drkoop.com/womens), is a heavily traveled site that offers trustworthy brand name awareness and goes far beyond merely offering women's health content. In addition to health information, this interactive Web service offers more than 90 on-line support groups; has regular chat sessions on topics such as ADHD, menopause, and prenatal care; and entices visitors with interactive learning tools, such as the Allergy Learning Lab. Consumers can create a "My Health" personal page by providing health and lifestyle information about themselves.

But think about what all these sites are offering: primarily, they offer information and content. That is fine if SuperNet Woman is doing research, but what if she wants to actually complete a health care transaction? What if she wants to schedule an appointment with the local obstetrician/gynecologist, listen to an audio stream about pediatric asthma from her child's allergist, or get a prescription refilled? National Web portals cannot execute such transactions today—your local or regional health care organization can. But if your company does not get organized quickly for e-commerce and e-care, the health and services content served up by national Web portals could attract SuperNet Woman away from your local health care organization. Further, although the national sites are prohibited from officially providing medical advice, who is to say that SuperNet Woman

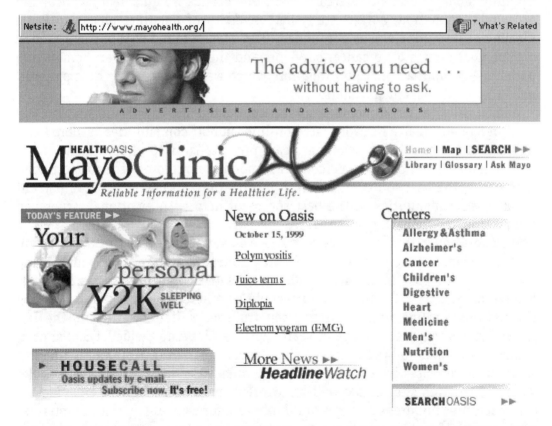

Figure 11–4 Mayo Clinic: A Recognized Health Care Brand. *Source:* Reprinted from Mayo Clinic Health Oasis (www.mayohealth.org) with permission of Mayo Foundation for Medical Education and Research, Rochester, MN 55905.

does not print the information in lieu of scheduling an appointment with a local physician? The result could be a gap in care delivery.

Court SuperNet Woman in cyberspace before the national Web portals expand further. Your health system, regional plan, or practice must attract these savvy Web surfers with interactive and practical information and e-services—or you risk losing them to the national women's Web portals.

ON-LINE SUPPORT GROUPS HELP WOMEN COPE

We have established that women seek relationships, in real space and in cyberspace. A growing list of on-line support groups has responded to this need and formed an intricate network of places for women to be heard as well as to become educated about the illnesses they or their families face. Although medical professionals originally feared that on-line groups would spread medical and other misinformation, a 1998 study by University of Delaware physician Paula Klemm negated this claim as unfounded.[18] Dr. Klemm found that participating in on-line chat groups gave cancer survivors and their families—even homebound patients—24-hour access to information, which was important to these patients' need to feel connected to others.

Additionally, a 1,000-member survey conducted by Tom Ferguson and Bill Kelly of Sapient Health Network rated on-line support communities as more helpful than either specialists or primary care physicians in 10 of 12 dimensions of health care.[19] Seventy-seven percent of respondents rated on-line support communities as the best source of in-depth information; 75 percent and 52 percent rated these communities as the best source of help with emotional issues and compassion and empathy, respectively.

It is no wonder that there are so many Web services devoted to on-line support. E-patients can log on anonymously 24 hours a day to receive feedback and support—or to post information—about a health condition they share with thousands of others. Particularly for people who are homebound as a result of their illness, on-line support groups can truly be a lifeline. Entering the key words "cancer, support, group" at search engine AltaVista yielded 1,520 sites in March 1999. Links to breast cancer, skin cancer, ovarian cancer, and lymphoma came up. Many sites have extensive list of links to additional information. For example, the Web site for the well-known real-space breast cancer organization Y-Me? features hundreds of pages of information for women and their families, as well as a list of additional resources.

Commercial companies have also created on-line environments for women. Avon, for example, has led a crusade against breast cancer since 1993.

AvonCrusade.com is the Web community where Avon provides information about its pink ribbon program about the disease (www.avoncrusade.com). Bio-Portraits, Inc. (Figure 11–5), a manufacturer of custom breast prostheses, serves up information about women's options after mastectomy. This Web service has an interactive feature that allows a woman to easily write her senator or representative and request that a breast prosthesis be reimbursable by all insurance plans, just as reconstructive surgery typically is. This feature is interactive and empowering, and allows women facing breast cancer (or those who are interested in supporting this cause) to have a collective voice. Such an opportunity was much more time-consuming before the Web.

In air space and cyberspace, women like to congregate to share information and experiences, and to offer advice. On-line support communities take the centuries' old tradition of these kinds of female gatherings to a new level, one where distance and time do not matter. SuperNet Woman can seek and receive support for any number of issues on line, at any time of day or night. Is your health care company taking advantage of building a relationship with SuperNet Woman via on-line support groups? Are there places for her to go to learn more about her child's allergies, menopause, and caring for her husband's health needs? A place

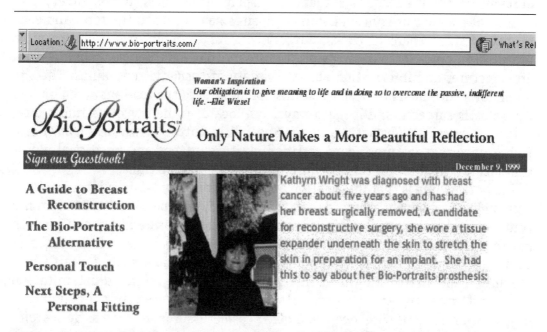

Figure 11–5 Bio-Portraits: Explore Surgical and Prosthetic Options Interactively. *Source:* Reprinted with permission from www.bio-portraits.com, © 1999, Bio-Portraits, Inc.

where she can share her own stories, too? Interactive, on-line support communities are appreciated and used by women. Consider adding a support group dimension to your company's Web service.

NIPS AND TUCKS

Each year, hundreds of thousands of plastic surgery procedures are performed in the United States, most of them on women. In both air space and cyberspace, women have been freed from the stigma that used to accompany plastic surgery, and they are purchasing more procedures than ever before. The Web offers women the ability to research the procedures in which they are interested, locate plastic surgeons in their area, and learn about the importance of board certification.

When it comes to information about cosmetic surgery procedures, the Web has plenty of it, on a variety of plastic-surgery-specific sites. Plastic surgeons are Internet pioneers in the physician community—many of them already have a Web site for their own practice and have had it for several years. Most of these sites are not transactional, however; they serve primarily as marketing ventures that display colorful photos and graphics, and promote the surgeon and his or her services. For a small fee, the American Society for Plastic and Reconstructive Surgeons makes it easy for a surgeon to display his or her own Web page.

Several plastic surgery commercial Web sites have come to the fore, and each receives its fair share of clicks. Surgery.com for example, owns the premium universal resource locator—www.plasticsurgery.com—and serves up before-and-after pictures and information about a variety of cosmetic procedures. The site also allows consumers to post questions about surgery that are answered on line by a plastic surgeon, and it has a physician locator to help visitors find a local surgeon. America's Cosmetic Surgery Specialists (http://www.acss.com/) is a Web service that features board certified plastic surgeons and a national physician locator, in addition to procedure information and pictures.

The bottom line is that information about this formerly taboo subject is widely accessible—and widely accessed—on the Internet. If SuperNet Woman, who has control over her discretionary income, decides to have cosmetic surgery, you can bet that she will research the procedures that interest her, as well as local surgeons' credentials. This empowered woman will not make such a health care purchase impulsively. She will do her homework and be informed before taking the final step toward surgery. How successfully are your health care organization's plastic surgeons—and other cosmetic surgeons such as dermatologists—positioned? An effective Web presence can promote not only the physicians, but ambulatory surgery centers and other facilities as well.

OLDER WOMEN ARE ON THE NET, TOO

Fifty-seven-year-old Brenda Wellington knew where to get more information after her elderly mother was diagnosed with Alzheimer's. "Her doctor was talking about a certain treatment, and I thought to myself, 'Well, I'm going to go and check this out." Brenda logged onto a variety of sites that offered comprehensive information about the disease, the drugs used to treat it, and how family members can cope. Mayo Clinic's Health Oasis (www.mayohealth.org) was a great resource for Brenda, "I joined an on-line support group that made me realize I wasn't the only one going through all this."

Brenda is one of a number of older women finding their way onto the Internet. A new study estimates that one of the fastest-growing groups on line is women over age 50. The study showed an increase of 50 percent in the number of American women over 50 years old using the Internet during the nine months ending in June 1998; there were 5 million of these users.[20] Many of these women go on line to e-mail their children as well as to surf the Net.

With Net access getting easier and easier—for example, the interactive television service WebTV does not even require a keyboard—older Americans have become less intimidated by the technology and are eager to see what it offers. The American Association of Retired Persons (AARP) has created a "Web place" that offers a myriad of health, financial, and technology information (www.aarp.org). National Web portals such as Excite.com offer a Seniors' Health channel that includes information on disease states such as Alzheimer's and interactive message boards.

With more and more senior women getting on line, what is your health care organization doing to reach them? Review your e-strategies. What is being done to cater to and deliver information and e-services to older women? Considering the health needs of this population, there are many pieces of information that can be delivered to keep these SuperNet Women healthy and well. A tailored e-newsletter about senior health and nutrition, a video Web feed that focuses on joint replacement surgery, or an interactive assessment that rates their nutritional wellness are all opportunities and good options.

DAUGHTERS BECOME EMPOWERED CAREGIVERS

For the 76 million Baby Boomers born between 1946 and 1964, caregiving has become the new midlife crisis. As has been the case in many cultures for thousands of years, when an elderly parent or relative is unable to care for him- or herself, it is usually the women in the family who provide the care. In the past, this caregiving was one of women's primary duties. But, Baby Boomers and other women now juggle full-time careers, household management, and often a family of their own. And because women in the Baby Boom generation typically had their children later in life than their mother's generation did, many women have found themselves "sandwiched" between elder care and child care.

In the United States today, about 75 percent of these caregivers are women. Fifty-seven percent are wives caring for their husbands; the rest are daughters looking after a mother or father.[21] The story that Marsha tells in Exhibit 11–3 is a common tale.

The Women's Bureau of the Department of Labor profiles the typical informal caregiver as an employed 46-year-old woman who spends 18 hours a week caring

---

Exhibit 11–3 Women Caregivers Come to Elderly Parents' Aid

Baby Boomer Marsha Zandbergen faced a situation many in her generation do. Her mother was beginning to have difficulty taking care of herself, and her eyesight started to diminish. "I'm an only child, so the responsibility was mine to care for her," Marsha says. A registered nurse, Marsha had also taken care of her father before his death.

Like 7 million other children who care for elderly parents, Marsha lived more than an hour away from her mother. In fact, her mom lived in Florida and Marsha lived in Arizona. So Marsha did what many caregivers do: she began to search for information on the Internet. "I started by going to Yahoo and typing in keywords such as 'Florida,' 'facilities,' 'hospitals,' and 'nursing homes,'" she says. "I just kept clicking until I found the information I needed."

And what kind of information did she find? Marsha located several Florida care facilities but she realized that her mother needed more care than they could provide. She also located specialists with offices close to her mother's home in Florida and researched medical products such as special eyeglasses to improve her mom's eyesight. "I thought you could just go to Walgreen's and buy magnifying glasses," says Marsha, "but there are magnifying glasses for working on the computer, for reading—all different kinds."

Marsha and her mother now share a home in a senior community in Sun Lakes, Arizona. Although it does take time for her to take care of her mom, Marsha says she's glad they chose Sun Lakes because there are areas for her mother to walk, exercise, have tea with friends, and get rides to and from the doctor's office.

Says Marsha, "There is a ton of information on the Internet about your options. All you have to do is start searching, ask your friends for recommendations, and be patient until you find what you need."

Courtesy of Marsha Zandbergen, 1999, Marshall Educational Publishing, Minden, Nevada.

for her mother. Often the elderly relative has at least one chronic condition, such as heart disease or osteoporosis. Despite myths to the contrary, families rarely abandon the terminally or chronically ill to institutions. Instead, women become caregivers—sometimes sacrificing their own health and finances, and often postponing retirement, to ensure that their loved ones live out their days with as much dignity, security, and peace of mind as possible.

Web services such as ThirdAge (www.thirdage.com), caregivers.com, or caregiverzone.com help women deal with the realities of taking care of a relative. Commercial Web service ThirdAge has a Caregiver Center that leads visitors through the issues they will face when an elderly relative falls victim to illness or a chronic condition. Checklists for how to talk about issues with the relative, resources for finding care, books on the subject of caregiving, and a series of links to other caregiving-related sites are available to visitors. Caregivers.com and caregiverzone.com are dedicated Web portals designed to deliver e-support.

Has your health care organization focused any Web attention on this growing health care need? Offering resources such as classes about caring for elderly relatives or options for local adult day care can be well received by SuperNet Women. Combining on-line support groups with local groups that get women to spend time caring for themselves as well as their loved ones is also important.

MOVE WITH THE TREND, NOT AGAINST IT: ATTRACT SUPERNET WOMAN IN REAL SPACE AND CYBERSPACE

Whether you are marketing in real space or cyberspace, targeting SuperNet Woman is profitable. You are probably already familiar with targeting her in real space; targeting her in cyberspace is unmapped territory. In fact, there is no better time than the present to focus your efforts on SuperNet Woman. E-commerce and e-communications in health care are still in their adolescence, and the opportunity is ripe for health care executives and providers to use their existing brand name and consumer trust at the local level.

Few Web services have yet taken the plunge regionally or locally, and that is where your health care organization, practice, or insurance company comes in. You already have a trusted brand—capitalize on it by structuring your Web service to connect women using products, services, and on-line support in both local real space and cyberspace. Follow the strategies outlined in Exhibit 11–4 and the recommendations below to target SuperNet Woman in your market.

1. *Focus on relationships.* Ask women to enter information about their health and lifestyle, build on-line discussion groups and communities, and bring them back with e-news they can use. Entice visitors by offering a prize—for example,

Exhibit 11–4 Six Strategies for Successfully Reaching Women on the Internet

1. Initiate a relationship: Welcome visitors with home page links—"What to fix for dinner?" Click here. "Free sample?" Click here. Ask women to register for customized navigation on repeat visits; 71 percent of the women surveyed said they would.
2. Nurture the relationship: Make it easy. Sixty-eight percent rated "ease of navigation" as their top priority; another 73 percent leave Web sites out of frustration. Use navigational functions based on lifestyle needs and interests, not product lines. For example, offer content about how to manage caretaking of elderly relatives or relationship issues.
3. Sustain the relationship: Eighty-one percent of women are motivated by updated content. And women, much more than men, are sharers and joiners. They love to talk and hear the opinions of others (91%). Build an on-line community around personal interests with chat rooms, expert forums, and lifestyle content.
4. Invigorate the relationship: Women Internet users are keenly interested in new products. Preview upcoming products or services on your site, or feature medical breakthroughs.
5. Deepen the relationship: Use on-line questionnaires and surveys to find about customers' interests and lifestyles. They'll tell you what they think. Seventy-eight percent of visitors will participate in a survey if the questions involve them personally or are thought-provoking.
6. Extend the relationship: Maintain ongoing contact with women via e-newsletters or customized faxes. To customize the content, ask about personal needs and interests, and deliver e-news or e-communication that suits the consumer's wants.

Courtesy of NetSmart Research, 1998, New York, New York.

"Take this survey and you could win a year's free membership to the hospital's state-of-the-art fitness center."

Offer an on-line weight management or journal service, such as DietWatch.com. DietWatch is the first diet program that integrates the power of a Web community with a personal nutrition and exercise diary. Owned by SoftWatch, Inc., DietWatch allows users to monitor their weight and nutrition via daily diaries and charting, and to communicate with others. Tips on exercise and health are also part of the community (Figure 11–6).

2. *Combine cyberspace and real-space outreach.* Your health care organization's competitive advantage over national Web portals is the fact that you have access to local services and businesses, and can integrate them into your Web service. Consider combining daily nutrition tips with a discount on selected produce items at a local grocery store. Or a coupon for a free consultation with one of your health system's dietary counselors. Promote local health-screening events

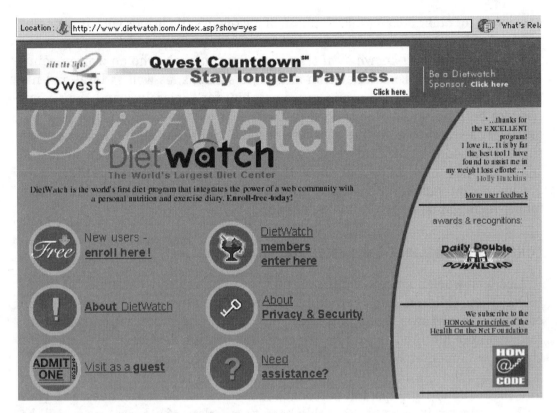

Figure 11–6 DietWatch: Web Community and Diet Program. *Source:* Reprinted with permission from www.dietwatch.com, © 1999, Mediconsult.com, Inc.

and clinics. Kroger Food Stores and Procter & Gamble, both based in Cincinnati, are targeting women by co-sponsoring mammograms at Cincinnati Kroger stores. Integrating events such as these into your health company's Web service brings Net life and real life together.

3. *Beyond health information to e-commerce and e-care.* Women are multifaceted consumers. Although health information is important, so are financial management, daily living, and relationship tips and services. Appeal to their varied interests by offering information and e-commerce services such as stock tips, family and stress management guides, recipes, and information about sexual relationships.

4. *Customize the information to different generations.* Young women have early career jitters and are often involved in rigorous sports activities. Women in their thirties are often caring for a growing family. Baby Boomers are becoming

caregivers for older relatives. Each phase of a woman's life brings with it different needs. Be sure to address each of them in some way on your Web service.

5. *Partner with well-known local brands.* In your market, who do women count on for information? Local television and radio stations, as well as local and national advertisers that sell products women buy for themselves and their families, are both potential Web service partners. For example, most major newspapers offer a searchable on-line database of job listings. Partnering with a service such as this adds significant value to your Web service, as well as an increased sense of community. And what about the local museum or science center? Integrating an interactive quiz with a promotion of these sites fits in nicely with family recreational activities and education.

CONCLUSION—DELIVER E-SERVICES FOR WOMEN

American women make a significant number of health care decisions for themselves, their children, and their ailing parents or relatives. As SuperNet Woman continues to empower herself on line, your health care organization cannot afford to ignore her. And as your health care organization devises its e-strategy for the future, SuperNet Woman should be a targeted e-consumer.

As you build e-services for women, remember to focus on relationships by offering e-support groups and personalized e-services. Do not condescend your visitor; SuperNet Woman has probably been to a variety of other sites and will be a discerning e-consumer. Transcend simply offering heath care information by focusing on a complete line of family management issues—such as finance, work/family balance, raising kids, and career. Building strong relationships, keeping things personal, and focusing on the things that matter will keep SuperNet Woman returning to your Web service time and again.

REFERENCES

1. J. Ledbetter, "Men Are from Mars, Women Are from AOL," http://www.thestandard.com/articles/display/0,1449,1750,00.html (18 September 1998), accessed 10 May 1999.
2. B. Tracy, "Survey Says Women Want Web Sites That Build Relationships," http://adage.com/interactive/articles/19970922/article1.html (September 1997).
3. T. Lugaila, "Marital Status and Living Arrangements," *The Official Statistics,* U.S. Census Bureau, 29 October, 1998, 1.
4. Lugaila, U.S. Census Bureau.
5. Lugaila, U.S. Census Bureau.
6. Lugaila, U.S. Census Bureau.

7. Lugaila, U.S. Census Bureau.

8. U.S. Bureau of Labor, 1998.

9. D. Phillips et al., "Quick Guide for Women Entrepreneurs," http://www.entrepreneurmag.com/page.hts?N=7395 (January 1999), accessed 10 May 1999.

10. "Working Women: Equal Pay—It's Time for Working Women To Earn Equal Pay, " http://www.aflcio.org/women/equalpay.htm, accessed 17 March 1999.

11. G. Espinoza, "Who's the Money Boss in Your Family?" http://www.womenconnect.com/layout/NoFrame/ICZones/Regions/regn_frame.htm?NavTo=/CARC/WORKLIFE&Goal=/Display/Content.htm&GoalID=A189374FA3F411D28A8A00C04F8EF354.

12. G. Espinoza, "Who's the Money Boss in Your Family?"

13. National Association of Investment Clubs, http://www.naic.org, accessed 17 March 1999.

14. "1998 Labor Day Report on Women in the Workforce," *Catalyst*, http://www.womenconnect.com.../FEATURES&Goal=%2FDisplay%2FContent.htm&GoalID=59E5CB41434211D28A8300C0 (7 September 1998), accessed 17 March 1999.

15. "1997 Ask a Working Woman Survey," http://www.aflcio.org/women/execsum.htm.

16. B. Tracy, "Survey Says..."

17. Intelihealth Survey, July 1998.

18. "Internet Helps Cancer Patients Cope," http://www.womenconnect.com.../HEADLINE&Goal=%2FDisplay%2FContent.htm&GoalID=A9FA0327202811D2A64E0010 (28 May 1998).

19. T. Ferguson and W. Kelly, "E-patients Prefer e-groups to Doctors for Ten of Twelve Aspects of Health Care," *The Ferguson Report* 1, no. 1 (1999): 1–2.

20. "More Older Women Surfing the Net," http://www.womenconnect.com...HEADLINE&Goal=2FDisplay%2FContent.htm&GoalID=EDDA69183D5411D28A8300C (28 August 1998).

21. "Caregiving Daughters Take Brunt of Stress," http://www.thirdage.com/news/archive/980330-03.html?rs (30 March 1998).

CHAPTER 12

Physicians Get On Line

Karen A. Zupko and Cheryl L. Toth

Dr. John P. Milner entered private practice in 1980. Over the years, Dr. Milner has experienced the chaos of the resource-based relative value scale (RBRVS), health maintenance organizations, capitation, and three different computer systems. Now, for the third year in a row, he has witnessed a decline in Medicare and managed care reimbursement. At the same time, managed care is creating more on-hold time and administrative burden than he ever imagined when he signed his first contract. These changes have put a strain on his practice.

As if the administrative hassles were not enough, last year many of Dr. Milner's patients began to arrive in the exam room armed with printed pages of health information from the Internet. While these patients proudly proclaimed that they had figured out their own diagnosis, drug options, and treatment regime, Dr. Milner realized that he had not yet read some of the information in his clinical journals.

CULTURE SHOCK

If you are a physician who is experiencing some of the same frustrations as Dr. Milner, welcome to the new millennium of health care. Empowered health care e-consumers and e-patients are taking a more active role in their care, and the Internet is brimming with information that can power the search. Access to information on the Internet is fast eliminating the "whatever you say" patient. Web channels such as regional Medformation.com and international Web portals such as America's Health Network, OnHealth.com, drkoop.com, and Mediconsult.com serve up information about health concerns from asthma to zoonoses, and physicians like Dr. Milner are realizing that this information affects which treatments patients will choose.

Dr. Milner recognizes the importance of keeping abreast of what is available to his patients on line, but given his existing schedule, he is probably wondering how he will find the time to check it out. He is already seeing more than 30 patients on the days he is not in the operating room. With an average visit length of 9 to 15 minutes, he barely has time to dictate the visit so that he complies with Health Care Financing Administration guidelines.[1]

But for his sake, and for the sake of his future practice success, Dr. Milner had better find the time. Futurists have long predicted this new world of health care—a world where physicians are facilitators of care and interact with patients electronically. With the 1998 explosion of the Internet as a viable platform for e-commerce, e-communications, and e-care that future is fast becoming a reality, and e-customers and e-patients are seeking information in greater numbers than ever before. But do not let this news spell doom and gloom. Frankly, the good news for physicians like Dr. Milner is that existing practices already have a competitive advantage over these new health information providers. This chapter outlines how physicians can harness this competitive advantage.

E-PATIENTS WANT THEIR OWN PHYSICIANS

Sure, e-consumers can find information on the Net, but how does this translate to diagnosis and treatment? What of the "taking care of patients" part of medicine? The fact is, right now e-patients have a couple of choices. They can get their e-care from cyberservices such as www.800doctor.com or Mediconsult.com (Figure 12–1). Or patients can get care from www.theirphysician.com—e-care from you, their physician.

We think most patients—and certainly all physicians—would prefer option two. But physician beware: there is not time to initiate endless discussions about whether the decision to get on line is the right one, whether the process costs too much, and so on. If you do not become informed about what is on line and start e-communicating with your patients in one form or another, fast, a portion of your practice is at risk of being siphoned off by cyberphysicians and on-line health information providers you have never met. And do not expect these cyberphysicians to refer the patient back to you. The Web is revolutionizing the way referrals are doled out. As Exhibit 12–1 explains, the referral process is being redesigned by consumers on the Internet. Savvy surfers can discover a specialty they have never heard of or a treatment that may not even be performed in their hometown.

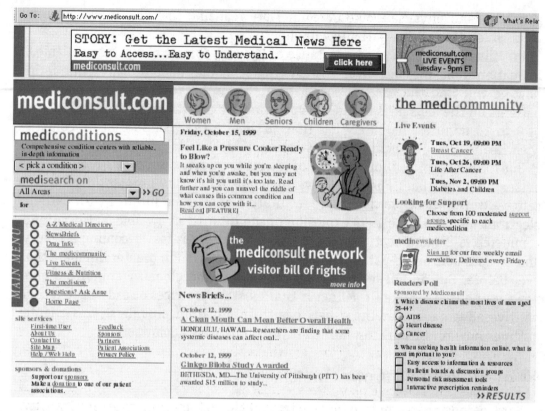

Figure 12–1 Mediconsult.com. *Source:* Reprinted with permission from www.mediconsult.com, © 1999, Mediconsult.com, Inc.

E-CHOICE—MORE THAN JUST A TREND

Most Americans agree that the gatekeeper model does not work. You cannot expect a human being (even if that human being is a physician) to be well versed in every condition from head to toe; to keep up with the latest clinical trials, new procedures, and drugs; and to see 30-plus patients a day. It simply is not possible. Never was.

Consumers across the country are marching into their employers' benefit manager's offices to announce that they want to see specialists whenever it seems necessary. The new health care consumer is empowered with information and will not stand for "mother may I?" care. Employers are responding by purchasing insurance plans that offer increased amounts of choice and point of service (POS) plans so employees can see a specialist, or *their* physician, when

Exhibit 12–1 Referrals Revolutionized

Most consumers and patients do not know what an interventional radiologist does. And they most certainly do not schedule an appointment with one until they have seen several other specialists. Internet technology and access to a worldwide network of computer databases and services are changing that.

At one time, a woman diagnosed with uterine fibroid embolization had one course of treatment: hysterectomy. Now she can type her diagnosis into an Internet search engine and learn about an alternative procedure performed by an interventional radiologist.

With the knowledge of this new procedure, she can schedule a consultation with a physician who performs the procedure, circumventing other specialists that she might have consulted in pre-Internet days.

Courtesy of KarenZupko & Associates, Inc., 1999, Chicago, Illinois.

they want to—even if they have to pay more. Oxford Health Plans, for example, had 86 percent of its enrollees in its POS plan in 1998.[2] Some companies are even experimenting with a voucher system that allows consumers to select any plan they want. If employees want to spend more, they can.

How does the Internet play into all this? As consumer choice is re-activated, mainstream Americans can seek care from the providers they choose. It was projected that about 100 million e-consumers would be on line by 2000[3]—and that more than half would seek health information on line. This means many more Americans will be empowered by direct access to health-related information and services on line.

PEGBOARDS, BILLING SYSTEMS, AND OTHER DINOSAURS

If somebody had told Dr. Milner when he finished his training how the practice of medicine would be impacted by a computer, he would have likely thought the person had gone into early dementia. The administration of health care started out simply and required only simple management systems in the 1970s and early 1980s. In fact, most offices used the "pegboard" system of billing management back then. The carbon-copy method of tracking a patient's charges, payments, and encounters, and billing statements worked fine during the age of indemnity insurance. Staff collected from patients, patients filed their own claims in most cases, and the money rolled in. Billing was easy to learn and involved little sophistication or automation.

Next, RBRVS came along, followed by managed care. Health maintenance organizations and preferred provider organizations paid only a portion of the physician's fee, requiring staff to record details such as payments, adjustments, and withholds. Managed care plans paid differently, had varying sets of benefit rules, and required authorization before most procedures could be performed. Capitation complicated things even further.

The long and short of it was this: a medical practice—like most businesses—could no longer function without a computer system. Business processes were just too complicated to manage without computers. As a result, physicians began to use some kind of billing software. Primarily created as automated versions of the pegboard system, these billing systems had features such as claims submission, account follow-up, and a daily transaction report. But now, as the health care system is poised to join other industries in the on-line race, these billing systems have become part of the reason physicians and health systems are held back from taking advantage of the full realm of e-commerce technology.

Why? As the need for automation evolved, multiple vendors jumped into the market and created independent systems, which have typically run on DOS, UNIX, and proprietary operating systems. Even today, it is estimated that there are more than 1,000 practice management information systems on the market—and this number is down from three years ago due to significant mergers and consolidation in the industry.[4] Many medical offices, hospitals, and health systems have purchased systems that will not serve them well in the year 2000 and beyond, are costly to replace, and have created significant fragmentation among providers, health systems, and payers. For instance, even within the same health community, patients may be required to complete a separate registration and clinical history form at each physician's office that they visit. This example, and others listed in Exhibit 12–2, illustrate the fact that health care providers have barely begun to take advantage of the technology available.

Attention all physicians: Internet technology and Web applications are revolutionizing health care e-communications, e-commerce, and e-care for professionals and consumers. Static "legacy" systems—systems that use proprietary or outdated operating systems—do not easily integrate with the Web platform. It is time for practices, hospitals, MCOs, and health systems to get connected using Web applications that offer streamlined connectivity and effective functionality.

AIR-SPACE PHYSICIANS LAG BEHIND CYBERPHYSICIANS

In general, the health care industry spends just under 2 percent of revenues on technology (other industries average 10 percent), and most medical offices have

Exhibit 12–2 Tasks Many Medical Office Staff Members Perform without Using Technology

---

- Pre-authorization process
- Referral authorization requests
- Determination of eligibility, benefit levels, and deductibles
- Setting up patient budget plans and following up
- Insurance claim follow-up
- Appointment and/or surgery scheduling

Courtesy of KarenZupko & Associates, Inc., 1999, Chicago, Illinois.

---

not kept pace with other industries in terms of purchasing technology, automating labor-intensive processes, and decreasing manual output.[5] For instance, although most practices file claims electronically to Medicare, Blue Cross Blue Shield, and other companies, tens of thousands do not use available clearinghouses for remaining claims. And most practices nationwide do not take advantage of electronic insurance payment posting (insurance payments posted directly into the practice's computer system, eliminating the need to have a staff person do so manually).

Thousands of physicians across America still schedule office visits and surgeries in a paper appointment book; use handwritten forms to track pre-authorization, eligibility, and benefit levels; and manage patient care from paper-based medical records. Despite claims that managed care improves efficiency in the health care system, the prolific growth of managed care has had the opposite effect: additional paperwork must be completed for many visits and procedures. It is important to point out, however, that even when automated solutions to paper-based systems are available in a practice's billing system, they often go unused. In many cases, physicians have bought a Porsche-like system, but their staff members are driving the system like a Dodge Neon.

Now enter the Web's e-technology. In a 1998 study by Cyberdialogue, 57 percent of physicians said that they believed that the Web can enhance physician-to-physician communication. But only 34 percent felt that way about physician-to-patient communication.[6] Thankfully, this assumption is changing. Healtheon Corporation, a leading Web enabler of physician practices, released findings in May of 1999 that showed that 85 percent of 100,000 physicians surveyed are using the Internet.[7] Late-adapter physicians take note. If the medical community were on its own island of automation, physicians might have time to research, consider, and come to a thoughtful decision about e-communication, e-commerce, and e-care. The fact is, many patients are still ahead of their physicians in this area.

Commercial health Web services are changing what it means for consumers to interact with health care providers. America's Doctor Online's "Ask-a-Doc" channel (www.americasdoctor.com) allows visitors to ask questions and receive immediate responses from licensed medical physicians—live, on line. But these physicians are not legally able to triage, teens cannot use the service, and a nurse could dispense most of the health information that the cyberphysicians give out. So while it may seem cool to wait on the clipboard to access a physician, it remains to be seen how far this form of e-care can really go with the legal, financial, and bandwidth barriers in the near future.

Opportunity knocks for local physicians! Why not give your e-patients an alternative to nameless, faceless cyberphysicians? As e-consumers become more familiar with services such as on-line physician chats, they will want to e-communicate with *their* physician. Setting up an e-communication strategy with e-patients now will ensure that your practice is ready when broadband cable allows audio and video streams to go directly into e-patient homes. Let your face, not the cyberphysician's, be the "good physician" on your e-patient's interactive television.

GO ON LINE WITH E-PATIENT COMMUNICATION

You are done seeing patients and, thankfully, this is not your night to take calls. You sit down at your home personal computer (PC) to check the value of your portfolio and to read the day's e-patient communications in your e-mail box. Click, click, click—done.

Sound farfetched? It is not. E-consumers send millions of e-mails every day. They use e-mail at work, and they use it at home. They e-mail parents, kids, and friends, and they expect to be able to e-mail their physician too. Progressive physicians have taken notice, and the May 1999 Healtheon survey revealed that 63 percent use e-mail daily and 33 percent use e-mail to communicate with patients.[8] E-communications with patients did not even register as a significant behavior when physicians were surveyed in 1997.

Before you jump to the conclusion that e-mail can only harm patient care, consider the many advantages of e-mail, including a reduction in call volume. If you are a primary care physician; pediatrician; or general ear, nose, and throat specialist, this is a significant advantage. Even if only 20 percent to 30 percent of your patient base is on line today, there is still an opportunity to decrease calls by directing them to e-mail or to frequently asked questions (FAQs) that are answered on your Web service. And remember that in the next several years that 20 percent to 30 percent of on-line patients will increase dramatically.

E-mail between patients and physicians is an idea whose time has come. Douglas Goldstein suggests that practices can push this two-way communication even further and support and monitor on-line disease and symptom assessment in their physician–patient Web services. At the very least, using e-mail for nonurgent medical issues is the logical next step for physicians who use the Internet for research or to communicate with colleagues. Mick Bauer, DO, from Tulsa, Oklahoma, knows the advantages of using e-mail and describes them in Exhibit 12–3.

Expect the number of physicians who e-communicate with patients to increase rapidly as physicians and managed care plans across the country explore the incredible potential of cyberspace interaction. For example, Kaiser Permanente uses an organized system of two-way communication between e-patients and e-providers that can save significant "telephone tag" time for nurses who call patients about lab results or do call-backs (Figure 12–2). It can also replace routine calls between primary care providers and specialists and reduce overall call volume for billing and general questions. E-patients can e-mail nurses and pharmacists and will soon be able to e-mail physicians. The service also allows e-patients to join discussion groups and make on-line appointments.

But like a new drug, e-mail has side effects, and not everyone is running out to sign up for an e-patient mailbox. Many older physicians think it will dehumanize the practice of medicine. Others worry that, without proper boundaries and protocol, e-mail will create more work. As a Phoenix internist laments, "I made several attempts to connect with my e-mail-enabled patients, but invariably they would begin e-mailing me back with unrelated questions and concerns. I have also been e-mailed an incredible amount of 'Internet medical information' with a request to comment on it."

E-mail also speeds up response time expectations. To meet them, physicians must schedule time during the day to read their e-messages—in addition to completing dictation, handling referral requests, and sorting through daily mail. And what about the legal risks for a population of professionals plagued with an ongoing threat of legal action from a variety of fronts? At least for now, litigation is limited, and guidelines are fluid. To be safe, make a conscious effort to watch what is being said in cyberdialogue in order to protect confidentiality.

Get wired for e-mail, and prepare for the wireless future and high bandwidth that are on the horizon. E-mail *will* change the communication among patients,

Exhibit 12–3 An e-Doc Speaks

Tulsa surgeon Mick Bauer, DO, communicates with his patients on line. "I get anywhere from 6 to 10 e-mails a day," he says. "I encourage my patients to send e-mail if they have questions after their consultation, and I also field all the messages from our practice's Web site." So far, Bauer says not many local patients use the Internet to communicate. But he does receive messages from consumers who have already identified their spine problem and are interested in having a fusion using bone morphogenic protein. "I get about two to three direct patient referrals a month, and most of them end up in the O.R."

Inquiries come in from places as close as Texas, Arkansas, and Oklahoma and as far away as Pakistan, Malaysia, and the Health Ministry of Yemen. "Some of the foreigners have gone so far as to send me their entire medical record in a ZIP file," says Bauer. Indeed, even his domestic e-mailers do not just limit themselves to a message. "They attach MRIs and bone scans for me to review," he says. "If they're a patient, that's fine. But if I've never seen them, well, there's no CPT code for that."

"What becomes tricky," Bauer says, "is responding to those patients who find our Web site and e-mail a question like, 'my husband has low back pain and our doctor says he needs surgery, can you give me more information?' Then I have to e-mail them at least one more time to get more information before I can begin to answer the question."

Other difficulties with e-mail: in several cases it has been established that once you have established e-mail contact, you have started the physician–patient relationship. "That could get sticky if the patient never comes into the office for an examination and something untoward happens," warns Bauer. As well, there are the limitations of the medium itself. "It can be impersonal for initial contacts—but after a face-to-face visit, it's great."

Bauer is an avid supporter of the new technology. "E-mail is becoming a bigger and bigger part of my practice. It doesn't take long to click it, read it, and respond." Bauer has set up templates for his common responses—as many physicians already do with transcription. His signature contains a disclaimer, just in case.

"I'm looking forward to the day the technology allows doctors to receive large files like MRIs and scans easily. It would be great if a referring physician could e-mail me with the message "You're consulting with my patient John Grey tomorrow; attached are his scans and my notes about his condition."

Courtesy of Mick Bauer, DO, 1999, Tulsa, Oklahoma.

physicians, and other providers—just as it has changed communication in other sectors. For nonurgent conditions, it is much more efficient than the telephone.

DECREASE COSTS USING E-COMMERCE AND E-TRANSACTIONS

Can you imagine a world where referral authorizations, surgery scheduling forms, and operative notes are not on paper? E-commerce could be the knight in shining armor that rescues health care from its paper woes. Just think of all the headaches that could be solved if your practice was Web enabled:

- piles of referral requests
- significant staff time spent on hold with insurance companies to follow up on a claim, obtain eligibility information, or request pre-authorization for a procedure
- paper-based claims submission to non-Medicare, Blue Cross, and Medicaid payers
- paper-based surgery scheduling procedures

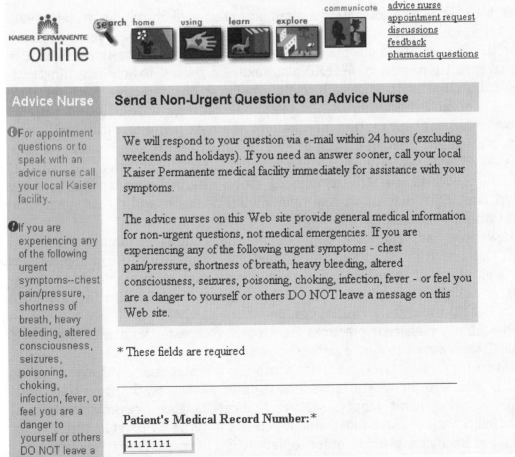

Figure 12–2 Kaiser Permanente. *Source:* Reprinted with permission from www.kaiserperma nente.org/membersonly/advice.htm, © 1999, Kaiser Permanente, Inc.

- regular and maddening follow-up of unpaid insurance claims because the payer "never received it" or it was rejected due to "patient ineligibility"
- continuous telephone messages and the need for nurse call-backs
- paper medical records and documentation

In 1998, e-commerce solutions to medical office paper hassles began to pop up on the Web. Netrepreneurs recognized the wide-open market and have made tremendous strides in offering new on-line services to customers. Health care Web sites have begun to move from a marketing focus to an emphasis on customer service. Companies are clamoring to be the Amazon.com of health care, by offering physicians, health systems, and payers the opportunity to improve efficiency by becoming Web enabled. Several of these companies are described below.

WebMD (www.webmd.com), for example, premiered its service in late 1998. At $19.95 per month—a fee that is waived for the first two years of use—WebMD offers access to on-line eligibility and benefit authorization and practice management information. WebMD also takes on several basic office functions, including after-hours voicemail. Using a network of interactive voice response systems around the nation, night telephone calls are answered and patients leave messages about routine information. The next morning, office staff members retrieve the messages. There is even a feature that integrates text-to-voice messaging and fax services on the same number. In addition, WebMD has partnered with Envoy—the commercial claims clearinghouse familiar to many physicians. ENVOYnet allows real-time eligibility checks and claims submission right from the desktop.

Healtheon, Inc., automates many of the paper- and labor-intensive processes that make health care administration inefficient. Some Healtheon applications are a bit ahead of the physician market; others, such as on-line claims submission and eligibility verification, are right on target. In 1999, Healtheon merged with WebMD to create a multibillion-dollar company that is clearly focused on Web-enabling physician practices from coast to coast. (Note: Healtheon and WebMD were slated to merge as this book went to press.)

Claimsnet (Figure 12–3) has gotten into the Internet claims submission arena and is a force to be reckoned with as it grabs e-claim profits from traditional practice management vendors such as Medical Manager (www.careinsite.com) and Medic. Each of these independent vendors is vying for coveted partnerships with key insurance plans in order to deliver vital transactions to medical practices.

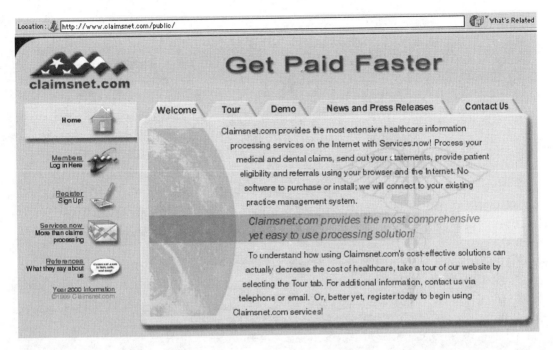

Figure 12–3 Claimsnet. *Source:* Reprinted with permission from www.claimsnet.com, © 1999, Claimsnet.com.

And there are other players too. At Officemed.com, medical office staff can perform secure real-time health care transactions. Officemed's customers range from large hospitals to single-physician practices. The company offers insurance eligibility verification and a real-time benefits inquiry against a patient's insurance plan.

Eliginet (Figure 12–4) is an on-line eligibility verification and referral authorization application. It eliminates long waits on the telephone and the need to leaf through the paper eligibility lists that are often outdated the day an insurance plan mails them to your office. Eliginet Web-enables complete eligibility files from your independent practice association (IPA) every day. Staff members simply type in a patient's name to obtain eligibility, coverage, benefit level, and sometimes deductible information.

More than just billing tools are available on the Web. Banking and financial services are scooping up on-line users—for both personal and business transactions. Check out your options at www.citibank.com, www.quicken.com (Figure

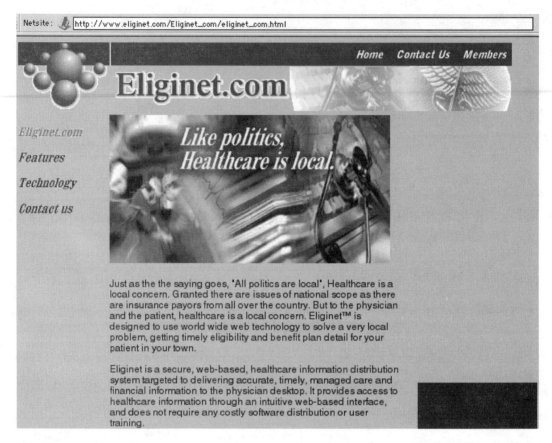

Netsite: http://www.eliginet.com/Eliginet_com/eliginet_com.html

Home   Contact Us   Members

Eliginet.com

Eliginet.com

Features

Technology

Contact us

Like politics,
Healthcare is local.

Just as the the saying goes, "All politics are local", Healthcare is a local concern. Granted there are issues of national scope as there are insurance payors from all over the country. But to the physician and the patient, healthcare is a local concern. Eliginet™ is designed to use world wide web technology to solve a very local problem, getting timely eligibility and benefit plan detail for your patient in your town.

Eliginet is a secure, web-based, healthcare information distribution system targeted to delivering accurate, timely, managed care and financial information to the physician desktop. It provides access to healthcare information through an intuitive web-based interface, and does not require any costly software distribution or user training.

Figure 12–4 Eliginet. *Source:* Reprinted with permission from www.eliginet.com/ Eliginet_Demo/Eligibility/Elg_Multiple/Elg_Results/elg_results.html, © 1999, Eliginet.com, Inc.

12–5), or www.wellsfargo.com. Already used by many physician offices, QuickBooks transactions can be easily uploaded on the Quicken Web service. The service also includes financial management tips, stock quotes, and customer information.

Office and medical supplies can be purchased on line and automatically shipped to your doorstep in no time. The www.officemax.com and www.staples.com services allow your office manager streamlined shopping by setting up personal lists and e-mail reminders.

Your challenge is to be thoughtful about your use of Internet technology so that it produces cost reductions and improved e-patient communication and care, not just more technology hassles. Do not go for just glitz and glitter—

determine which Web applications can solve the problems that plague your practice most.

BUILD AN E-SERVICE, NOT A SITE

E-patients are surfing the Web, and transaction costs can be decreased significantly by using Web applications to run your business. Should you be thinking about launching a Web site at this point? No. Smart physicians will invest in a Web *service*, not a Web site.

What is the difference? A Web *site* is a static application that could more accurately be termed "brochureware." Essentially, a medical practice takes its

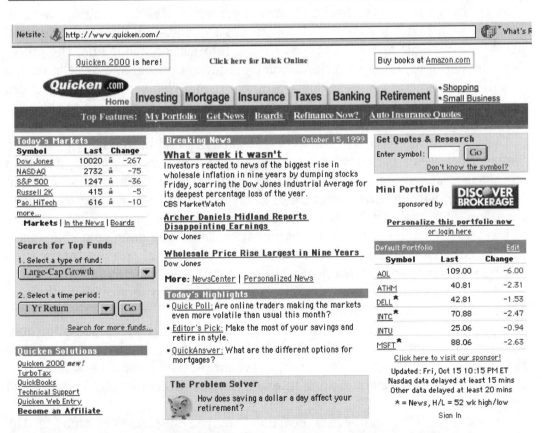

Figure 12–5 QuickBooks. *Source:* Reprinted with permission from www.quicken.com, © 1999, Intuit, Inc. Quicken® is a registered trademark of Intuit, Inc.

existing print collateral and posts it on the Web. Maybe the practice even lists a set of hyperlinks to other sites as a "service" to its patients. In 1999, brochureware was the most common form of Web site for most medical practices, but brochureware is flawed in two ways. First, e-patients have no real reason to return to a static site where only office hours, a curriculum vitae, and pictures of the office are posted. Second, if your practice has spent time and money developing an on-line presence, why hyperlink to other Web sites that may be your future competitors?

Brochureware does little to excite patients or bring them back to your site, and "flat text" about the practice offers little health information. Think communication, not marketing—transactions rather than individual encounters.

A Web *service*, at its most basic level, e-communicates a variety of timely information, promotes the practice and its services within the community, and gathers valuable information about the patients served. Figure 12–6 shows the Web service of Dr. James Nachbar, an early user of Web technology. Back in 1995 he launched his Web site. It continues to evolve into a service-focused place for e-patients and e-consumers to find information about him, the procedures he performs, do registrations, complete forms on line, and get the results of patient satisfaction surveys. Establishing a strong Web service with advanced e-services and useful content allows your practice to reach out more to the communities you serve.

The e-healthcare revolution is about interactivity and better service, and the Web technologies e-patients expect from you are those used by other industries to engage the user. Brochureware, with its lengthy narratives and laborious need for scrolling, will lose the attention of savvy e-patients and e-consumers every time. But if you realize that your Web site is nothing more than brochureware, do not worry. Take pride in the fact that you are a maverick among your colleagues, just for getting on line in the first place. Your "phase one" site put information on the Web, creating a basic on-line entry point to your practice.

Set your sights now on developing an interactive Web service that allows e-patients two-way communication with you and your staff as well as the ability to navigate through information and surveys. Cultivate "sticky" e-patients (ones who come back regularly) by offering health information, purchase, and transaction opportunities that entice them to stay awhile—and come back later. The key is to offer consumers greater interactivity and access to real services and information.

For example, Heartland (www.heartland.com), a 30-physician group in the Midwest, serves up two-way communication with patients, lab, and pharmacy as well as frequently asked questions on its Web service. Visitors can download

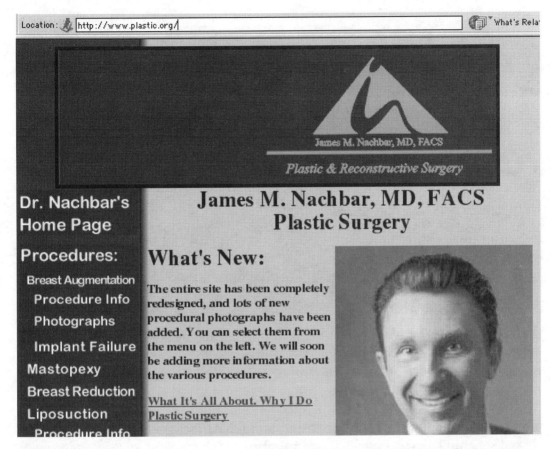

Figure 12–6 Dr. Nachbar's Home Page. *Source:* Reprinted with permission from www.plastic.org, © 1999, James Nachbar, M.D.

registration forms and the practice's financial policy statement, take interactive satisfaction and health surveys, and get the latest in health information and breaking medical news. Heartland plans to offer on-line e-care monitoring so providers can interactively manage chronic conditions such as diabetes.

Figure 12–7 shows Tulsa Orthopedic Surgeons' Web-enabled slide show of a carpal tunnel surgery. Information about and pricing for the procedure is provided on the practices Web service, as well as diagrams of laparoscopic spine surgery. Live pictures are coming soon. The latest news about one surgeon's participation in a clinical trial is also featured. This three-person group of surgeons has been on the Web since 1996.

As these groups of physicians have learned, interactive on-line communication and customer service improves communication between patients and medical

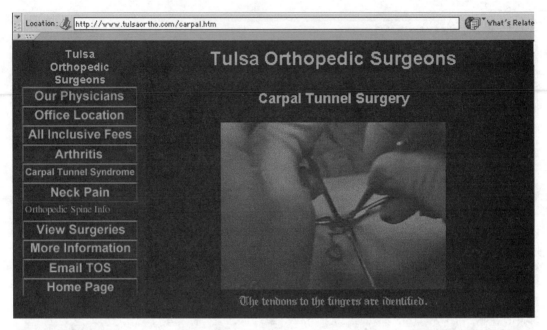

Location: http://www.tulsaortho.com/carpal.htm   What's Relate

Tulsa Orthopedic Surgeons

Tulsa Orthopedic Surgeons

Carpal Tunnel Surgery

Our Physicians
Office Location
All Inclusive Fees
Arthritis
Carpal Tunnel Syndrome
Neck Pain
Orthopedic Spine Info
View Surgeries
More Information
Email TOS
Home Page

The tendons to the fingers are identified.

Figure 12–7 Tulsa Orthopedic Surgeons. *Source:* Reprinted with permission from www.tulsaortho.com, © 1999, Tulsa Orthopedic Surgeons.

professionals, makes transactions easier, and builds recognition of your practice "brand" within the local medical community.

BEGINNER'S GUIDE TO BUILDING AN E-SERVICE

Before any practice launches itself into cyberspace, it must assess the local e-consumer market. Survey a small sample of patients to determine what kind of e-services they want. Questions could include the following: Do you use the Internet to access health information, and, if so, what type of health information do you access? What kind of health information or transactions would you like to receive via the Net? Can we send you "News You Can Use" e-mail alerts on health developments, services, products, and information? Exhibit 12–4 is a sample survey that you can customize for your own practice.

At a minimum, your practice can offer basic interactive services such as an online registration form, your financial policy, and the ability to request an appointment. Even if initially this appointment request is simply an e-mail to staff members that triggers them to call the e-consumer and fulfill the request, it at

Exhibit 12–4 Sample Survey

To improve our communication with patients, our practice is considering an interactive Web service and e-mail communication options. By answering these questions, you will help us develop new on-line services that serve you best. Thank you for your input.

1. Have you searched for health information on the Internet?   Yes   No

2. If you search for health information on the Internet, what are the three sites you visit most? www._____   www._____   www._____

3. Do you have an e-mail address?   Yes   No

4. Is this e-mail address personal or work related? _____

5. If we can reach you with health or medical information via your e-mail address, please provide it: _____

6. Would you communicate with your doctor via e-mail if that option were available?   Yes   No

7. Would you like to receive, via e-mail, regular e-zines from your doctor containing the latest medical information he or she has read?   Yes   No

8. Have you ever joined an on-line support group?   Yes   No

   For what condition? _____

9. What is your modem speed?   14.4K   28.8K   33.3K   56K   56K+   Don't know

10. Which browser do you use?   Explorer   Netscape   AOL

11. Which on-line features and transactions would you use, if they were available?

   ____ E-mailing the doctor or nurse

   ____ Scheduling appointments

   ____ Obtaining health information and tips

   ____ Obtaining nutrition information

   ____ Finding out schedules of local health fairs

   ____ Updating your account

   ____ Requesting prescription refills

   ____ E-mailing the billing office

   ____ Learning about health care books and products

   ____ Accessing lab results

   ____ Learning about breaking medical or drug news

   ____ Obtaining information about the doctors

   ____ Using discussion and support groups

   ____ Getting answers to medical questions

Source: Copyright © 1999, Douglas Goldstein.

least begins to get consumers in the habit of scheduling via an on-line access point. Although these few interactive features are still considered low on the interactivity scale, we would call this endeavor a *Web service* (instead of a *Web site*) because it does include ways for consumers to interact and communicate with the practice and allows office staff to gather and process information. The data can then be used to target specific populations, tailor the Web service, or improve the practice's newsletter content.

Central Valley Ear, Nose, and Throat has moved beyond brochureware to Web service. The practice has five office locations in the Central Valley of California, and its Web service (Figure 12–8) includes comprehensive information about each physician, new procedure breakthroughs, office locations, and staff. A schedule of seminars given by the physicians and nurses is available, and visitors can complete an on-line form to register for them or to schedule an appointment.

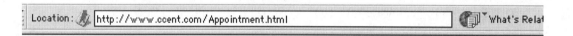

Location: http://www.ccent.com/Appointment.html   What's Rela

Welcome to the CCENT Appointment Desk

TO OBTAIN AN APPOINTMENT

WITH ONE OF THE PHYSICIANS

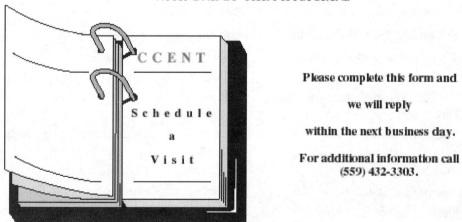

CCENT

Schedule a Visit

Please complete this form and

we will reply

within the next business day.

For additional information call
(559) 432-3303.

Figure 12–8 Central Valley Ear, Nose, and Throat. *Source:* Reprinted with permission from www.ccent.com/Appointment.html, © 1999, Central California Ear, Nose, and Throat.

Each of the practice's specialty areas—general ear, nose, and throat; hearing services; speech and language center; and aesthetic surgery—is described in detail, and the practice also announces job openings on the site.

Once you determine that consumers in your patient base are ready for your Web service, it is time to get to work. There are a number of e-tools on the market to help you build your e-service. HTML editing software such as Microsoft's FrontPage, Adobe's PageMill, or NetObjects' Fusion is available for a very reasonable price at local retailers. Some of these retailers even offer classes in how to use the software.

The Image Cafe Store (www.imagecafe.com) offers inexpensive, professional-looking Web sites that do not require technical knowledge or additional software. Most sites can be purchased for about $300, and are easily updated by you or your office manager once they have been launched. Even some specialty societies have gotten into the Web service act. The American Society for Plastic and Reconstructive Surgeons offers a brochureware page for its members at a nominal cost. The Pediatric Physician Alliance helps its affiliated physicians get on line. As this book went to press, the AMA was rolling out Web applications to support physicians in putting up patient Web sites.

As the saying goes, you get what you pay for. This saying holds true with e-tools and "packaged" Web site motifs. Certainly, there are low cost options available. But will they help your practice transcend brochureware and create fully functional e-services? Who will maintain the services once they are up and running, and how will you ensure that credible medical information is posted and secure transactions function right? Be clear about whether the options you are considering are e-service focused or are simply brochureware.

e-Information about the Practice and Physicians

As you think through the basic Web service design and development, include e-information about the practice and physicians, information about the services you provide, e-newsletters, on-line surveys, and forms in your level one Web service. The following list outlines some of these basic items you should include on your level one Web service.

- registration
- history and physicals on line
- location, office hours, and how to reach you—the basics
- clinic and satellite information, maps (linking to www.maps.yahoo.com is a good way to go)
- individual pictures of physicians looking friendly

- professional information about each physician and provider
- information about the specialty
- conditions the physicians treat—in lay terms
- on-line version of your registration form
- FAQs about the practice's financial and office policies
- appointment request via e-mail
- plans with which the practice has contracted

e-Tip: Resist the Temptation To Just Put Up "Flat" Text

You might start, for example, with a picture of each physician with his or her name underneath. When the consumer clicks on the picture, a brief summary of the physician's credentials and philosophy comes up. At the end of this summary are a series of hypertext links such as "What patients say about Dr. Brown," "Dr. Brown's training," and "Contracted health plans." Displaying the information in an interactive format allows consumers to click on the specific information they want—without scrolling down endless lines of narrative.

e-Tip: Making this section comprehensive will reduce telephone calls to office staff and free up time for improved internal practice marketing activities—like looking at the patient in the check-in window and saying hello.

OTHER FEATURES TO ADD TO YOUR WEB SERVICE

e-Newsletters

A monthly or quarterly e-newsletter with health tips for current and prospective patients is an extraordinary way to communicate with patients. Include a section with information on your practice, including news such as flu shot schedules, school physical dates, and other timely topics. E-newsletters can help build patient retention and improve compliance with treatment recommendations; www.e-zines.com provides step-by-step instructions on creating an attractive, informative, and successful e-newsletters. The site's tips and tools are easy to use, even if you are a novice. For less than $100 per year, e-commerce sites such as Listbot (www.listbot.com) allow easy creation and management of your mailing list and can send newsletters of up to 7,500 words. You can include up to 20 modifiable demographic questions, and the software saves the mailing list in a centralized database, accessible at any time.

e-Surveys

Surveys are a lot less complicated than you might think. Leading patient satisfaction survey company Point of View Survey Systems has an excellent Web-enabled survey system (Figure 12–9). You simply pay a fee to attach it to your service. You adapt your existing survey questions, and e-patients complete the survey form on line. The survey results are password protected to ensure the patients' privacy at all times. Point of View can also help you assess your patients' health risk using SF-36 and other outcomes measurement tools.

e-Forms

Decrease paper hassles in your office and streamline the check-in process. Beyond simply posting a registration form for patients to download, you can create on-line forms that push all the data entered via e-mail to your staff. Create

Location: http://www.povss.com/marketing/ice_cream_swirl/vsq.html   What's Relat

High levels of Patient Satisfaction and Physician Responsiveness are critical to Medical services growth now and in the 21st Century.

The following survey is meant to be a sample of how questions for Patient Satisfaction might be seen visually on the POVSS 'NetSurvey and how simple the process of completing and sending the 'NetSurvey can be.

This survey measures Patient Satisfaction in the clinical setting and the patient may enter an identification number if tracking is important. Physicians/clinicians can be scored individually. The Visit Specific Questionaire (VSQ) is a public domain survey adapted from Health Outcomes Institute, Bloomington, Minnesota and offered on 'NetSurvey by POVSS.

Please answer the following questions by clicking your mouse on the response.

	Excellent	Very Good	Good	Fair	Poor
How long you waited to get an appointment	O	O	O	O	O
Getting through to the office by phone	O	O	O	O	O
Length of time waiting at the office	O	O	O	O	O
The technical skills (thoroughness, carefulness, competence) of the person you saw	O	O	O	O	O
The personal manner (courtesy, respect, sensitivity, friendliness) of the person you saw	O	O	O	O	O
The visit overall	O	O	O	O	O

Figure 12–9 Point of View Survey Systems. *Source:* Reprinted with permission from www.povss.com, © 1999, Point of View Survey Systems.

true on-line registration forms, self-completed clinical history forms, and so forth so patients can print them and complete them prior to arriving in your office. Staff then receive an e-mail with all the information needed to register the new patient in the computer and create a chart.

e-Tip: Start requesting patient and family e-mail addresses on in-office patient registration forms and anywhere else you ask patients to provide their telephone numbers.

Take advantage of this e-mail database and use it to push information out to your patients via frequent e-alerts that are delivered directly to their e-mail boxes. These e-alerts can drive usage back to your site and direct patients to timely information, updates, and news. It is a low-cost avenue for encouraging health and wellness among the populations you serve as well as promoting your practice and the services you offer.

DEVELOPING AN ADVANCED WEB SERVICE

Do more administratively on line, and you will improve patient satisfaction and lower practice operating costs. Once you have a handle on the fundamentals of an interactive Web service, a stronger Web presence can allow an even greater influence over your e-community. A more robust Web service will not only offer increased functionality and interactivity to patients and their families but also mean that your practice can reach and positively affect the lives of more people—especially those living in more remote communities. And this advanced e-service can reduce the number of calls handled by office staff and ultimately lower your operating costs.

Your practice can lead the way in demonstrating how this robust Web service reduces costs, educates patients, and builds community trust and loyalty. Using the level one Web service as a foundation, offer your e-patients and surrounding communities an e-service with greater functionality and interactivity. This next level of Web service offers even more services that save patients time and save time and money in the practice. An advanced Web service builds on the level one e-service, as well as features such as e-newsletters and e-surveys.

Delivery of Lab Results and Tests via e-Mail

Rather than telephoning your office for lab results, e-patients log on to a secure, password-protected area of the site to pick up the lab results of noncritical tests. This interactive service can include "pop-up" educational boxes explaining what the lab values measure and what they mean. If a patient has values close to or outside of the norm, educational material (e.g., diet and exercise tips) is delivered immediately on line.

Two-Way Communication with Office Staff—for Billing and Medical Questions

Offer e-patients access to you or the nurse for straightforward medical questions and to the billing staff for questions about their account. Two-way communication is a password-protected way for staff to save significant time on communications such as nurse call-back "telephone tag." It can also improve productivity by reducing constant telephone interruptions. Staff can better organize their time by sending e-mail or telephone responses during downtime.

Access to Disease- and Condition-Specific Information

Include a search feature so consumers can access disease- and condition-specific information for the most common diseases and conditions such as diabetes, pregnancy, heart disease, allergies, women's health issues, children's health issues, seniors' health issues, and more. Coordinate your Web service with on-line monitoring services such as Patient Infosystems (www.healthdesk.com) to help manage e-patients with chronic conditions.

Automatic Appointment Reminders via e-Mail

Be sure those joint replacement patients keep coming back and women over 40 get regular mammograms. Reduce the number of times patients forget appointments. Push automatic appointment reminders via e-mail. These reminders can also be customized to provide fasting information for lab tests and other specific information related to the patient's appointment.

Patient Bulletin e-Boards

Why have your patients go to www.800doctor.com when they can visit www.yourpractice.com and join on-line discussion groups about their condition? This feature provides a forum for patients to communicate with one another on specific or general topics. It may also include a Web feature that offers moderated chat with selected physicians or other medical professionals. Also included with this feature can be helpful health tips, assistance with dietary compliance, recipes, useful links, and more.

Disease- and Condition-Specific e-Mails with Text, Audio, and Video

Patients suffering from chronic diseases or conditions can manage their conditions more effectively using information, news, and services e-mailed directly to them. These e-mails would send patients to your practice's Web site for more information or alert patients to upcoming classes and other community events related to their condition.

The costs for these advanced services vary. Check with your hospital's Web services team to determine which might be feasible for your practice.

TAKE ACTION! 10 TIPS FOR SUCCESSFULLY WIRING YOUR PRACTICE

Be the first in your medical community to go on line for e-patient communication, e-services, and e-commerce. Follow these 10 tips as you develop an interactive e-patient service in your practice.

1. *Find out how many of your existing patients are on line.* If you practice in a city where many people are connected to the Internet—Washington, DC, San Francisco, Chicago, Los Angeles, Phoenix, and so on—the answer is already clear. If you do not, survey the patient base to determine interest in interactive communication and e-care delivery.

2. *Try the Net on for size.* Get an e-mail address and jump on line. If you have not done so already, you need to see what all the fuss is about. Buy a book at www.amazon.com or office supplies at www.officemax.com. Get on a mail-order coffee club at www.starbucks.com and sign up for an e-zine at www.fool.com. Pay particular attention to the use of interactivity, color, design, and writing style at the Web sites you like most.

3. *Get hip about health information and support groups on line, and sanction those Web services that you deem credible.* Savvy physicians will offer their patients a written (or e-mailed) directory of sanctioned, credible Web services. Check out www.mediconsult.com, www.drkoop.com, www.askdrweil.com, and www.thriveonline.com. Find out what these services are promoting as "health information" in your specialty. Go to major search engines such as www.yahoo.com or www.excite.com and type in your specialty, or a few of the diagnoses you treat most often, and see which sites come up. You should be aware of at least the first 10 sites listed—your patients have probably been to them.

If you manage patients with breast cancer, pancreatic cancer, diabetes, asthma, and other chronic conditions, be aware of the proliferation of on-line support groups. Visit them to see what is being talked about. Print a list of the best ones and offer it to patients who suffer from the condition. Do not forget that many of these patients have limited mobility. Connecting them to the "outside world" via the Internet can be helpful.

4. *Prepare the troops.* The Internet fundamentally changes how a practice operates and is a threat to "the way we've always done it." The .com revolution will alter staff members' lives even more than the office's first computer system did,

and it is up to you to adequately prepare them for the shift. You know the typical reaction to change in practice systems: denial and fear. But this change cannot be ignored; your patients are, or soon will be, demanding it. Be clear with staff about where you plan to steer the practice, and consider investing in a training class for them if they do not already access the Internet at home.

5. *Install an Intranet and get the whole staff surfing.* "But they won't get any work done because they'll just surf the Web," you say. Nonsense. The Internet is just as important an information pipeline as the telephone wire, and it is the rare practice that has difficulty with staffers yapping on personal calls for hours at a time during the business day. On the contrary, you cannot afford *not* to get the practice on line. How else do you expect staff to access on-line eligibility and referral authorization, purchase medical supplies, and access practice management information in the future? Begin by installing an Intranet—a Windows-based network that connects all the PCs in the practice with each other privately and also has a ramp to the Internet.

6. *Initiate e-communications and e-services for your e-patients.* Get your Web service started using the tips presented in this chapter. Offer e-mail as a valid way to communicate (for nonclinical reasons, unless yours is a secure site) with you and your office staff.

7. *Explore e-commerce solutions to age-old hassles.* Prepare for the future! Phase out those old paper appointment schedules, chart number log books, and nonautomated account follow-up systems. In the new millennium, successful practices will let technology work with them by initiating automated solutions to paper-intensive systems. Surf on over to ePhysicians.com or OfficeMed.com and get pricing for eligibility and claims submission. Open an account with OfficeMax and order office supplies on line. Instruct your manager to access the Quicken site for on-line banking services and the latest financial information and news. Ask staff to visit Modern Physician (www.modernphysician.com) and print the latest practice management articles. It is all available today, but you have to be wired to get it!

8. *Decide whether your legacy system can "grow up" and get Web connected.* While you are getting the practice wired to the Net, evaluate how far your current practice management system will make it into the new millennium. At a minimum, it must maintain unlimited payment schedules and adjustment categories, and enable staff to post by line item, or you will continue to get eaten alive by managed care plans. The system should also have a stellar appointment scheduler and a relational database report writer. Also, the vendor should at least be talking about a relationship with an e-records company and voice-activated dictation.

9. *Check out continuing medical education (CME) and practice management information on line.* Many specialty societies now offer on-line CME—check yours to find out. Medscape (www.medscape.com) is brimming with useful management information. Sign up for its "Money and Medicine" e-newsletter. The Medical Group Management Association has useful information on its service, www.mgma.com. You can also print the latest practice management articles through the on-line publications of magazines such as *Modern Physician, Medical Economics,* and *Modern Healthcare.*

10. *Plan for technology investments now.* We know the typical accountant's advice—drain the accounts at the end of the year and take it all before Uncle Sam does. Challenge yourself to new-age thinking! Instead of taking it all home, invest earnings in your practice's e-technology needs, which include all dimensions of e-communications, e-commerce, and e-care.

REFERENCES

1. "The Internet as a Driving Force of Societal Change," http://www.intel.com/intel/e-health/internet.htm.
2. J. Kleinke, "Power to the Patient," *Modern Healthcare,* 23 February, 1998, 66.
3. "Almost 80 Million Americans Online," http://www.cyberatlas.com/big_picture/geographics/quest.html (5 March, 1999).
4. Eliginet, Inc., *Business Plan* (Chicago, IL: 1998).
5. C. Clark, *Healthcare Information Systems* (1995), 679, quoted in M.L. Millenson, *Demanding Medical Excellence* (University of Chicago Press, 1997), 91.
6. T. Miller and S. Brown, *HealthMed Retrievers* (New York: Cyberdialogue://findsvp, January 1998), 10.
7. "Healtheon Corporation Internet Survey of Medicine," http://www.AOLNews.com (6 May, 1999), accessed 9 March 1999.
8. "Healtheon Corporation Internet Survey of Medicine."

CHAPTER 13

Medical Extranets

Cheryl L. Toth, Matthew B. Calish, and Douglas E. Goldstein

THE IDEA that the American health care system is in need of improved efficiency and communication channels is generally accepted by most Americans. If one views the entire system as a sick patient seeking medical treatment, the chart notes for the "office visit" would likely look like this:

PATIENT NAME

The American health care system.

PRESENTING COMPLAINTS

Paperwork backup and protocol confusion. Bleeding physician and hospital profits and losses due to rising overhead. Irritability of patients. Lack of communication between elements of system.

HISTORY

Fragmented communication within the provider community, underutilization of technology and automation in the patient care and administrative processes, and years of distrust between providers and insurers have caused the patient's condition to worsen. Consumers, physicians, and hospitals have finally said "We've had enough."

EXAMINATION

The following acute symptoms were observed:

- outdated and underused technology in physicians' offices and hospitals
- thousands of variations to managed care contract guidelines
- cumbersome referral and pre-authorization requirements in physicians' offices and hospitals

- inability of clinicians to collaborate across hospital, physician practice, and specialty lines
- costly, labor-intensive, and paper-heavy processes associated with lab work, prescriptions, medical records, and other pieces of information
- hospitals and medical offices pressured by increased overhead and decreased reimbursement

MEDICAL DECISION MAKING

Diagnosis. A classic case of poor communication, underautomation, and expensive overbureaucratization.

Treatment Plan. Using the Internet as a platform and a Web application called an Extranet, connect health systems, health plans, providers, and patients. Save money, save time, reduce paperwork nightmares, and foster e-communications networks—all from the desktop.

Prescription for Change. If the American health care system arrived in an ambulatory care setting, the specialist treating it would probably code the patient a 99245. Its problems are decidedly comprehensive, and "medical decision making" is high risk, given the complexity of systems and long history of redundant, labor-intensive processes and mistrust among health system participants.

Enter e-commerce. Savvy health care organizations have begun to discover that deploying Internet technology can improve the giant, bureaucratic mess called "health care administration." Eligibility verification, referral authorization, clinical collaboration, demand management, emergency department authorization, and hundreds, potentially thousands, of other types of health care communication and transactions can be automated via Web-enabled technology.

Imagine—a check-in process at the hospital or physician's office that does not require four different forms. A communication channel where providers can communicate, confidentially, about patient care. A streamlined, electronic way to request authorizations and referrals. These revolutionary shifts will do more than just improve the unwieldy processes of managed care. They will assist staff on both the payer and provider sides by decreasing or eliminating the mounds of paperwork that have driven health care processes for many years.

It is not just hospitals and providers who will benefit. Health insurance companies also incur significant costs to push paper. According to a 1999 Sherlock benchmarking study, the average per member per month insurance plan administrative expense was $16.59—$4.97 of which goes to marketing and actuarial expenses.[1] These costs drive up overall health care expenses just as the gluttony of medical office paperwork and proliferation of duplicate tests do.

The Extranet panacea can reduce many of these costs by connecting insurance plans with patients and providers.

WHAT IS AN EXTRANET?

An Extranet is a Transmission Control Protocol/Internet Protocol network that is a *private* communications and customer service channel between affinity groups such as a health system and physicians, physicians and a health plan, or any combination of health care trading partners. In short, an Extranet is a secure channel between known strategic partners, customers, and organizations that want to reduce operating costs, streamline transactions, be more productive, and improve overall quality. The Extranet uses a combination of wide area networks and the public Internet to move data and information from place to place.

One way to think about an Extranet is to compare it to today's cable system. Just about everyone has basic cable, but if you want premium channels you have to subscribe and pay for them. This privileged access ensures that only those who subscribe to these premium channels have access to them on their television. Similarly, a "premium channel" Extranet is a private, secure, targeted channel with services tailored to the needs of a specific industry segment and customer. It is sort of like subscribing to the menu of extra cable channels such as Home and Garden or the SciFi Channel. Within the confines of an Extranet, sensitive or confidential information is data warehoused in a secure area—away from the public Internet. In order to access the Extranet channel, users are required to enter a username and password, or there are other security mechanisms.

The number of potential Extranet applications is limitless. In a nutshell, if it is being done today by fax or telephone, then it is likely that money and time can be saved by converting these real-space and telephone-space transactions to Extranet transactions. Initial applications being rolled out on Extranets are listed in Exhibit 13–1. The big advantage of Extranets in the health care system is that because they utilize Web browsers, they cut across different operating systems—such as Windows, UNIX, or Macintosh—and allow any authorized Extranet user to access the information on the Extranet server.

Extranets offer enormous benefits to health care organizations. They are revolutionizing the way physicians, hospitals, and health plans run their operations. The overhead reduction and economies of scale that Extranets provide are significant. The "hassle factor" and inefficiency of managed care contract adminis-

Exhibit 13–1 What an Extranet Can Handle

- On-line claims submission
- Claims payment and reporting
- Eligibility verification
- Referral authorization
- Database of providers and credentials
- Clinical guidelines
- X-ray and lab results
- Prescriptions
- Health insurance purchases
- Electronic medical forums by disease state or condition
- Secure e-communication of confidential information
- Clinical discussions with leading experts
- Continuing medical education programming
- Consumer health education and compliance monitoring
- Immediate access to near-binding quotes for e-consumers
- Gateway access to the public Internet

Source: Copyright © 1999, Douglas Goldstein.

tration and management reporting can virtually be eliminated because it can be automated on the Web. Extranets are not only excellent business-to-business tools, they are tremendous relationship builders because of the way they facilitate clinical and informational integration.

EXTRANETS VS. ELECTRONIC DATA INTERCHANGE (EDI)

Do not confuse Extranets with electronic data interchange (EDI). EDI is actually an early version of an Extranet—the flower before the fruit, if you will.

EDI enables physicians' offices and hospitals to transmit data (such as claims or enrollment applications) or receive data (such as remittance advice or payments) *electronically*. EDI is a fast and relatively inexpensive way to carry on day-to-day business, and it streamlines business processes and reduces operating costs. Exhibit 13–2 outlines some of the ways EDI improves efficiencies. The technology used by EDI is typically a local area network and a dial-up connection.

Practice management and management services organization (MSO) information system companies such as Medical Manager (www.medicalmanager.com), Medic (www.medcmp.com), PCN Healthnetwork (www.pcn.com), and other leading practice management and MSO software vendors have offered EDI services for years. The functions of these EDI applications, however, have typically been limited to claims submission, connectivity with the hospital to access operative reports and admission data, and electronic payment remittance, among other functions.

But, EDI is not a true Extranet. EDI's early form of "e-commerce" stopped far short of being a complete, multifunctional, on-line service using Web technologies. A *true* health care Extranet supports many functions and applications related to the business and clinical aspects of health care delivery—not just claims submission and hospital information look-up. Extranets offer interactive, real-time transactions among multiple business partners. Integration of e-patients and e-consumers, providerwide e-communications, disease management e-care applications, and more are what round out an Extranet. For example, Extranets make the following scenarios possible.

- Using the Extranet, a cardiologist can retrieve laboratory information, admit a patient, and obtain access to a clinical guideline.
- A rural primary care physician with a patient to transport to the regional medical center can authorize a referral to a specialist and send the patient's medical records via an encrypted channel.
- Health insurance plans can reduce administrative costs to the point where e-consumers can shop and purchase any health insurance plan, on line, regardless of their employer.

Exhibit 13–2 How EDI Transactions Make a Difference

- EDI reduces high administrative costs and delivery delays. Physicians save, on average, $1.50 or 35% per claim versus paper.
- EDI means faster processing and access to data. Physicians save an average of 30 days in collecting accounts receivable for electronic claims, or improve cash flow by 52% over paper claims.
- EDI increases operating efficiency. Physicians report 21% less rejection for initial claims and 20% fewer follow-ups.

Source: Data from Thomas Edison College and New Jersey Institute of Technology Study, 1995, and www.connecticare.com, © 1999, Connecticare.com.

- A pulmonologist can electronically monitor severe asthmatics by evaluating the pulmonary function test results the e-patient enters on the computer daily.
- Office staff receive fewer rejected claims because eligibility and benefits are obtained prior to sending the claim.

Fasten your seatbelts. When Extranets are linked to comprehensive data warehouses that include ambulatory, hospital, pharmacy, and home care claims information, the unleashed power of virtually connected networks to assess and analyze clinical information will change the administrative course of the American health care system.

Think about it. In just two short years the Internet has gone from "Hey, isn't this Web site cool?" to a serious e-business commerce tool. Over the next five years, Extranets will be the premier technology used to deliver clinical and information integration for more effective capitation and risk management through an Internet-based e-commerce channel. Virtual connectivity will become vitally important when it comes to managing two-way communication between providers and e-patients, handling discounted fee-for-service and capitated contracts in an independent practice association (IPA) or network, and truly keeping patients well via on-line disease management tools and applications.

Here is some e-advice: save time, save money, and reduce staffing costs and burdensome paperwork. Get an Extranet.

IMPROVING EFFICIENCY AND E-CUSTOMER SERVICE

Extranets promise to significantly reduce the amount of faxing, telephone calls, and printed communications. With a click of a mouse, this information can be delivered via bytes of data moving at high speeds through the Extranet and delivered directly to the computer desktops of physicians, health care executives, and staff. No paper, no printing, no mailing, no certified or express mail charges—and a decrease in unnecessary telephone interactions. This is not *Star Trek* technology. It is here today, and it will reduce practice and hospital overhead tremendously.

Think about the hundreds of thousands of pieces of paper and transactions that can be eliminated from physicians' offices and hospitals: referral authorization process, lab results retrieval, surgical scheduling, hospital admissions, standing orders, prescriptions, patient registration, paper claims, explanation of benefits (EOBs)—the list goes on and on. Extranets revolutionize the labor- and paper-intensive administrative process of health care by connecting virtual partners and automating outdated, repetitive, and inefficient information distribution channels.

When paperwork becomes more streamlined, patients will smile. How many times have you been frustrated by being asked the same questions, over and over, for each new physician visit or hospital stay? An integrated Extranet will ultimately allow providers to share this information so that when you show up at the ear, nose, and throat physician's office, your primary care physician will have already sent your registration data and pertinent medical history over the secure Extranet channel.

Here is another customer service nicety: e-consumers will be able to access information themselves. E-patients will be able to order their own prescription refills, access medical records, and obtain disease management information. Health insurers see this empowered e-consumer as a new e-customer. Self-service on the Web offers an incredible advantage over only being able to offer consumers one or two insurance products, which at this point are offered via employers. An Extranet would allow e-consumers to access literally all of a health plan's products—and the plan would not have to pass on the administrative burden of managing them to employers.

Extranets are already creating efficiencies like these in other industries. Ford Motor Company has set up a customer service Extranet so dealers can access the complete repair history of an individual automobile and customer preference, anywhere in the country. Mobil Corporation has created an Extranet application that streamlines the purchase order process from over 300 distributors around the world. On-line brokerages such as Charles Schwab (www.schwab.com) allow customers secure, password-protected access to trade securities, the ability to obtain research from Schwab's partner companies, and the ability to manage their portfolio.

Ready to revolutionize your organization with an Extranet? Read on to find out how successful health systems and physician organizations are meeting the challenge.

EXTRANETS FOR VIRTUAL PHYSICIAN INTEGRATION (VPI)

A major focus of Extranet applications is the virtual integration and clinical connectivity between independent physicians—who may be part of an IPA, MSO, or health plan provider panel—and business partners such as plans, labs, pharmacies, and suppliers. A highly fragmented group, physicians are ripe for virtual integration via Extranet technology. As Figure 13–1 shows, a VPI Extranet connects these physicians with services such as lab ordering and report retrieval—as

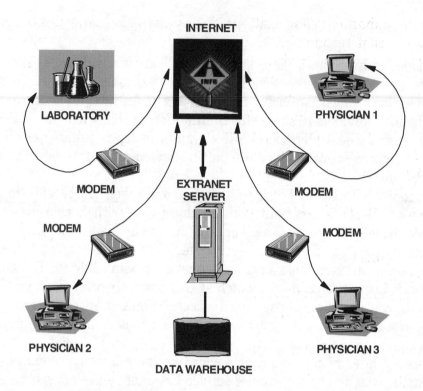

Figure 13–1 The VPI Network. *Source:* Copyright © 1999, Douglas Goldstein.

well as with each other. The data are pushed across the Internet via an Extranet server that is connected to each partner by a modem. Confidential information is securely stored in a data warehouse—not on a server that is accessible to the public Internet.

The strategy behind virtual integration is to partner with physicians by delivering information connectivity and improved managed care performance by reducing the inefficiency of current telephone interactions that waste the time of physicians and office staff. Physician-to-physician telephone calls that interrupt busy clinics (and annoy patients), duplicate registration of patients that travel between provider offices, and referral requests and authorizations can all be facilitated electronically on an Extranet. VPI applications can provide secure connectivity among physicians in a health system, network, or health plan.

Several companies are jumping into the VPI market. Healtheon, Inc. (www.healtheon.com), was one of the first to attempt taming of the fragmented physician market "beast." In 1996, Silicon Valley veterans Jim Clark and Pavan

Nigam saw an opportunity for health care providers and companies to take advantage of Internet technology. They saw a wide range of problems: most processes and transactions in health care were duplicative and paper based, resulting in wasted effort, frustrated users, high labor costs, and delays in care.

After a bumpy start (Healtheon's technology wizards initially underestimated the extraordinary variation in practice management systems, lack of technology knowledge among staff, and complexity of health care transactions), Healtheon secured a $25 million joint venture with Brown and Tolland, a large IPA in California, to implement Internet connectivity for physician referrals, coverage eligibility, authorizations, and claims. According to information listed on its corporate Web site, in 1999, Healtheon boasted the following transaction and partnership statistics:

- 67,000 physicians
- 450 payers
- 25 million administrative EDI transactions
- 25 million clinical transactions
- 200,000 contracted lives
- 5 million transactions per month

In May of 1999, Healtheon announced it was merging with WebMD (www.webmd.com), another VPI company. The Healtheon/WebMD merger created a company with a multibillion-dollar market capitalization.

Other companies, such as Pointshare[SM] (Figure 13–2), are deploying Extranets to link various health care providers along the delivery system continuum. Pointshare focuses on health systems and physicians in the Northwest. Its Extranet package provides access to the health care community and confidential communications between providers. Clinical Messaging for Hospitals automatically delivers patient test results and other mission-critical patient information from community hospitals, reference labs, and imaging centers to remote physician practices. Emergency room reports, lab results, imaging results, discharge summaries, admission notifications, operative reports, and inpatient consultations arrive instantly in physician offices, eliminating the delays and costs of U.S. mail, courier, and medical staff mailboxes. Administrative staff no longer have to waste time on mundane clerical tasks like "pulling" information from disparate sources; opening, sorting, prioritizing, and routing mail; pulling charts; hunting for loose copies of faxed consultation reports; and waiting on hold for laboratory results.

VHA Inc. (www.vhasecure.net) is a nationwide network of 1,400 community health systems. The system has spent $25 million to build VHAseCURE.net—an

Extranet that links VHA member hospitals and physicians, consumers, and hundreds of suppliers. The Extranet has two levels of member services. The basic level allows for Internet access, supply management, research services, and other capabilities. The next level, which has an additional usage fee, offers electronic commerce, electronic medical records, pharmacy management, and other services.

Extranets that virtually integrate health care providers and trading partners will guide physicians in harvesting the benefits of new information and communication technology to improve quality, enhance access, and increase revenue and profitability. Extranets will also significantly increase effective managed care delivery and substantially enhance the ability of the aligned medical network to manage capitation effectively. Why? Because this kind of connectivity allows everyone in the care community to sing from the same song sheet.

Extranet e-Case Study: Eastern Ohio Physician Organization

Eastern Ohio Physicians Organization (EOPO), an IPA in Youngstown, Ohio, has built an Extranet and hopes to save the 350 physicians in its network time and money (Figure 13–3). With development costs of approximately $200,000, EOPO's Extranet is being continually refined to reflect the needs of its medical practice subscribers.

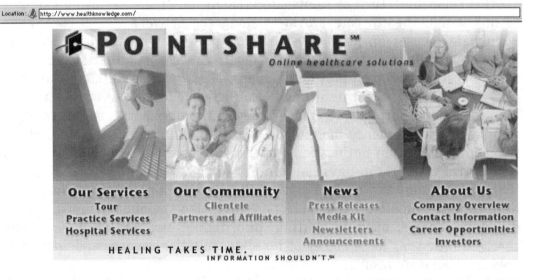

Figure 13–2 Pointshare℠. *Source:* Reprinted with permission from www.pointshare.com, © 1999, Pointshare℠.

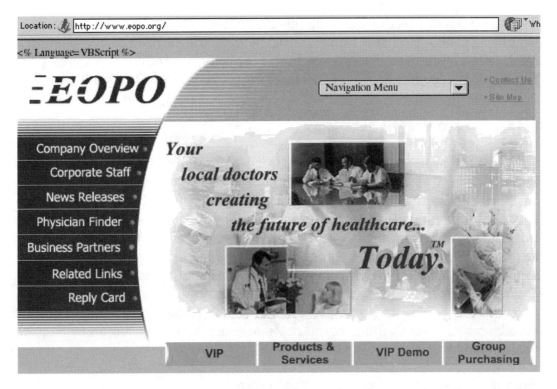

Figure 13–3 EOPO. *Source:* Reprinted with permission from www.eopo.org, © 1999, Eastern Ohio Physicians Organization.

EOPO saw a significant need to reduce time-intensive paperwork in physicians' offices, so the IPA automated eligibility and referral authorizations first. EOPO's Extranet offers an eligibility search engine that includes approximately 60 percent of the region's payer market. With a few mouse clicks, office staff can verify eligibility at the time of patient check-in, which eliminates the need for placing lengthy telephone calls to managed care plans. Referrals to specialists are easy too. The primary care physician completes an on-line form, and the request is sent via e-mail to the IPA for approval. The IPA then sends the authorization over the Extranet, directly to the specialist.

EOPO has been innovative in the area of transcription services by offering a cost-effective solution to a typically expensive office function. Physicians dictate into a telephone line, and the digital recording is transcribed by EOPO employees. Documents are then e-mailed to the physician or office for corrections and printing.

Other Extranet functions include on-line claims submission to more than 600 insurance plans, a central calendar that allows offices to schedule operating room time on line, and a physician finder for e-consumers. EOPO plans to push lab and pharmacy information to medical offices soon.

EXTRANETS FOR HEALTH CARE PLANS

There have been tremendous strides in on-line service offerings to customers as health plan Web sites have moved from a marketing focus to an emphasis on customer service. Two and three years ago, most Web sites offered limited value-added information with a myriad of hyperlinks to other health care sites. This was a flawed strategy; the link sent the consumer out of the Web site to another location. If an organization is going to spend money developing on-line service functionality, why export visitors to another consumer-sponsored site?

Health plans have since wised up, and they now offer Extranets that focus on e-consumers, e-patients, and e-providers. A variety of transactions, from on-line enrollment to claims adjudication and more, are becoming more common on health plan services.

Extranet e-Case Study: Aetna U.S. Healthcare

Several years ago, Aetna U.S. Healthcare launched its consumer-oriented Web service, which included "DocFind," membership information, and information on employee and provider services (Figure 13–4). Nothing else.

Then in August 1997, the plan really began to cook. It served up a pilot of its newest on-line product, EZenroll™—an easy, on-line enrollment service for e-consumers that also complied with disparate state regulations and promoted accurate and complete enrollment form submission. A member simply enters his or her address and state and EZenroll automatically displays the correct enrollment form based on the member's address. Barring errors in entering the address, state compliance is automatic.

EZenroll was designed to be self-monitoring. If any information is incomplete or inaccurate, the system does not transmit the form. Instead, it indicates which areas are incomplete or inaccurate and directs the member to complete or correct these areas before the form can be accepted. Once a clean form is submitted, EZenroll scrubs the data and automatically creates identification cards and other membership materials and readies them for mailing to the member. Sounds too good to be true? EZenroll became available to all members in October 1997 and is used by more than 20 employer groups.

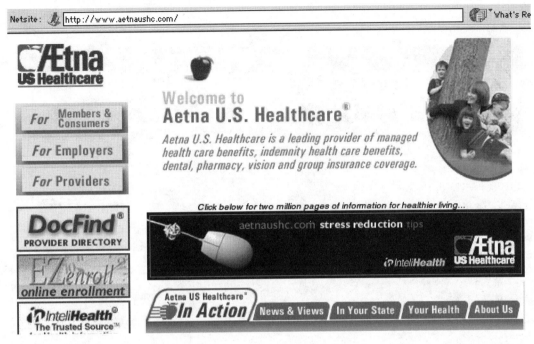

Figure 13–4 Aetna U.S. Healthcare. *Source:* Reprinted with permission from www.aetnaushc.com, © 1999, Aetna US Healthcare.

Fast forward to 1999, and Aetna U.S. Healthcare is still innovating. Now members can access value-added health care information through an alliance with "Doc Line" and links to its virtual partner, InteliHealth (www.intelihealth.com). E-patients can change their primary care physician or other enrollment information and search for a physician that meets specific criteria.

And providers are not left out either. E-Pay is an e-commerce solution that promotes an electronic referral, encounter, and claim system that allows processing and payment of clean claims within 15 days.

Aetna U.S. Healthcare hosts its Web service on a UNIX-Sun computer platform. It uses Web Objects software to create the EZenroll forms and database.

Extranet e-Case Study: Blue Cross Blue Shield of California

Systems integrator Sash Communications recently helped Blue Shield of California develop a platform for health insurance application approvals over the Internet using off-the-shelf applications (Figure 13–5). The system cost approximately $2.25 million and took six months to build.

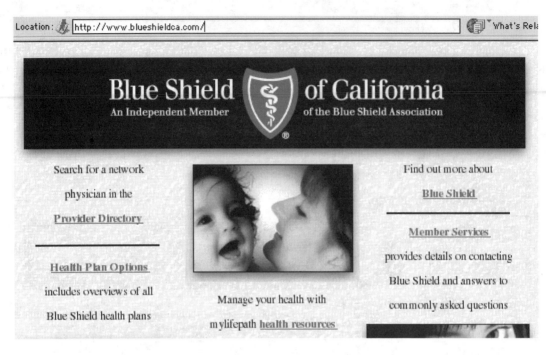

Figure 13–5 Blue Shield of California. Courtesy of www.blueshieldca.com, 1999, Blue Shield of California.

Sash worked with key Blue Shield employees to automate the insurer's work flow processes into a Web application process—not an easy task by any means, since these processes are full of "if, then" scenarios. The result: Blue Shield's Extranet has a modular design that runs a series of small programs called engines that determine whether an applicant is qualified when he or she submits an application on line. The engine rules make sure all fields are properly completed—which decreased the application turnaround time for the insurer. The old-fashioned paper process produced first-time application returns of 20 percent because of incomplete information.

Blue Shield's brokers can access the Extranet as well. Their transactions are secured through a combination of encryption, digital certificates, password access control, and firewalls.[2]

Connecticare (www.conecticare.com), Oxford Health Plans (www.oxhp.com), and Group Health Incorporated (Figure 13–6) are among the many other plans serving up Extranets for members, providers, and other business partners.

Connecticare, a health maintenance organization serving Connecticut and Massachusetts residents, uses an Extranet to support greater connectivity between physician panel members and the plan. Electronic claims submission, e-communications, on-line eligibility verification, and electronic funds transfer are some of the features it offers providers. In 1999, the company began to offer electronic remittance advice, an electronic alternative to receiving an EOB in a paper format, and claims status reporting, which offers the capability to electronically check the status of claims at any time after submission. Connecticare also offers members services on line. E-members can register for health education workshops, find out about local fitness centers that offer discounts, search for providers, and read Connecticare's award-winning newsletter.

Oxford Health Plan allows office staff to check the status of claims on line and check patient eligibility and benefits. Members can view their claim status as well as make address changes, notify Oxford of emergency department visits, and change their primary care physician.

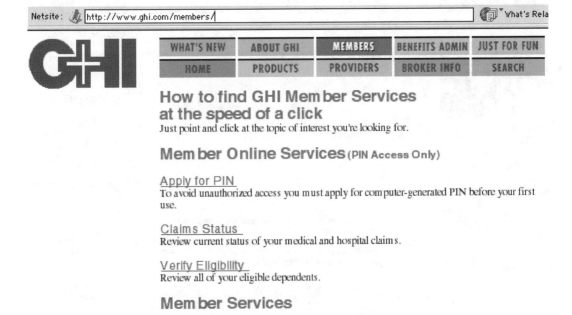

Figure 13–6 Group Health Incorporated. *Source:* Reprinted with permission from www.ghi.com/members/, © 1999, Group Health Incorporated.

Group Health Incorporated, which serves all of New York, offers on-line eligibility and claim status queries, downloadable claim forms, on-line members services, and health and wellness information.

EXTRANETS FOR BETTER HEALTH AND WELL-BEING

Connecting information, education, and e-support services can help e-consumers and e-patients improve their own health and well-being. Although national portals such as OnHealth.com, America's Health Network (www.AHO.com), and HealthCentral.com offer the e-information part and aim to empower consumers to take charge of their own care, they cannot offer the security of one-to-one transactions or e-communication. Several Extranet companies have taken advantage of this e-security gap and provide connectivity among e-patients, e-providers, health plans, and health systems.

Abaton.com (Figure 13–7) provides Web solutions for health systems, medical practices, and pharmacy benefits managers. The company has a strategic and

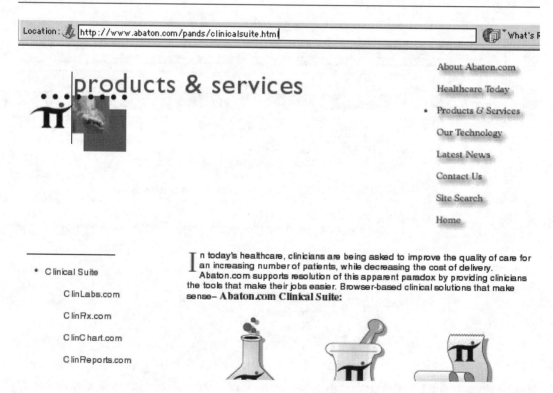

Figure 13–7 Abaton. *Source:* Abaton.com, Inc. © 1999. Reproduced by permission.

financial partnership with the Intel Corporation. Abaton's application minimizes the number of steps for delivering care and offers two-way communication between clinicians and providers. E-patients can obtain lab results and personal clinical reports on line. Nurses can schedule their own to-do lists and automate prescription refills.

Optum is another market leader that provides comprehensive information, education, and support services that can improve the quality of life for e-patients. Optum offers services in telephone space and cyberspace, and its Health Forum solution (www.healthforum.com) uses the Web to help e-patients make appropriate daily health decisions and become more effective managers of their own well-being.

The key features of Health Forum include a personalized home page that delivers the health news that consumers choose, the ability to e-mail a question to a nurse (nonemergent), access to plan benefits, and a searchable database of health and well-being information.

FEELING A LITTLE INSECURE?

As the use of Internet technology has grown in the health care industry, providers and patients continue to express concern about security on the World Wide Web. Patient advocates and patients themselves believe privacy will be intruded upon if health care providers and systems begin to put health and medical care on the Web. While it is true that an Extranet plan must address numerous security concerns, particularly around sensitive patient data, these concerns are not insurmountable. And although many professional societies and government agencies are cautious, the benefits of enhancing medical care delivery and improving process efficiency far outweigh the security risks.

The challenge as you create an Extranet is to be sure that you have prepared properly to protect the data. First and foremost, the Extranet must be protected by firewalls and security protocols to ensure that confidential information stays within the designated members of the alliance. So, even though the Extranet is running on the Internet, your confidential patient data are securely tucked away behind a virtual blanket of security. Other e-tools, such as authentication and encryption, also are critical to assuring visitors that the Extranet environment is private.

For additional protection, a secure sockets layer (SSL) can be put in place. Designed by Netscape, SSL protocol facilitates secure transmission of private documents over the Internet. SSL uses public-key encryption to exchange a session key between the client and server. This session key is used to encrypt the http transaction (both request and response). Each transaction uses a different session key so that if someone manages to decrypt another transaction, that person will need to spend as much time and effort on the second transaction as he or she did on the first.

BEWARE OF WATCHDOGS

As this book went to press, the American Medical Association did not have a formal position on using electronic Internet technology, pending completion of a large study. It does, however, emphasize that even with a patient's written consent to transmit his or her information via the Internet, it is still the responsibility of the caregiver to ensure the confidentiality of the information. (Sounds like the familiar problem of managed care plans that do not pay for a procedure but hold physicians accountable if they do not perform it when it is medically necessary.)

In January 1998, the American Medical Informatics Association came out with guidelines for physician-to-patient communication on the Internet. Exhibit 13–3 lists some of these guidelines. Several leading health care institutions are taking the guidelines to heart and moving full speed ahead with Extranets that carry at least some confidential information about patients. For a complete copy of these guidelines, go to http://www.amia.org/pubs/pospaper/positio2.htm.

Exhibit 13–3 Sample Guidelines for Physician-to-Patient Communication on the Internet

- Consider obtaining patient's informed consent for use of e-mail. Written forms should
  —Itemize terms in communications guideline
  —Describe security mechanisms in place
  —Indemnify health care institution for information loss due to technical failures
- Use password-protected screen savers for all desktop workstations in the office, hospital, and home.
- Never forward patient-identifiable information to a third party without the patient's express permission.
- Do not use unencrypted, wireless communications with patient-identifiable information.
- Double check all "TO:" fields prior to sending messages.
- Commit policy decisions to writing and put them in electronic form as well.

Source: Copyright © 1999, Douglas Goldstein.

Security issues can get sticky but are not without solutions. Columbia-Presbyterian Hospital of New York, for example, developed a program that automatically prints out mailers to remind patients to take their medication. At the time the mailer is printed, Internet technology is used to notify the patient's physician. Columbia-Presbyterian's goal is to develop a system that is accessible to anyone with a personal computer. To ensure that these transactions are confidential, the hospital has employed a three-tier security protocol: message encryption, secure sockets, and electronic identification card. Columbia-Presbyterian hopes to develop a system for e-patients to review their records on line.[3]

Johns Hopkins Hospital in Baltimore uses an Intranet to connect various departments within the hospital so that they may share patient information. The University of California San Diego Medical Center is developing Web-based access to clinical patient information. The Patient-Centered Access to Secure Systems Online will be available for physicians and e-patients.[4]

Anxious providers and health care executives, rest easy. A variety of security tools are available, and using a combination of them makes for a secure Extranet environment that is difficult for hackers to penetrate. Also, as Internet use increases, Americans will continue to become more and more comfortable with on-line transactions. Look at how often credit cards are now being used to make on-line purchases and how on-line trading has exploded in the last two years. As more e-patients become e-consumers, they will soon look back and wonder, "How did we ever get by when we had to actually call the physician's office for that information?"

SUPPLY CHAIN COMPRESSION: HEADS WILL ROLL

All this Extranet stuff sounds great, right? Lower costs, greater efficiency, e-commerce solutions for nearly all paper-based processes and systems. But wait. What's going to happen to those vendors in the supply chain that push all that paper? What of the "middlemen" and distributors who take a cut just for getting a manufacturer's product or service into the minds and hands of customers? The added organizational layers and percentage markups of distributors and high-commissioned sales representatives could go the way of the dumb terminal. Although some jobs will remain, they may evolve into training or service positions—not the high-paying positions that exist today. Exhibit 13–4 lists some of the job positions that are at risk.

Although sales forces and distribution networks have to date been the only way manufacturers got their products to end users, the Internet stands to drastically change that. The Internet will become the distribution system. Web-en-

Exhibit 13–4 Positions at Risk of Being Eliminated by e-Technology

- Practice management system vendors
- Medical device distributors and salespeople
- Health insurance brokers and agents
- Pharmaceutical detail representatives
- Purchasing department administrators
- Medical supply salespeople

Source: Copyright © 1999, Douglas Goldstein.

abling product and service information and pushing it to e-consumers cost virtually nothing. No salaries, no commissions, no benefits, no expense accounts. Why would manufacturers pay commissions when they can deliver their products directly to e-customers, on line, essentially for free?

Take a look at the travel industry. For years, travel agents mediated between consumers and airlines, hotels, and rental car companies. But now, three-quarters of the top 75 airline, hotel, and car rental companies reach e-consumers directly, on the Internet.[5] On top of slashed commissions, travel agents have seen their distribution exclusivity destroyed and are beginning to seek new lines of business, such as corporate meeting planning, or to charge customers for their services. Many travel agencies are going out of business.

Real estate agents and insurance brokers face a similar future. Point your browser to www.century21.com or www.remax.com, and you can search for properties by city, price, and amenities. Go to www.prudential.com, and you can read detailed information about every insurance product Prudential sells. If the e-consumer does all the work, what happens to the value of the agent? How can he or she justify commanding a commission when the e-consumer did everything? Agents and brokers will have to earn their keep by shifting to after-sale benefits (in real estate, for example, coordinating the moving company or recommending landscaping), or e-consumers will not pay. And who would blame them?

As e-consumers begin to self-serve in greater numbers, products will become commodities. When e-consumers can access LifeQuote to compare life insurance prices from 50 different companies, or PriceScan to compare prices for computer equipment and software, all bets are off for supply chain intermediaries. Prices will fluctuate in real time, driven by e-consumers; and fewer transactions, faster, with fewer layers of bureaucracy, will mean fewer players in the game.

FINAL TIPS, TACTICS, AND TALES

With the pace of change in technology driving costs down, it pays to carefully evaluate the potential applications of an Extranet in your health system or organization. Run a cost benefit analysis to determine how the costs of conducting cyberspace transactions compare with the costs of conducting real-space transactions. Use a team of people from different parts of the organization—administrators, clinicians, information technology folks, front-line staff from medical offices and the hospital—and do not forget to include patients in the mix. As with many information technology projects, the time and attention needed to implement the project is always longer than anticipated. As you begin to design, develop, and deploy your organization's Extranet, plan your activities carefully.

Look Before You Leap. In the rush to become the Amazon.com of health care Extranet companies, a variety of vendors have come to the fore with Web applications. Healtheon/WebMD, OfficeMed, and others continue to roll out newly packaged applications, but let the buyer beware. These early adapters often sell 1.0 version releases that must be considered carefully before a health system with 20 sites and 100,000 covered lives purchases them.

Measure the Size of Your Existing "Pipes." The type of data that can be moved effectively on an Extranet depends on bandwidth and the speed of your organization's dial-up connection. The size of the "pipe" (bandwidth) or the "nozzle" (hardware) that the pipe is connected to also affects the ability to move data or graphical information.

For instance, an on-line video consultation between a primary care physician and a specialist does not work on a 28.8 Kbps dial-up connection, but it does work on a 128 Kbps or WAN connection. Which applications your Extranet pushes through the pipeline must be carefully analyzed to determine the best combination of communication channels to move the volume of transaction data that is anticipated.

Beware of the Cultural Barriers to Entry. Even if an Extranet is the right thing to use today, a big barrier to success can be the individual users (i.e., hospital and physician office staff) themselves. In the past, health care workers and physicians have often had a "this is the way we've always done it, why change?" attitude. Your challenge as an organization is to involve staff members—who, by the way, will use the Extranet more than anyone else—and share specific information about how an Extranet will make their jobs easier. These employees' willingness to use computer software programs and ability to feel comfortable interfacing through cyberspace—instead of talking on the telephone or sending out a bill through snail mail, as they have done for the last 20 years—are contingent on your ability to sell them on the concept of change.

Make Flowcharts of the Processes and Transactions That an Extranet Could Improve in Your Health System before Deciding What To Buy. Start by making flowcharts of the current processes and costs associated with delivering the service in telephone space or real space. Consider the staff, physicians, and managers that will need to be involved to ensure the Web-enabled solutions to these processes will actually benefit them.

Think about Your Extranet in Bytes. Developing a full-blown Extranet is like devouring a multicourse dinner. Decide which set of applications will be the appetizers and pick those that will whet the appetites of your business partners most. Then move on to a phase two rollout—the "entree." Then decide what will be the dessert that tops it all off. Extranets are an evolving process. Take each course separately, and you will end up with a better result.

Be Clear about Costs and Logistics. As you plan your Extranet, you must determine who will be in charge, how the Extranet will be staffed, and how much software, hardware, talent, and training will cost. It is also critical to determine the combination of internal staff time and outside consulting support necessary to design, program, and deploy the application. The overall cost of an Extranet effort is totally dependent on its functions and the number of users, but the examples in this chapter would range from several hundreds of thousands to $25 million or more to implement.

CONCLUSION—THE HEALTH CARE E-COMMERCE WAVE

So what of the sick patient introduced at the beginning of this chapter? The American health care system has begun to get well through the e-commerce cure.

Initial Treatment Plan

Web-enable business functions such as eligibility verification and claims submission, where return on investment is clear and can be realized quickly by physicians and those who manage them.

Ongoing Treatment Plan

Continue using Web applications to cut paperwork, improve efficiencies, and lower costs. Strive for full integration and e-connectivity among physicians, health systems, insurers, and patients.

As hospitals, insurers, and physician organizations devise creative strategies to replace traditional transactions with secure cyberspace transactions, health care commerce will be transformed. Extranets will slash the costs of conducting business, save time, and boost convenience for e-customers, e-members, and e-patients. Evolving traditional business activities from their current labor-intensive and fragmented status to full e-connectivity can immediately reduce some costs and improve efficiency. The real e-commerce benefits, however, will come from the second- and third-generation e-commerce solutions, which include full e-connectivity with all health care business partners. These applications will produce even greater economic value for e-consumers and e-patients by enabling more contact between them and e-providers.

Health care organizations that streamline real-space and telephone-space transactions using an Extranet will have significant advantage over those that do not. Because of the rush to be first, expect to see a battle for control over the physician desktop interfaces, but do not take a wait-and-see attitude, or you will most certainly lose the advantage in your region. And you will continue to spend a lot of money on administrative tasks that could be less expensive.

There are limitless applications of Extranet services and e-commerce solutions that can improve productivity, enhance communication, and increase quality. Health care executives and physicians must realize, however, that e-commerce is more than just technology. It is an entirely different way of conducting business. As your organization implements e-commerce tactics, you will need to challenge the way you think and the way operations are structured. The only limits on Extranets have little to do with technology and everything to do with the ability of your health system employees and stakeholders to innovate and deploy solutions and resources.

REFERENCES

1. Electronic Commerce for Health Insurance Choice, *P.U.L.S.E. Analysis* (Sherlock Company, 1999), 1.
2. L. Sherman, "Health Care Company Speeds Up the Process," *Inter@ctive Week* (5 October 1998), 36.
3. D. Goldstein et al., *Patient Confidentiality and Security on the Internet* (Alexandria, VA: Radiology Associates, 1998), 4.
4. Goldstein et al., *Patient Confidentiality and Security,* 4.
5. J. Evans, "Travel Agents Feel the Squeeze," *Washington Post,* 27 December 1998, A1, A16.

CHAPTER 14

Pharmaceutical Companies Ride the e-Power of the Net

Steven Sutor

YOUR PHYSICIAN just diagnosed you with diabetes. You are 40 years old and stunned. You do not remember much of what the two of you talked about when you were in his office—except giving up the foods you like and maybe going blind one day. Where can you turn to get the information you need?

You are 67, and you have just been told you had a "mini stroke," whatever *that* means. The physician gave you some brochures and talked about it like it was no big deal—"it happens all the time," he said. Well it has never happened to *you* before. How can you find out more?

You did not know what the discomfort was, but now the clinic says it is a sexually transmitted disease (STD). Three people saw you in about 15 minutes—after you waited over two hours—then gave you a pamphlet that is not very clear. Does your boyfriend have it? Can your little girl catch it somehow? How can you ask these kinds of questions when everyone is in and out of the room a dozen times?

For the first time in the history of health care, you can turn to a multibillion-dollar international pharmaceutical manufacturer for the answers to the above questions and more.

That is right: the companies that make drugs for diabetes, stroke, and STDs have first-rate information about your disease. And these pharmaceutical companies are ready to tell you just about everything you want to know. In fact, these pharmaceutical companies have so much information that it would take dozens of expensive, time-consuming office visits to get all of it the "old-fashioned" way—from your physician.

How do you get to this pharmaceutical firm? Click on the Web. What site, what company, you wonder? Every company that manufactures prescription and over-the-counter medication and expects to survive—to thrive—in the new millennium.

IT IS AN E-REVOLUTION

Pharmaceutical manufacturers are shaping a *revolution* within an *evolution*, an irreversible new paradigm in health care, by acknowledging and harnessing the power of the Net to reach the "new" patient, the health care e-consumer.

The *evolution* is in health care itself, moving rapidly away from unqualified reliance on the historic, didactic relationship between the physician and the passive patient. The *revolution* has pharmaceutical manufacturers bypassing the traditional prescriber and going right to the end user. This revolution is truly changing the face of health care, and e-commerce and Web technology have made it possible.

Pharmaceutical companies are siphoning money and influence from managed care organizations, pharmacists, and physicians as the companies help to create the new, empowered health care e-consumer. And this revolution is not going away; it is not going to be legislated away, and it is not going to fail. E-patients have tasted the power of disease-specific knowledge and have seen what will happen when they go to the physician and demand a product: they know they are likely to get it.

Using the Web as their tool, drug manufacturers are narrowing the gap between the information offered to prescribers and that offered to consumers. In fact, many firms no longer have secure sites for physicians, feeling that it is inappropriate to keep information from the health care consumer. Both providers and patients can follow the same e-path through the site and draw their own conclusions. In addition to the economic impact, the impact on the physician–patient relationship is enormous, creating what Dr. Debra Roter of the Johns Hopkins School of Public Health calls the consumerist medical interview.

This shift is generating enormous informational power for health care consumers—power that allows e-patients to actually influence prescribing habits. Managed care plans are struggling with a significant increase in drug benefit costs and are looking for the standard quick fix. Physicians are feeling threatened. But direct-to-consumer (DTC) marketing and the sales generated by it are here to stay.

This chapter focuses on how pharmaceutical manufacturers are using the Web to influence, educate, and engage not only those who currently prescribe their products—the traditional physician audience—but the new breed of e-patient. The chapter takes a close-up look at how pharmaceutical companies use the Web to connect with patients, creating health care e-consumers in the process, to permanently change how Americans ask for, access, and consume pharmaceuticals.

EXPERTS AT PROMOTION AND COMMUNICATION

That pharmaceutical firms are aggressively harnessing the Web should not come as a surprise. The dominant firms have investigated and participated in most major and minor communications trends over the years. For example, pharmaceutical sales representatives—detailers—have used laptop computers for at least 10 years. Loaded with PowerPoint slides and graphics that allowed substantial amounts of information to be shared with prescribers, these presentations left little room for factual error. Video-based intracompany meetings, transmitted by purchased satellite time, have been a standard since the late 1980s, when a drug company wanted to introduce a new product internally, announce Food and Drug Administration (FDA) approval, "meet" with regional directors, or simply rally the troops. Finally, most medical trade journals—print-based communications, delivered directly to the physician's office—are almost completely supported by pharmaceutical advertising.

What all of these marketing, promotion, and sales activities have in common, though, is that, outside the firm itself, they are directed to the traditional audience, the prescriber, around a traditional message: "Provide our product to your patient." As pharmaceutical companies ride the power of the Net, however, that system is changing.

DTC ADVERTISING EXPLODES

The audience and the message began to evolve several years ago, when DTC advertising was explored as a new marketing avenue. In the early 1990s, product awareness was the goal, and print was the medium. At first, DTC was something of a throwaway dollar for the pharmaceuticals; it was what was left from promoting product to the prescriber. Then physicians and managed care organizations began to notice that patients were actually asking for the drugs that they had seen advertised.

In 1992, a prescription product was advertised on television for the first time. It was a nicotine patch. The American Association of Advertising Agencies noted that the ad resulted in such demand that it exceeded supply of the patches. According to *American Demographics*, "Fully one-third of the 163 million adult Americans who have seen or heard a DTC television, print, or radio ad have spoken to their physicians about the medication."[1] And according to the *Journal of the American Medical Association*, as many as 12.1 million consumers have requested and received a prescribed drug as a direct result of seeing a DTC advertisement (see Figure 14–1).[2]

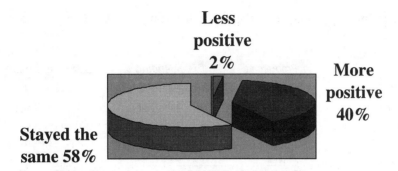

Figure 14–1 DTC Advertising: Impact on 163 Million Adults. *Source:* Data from A.F. Holmer, Direct-to-Consumer Prescription Advertising Builds Bridges Between Physicians and Patients, *Journal of the American Medical Association*, Vol. 281, p. 380, © 1999, American Medical Association.

Is DTC effective? IMS Health, the world's largest pharmaceutical data organization, notes that patient visits to physicians for osteoporosis nearly *doubled* in the one-year period following the debut of DTC advertisements for a new drug for the condition.[3] In unpublished data from December 1998 by Andrew Witty of Glaxo Wellcome Inc., 49 percent of the people who called a toll-free number in an ad for genital herpes saw their physicians about the condition within three months. It should also be noted, however, that 51 percent of those who saw the physician did not actually receive a prescription, even though it is likely that they asked for one. But that means that 49 percent did get a prescription. And that is 49 percent more than before DTC.

How much new business does DTC drive? Table 14–1 shows the 1998 top 10 DTC spending amounts per drug compared to same-drug spending to reach prescribers. These figures are a clear indication of the importance of DTC advertising. For all but two of the drugs listed in the table, firms spent more on DTC advertising than on advertising to subscribers. It is the revolution of patient as prescriber.

And while there have been no definitive studies to prove that there is a link between DTC and sales, according to *Med Ad News*, spending on prescription pharmaceuticals was up 42 percent in the United States in 1997 (latest figures available), with the United States accounting for a full 33 percent of the world market.[4] Coincidence? Not likely. As the pharmaceuticals reach out to prescribers and to consumers, spending and the U.S. market share will continue to grow.

Certain "disease" categories were all but invented through DTC advertising. Take nail fungus, for example. It was a negligible condition prior to pharmaceutical advertising. The rise in prescriptions for antifungal medication, however,

Table 14-1 The Top 10 Pharmaceuticals in DTC Spending in 1998 (Compared to Same-Drug Spending for Professionals)

Company	Product	DTC Spending	Spending for Professionals
Schering-Plough	Claritin	$66,707,000	$37,110,000
Bristol-Myers Squibb	Pravachol	$55,883,000	$29,666,000
Glaxo Wellcome	Zyban	$35,765,000	$13,599,000
Pfizer	Zyrtec	$34,191,000	$28,383,000
Eli Lilly	Evista	$31,513,000	$30,719,000
Hoechst Marion Roussel	Allegra	$30,872,000	$33,443,000
Merck	Propecia	$28,556,000	$12,058,000
Astra	Prilosec	$28,042,000	$24,600,000
American Home Products	Premarin	$25,472,000	$18,549,000
Lilly	Prozac	$25,328,000	$29,674,000

Source: Data from A. Holmer, Direct-to-Consumer Prescription Drug Advertising Builds Bridges Between Patients and Physicians, *Journal of the American Medical Association*, Vol. 281, No. 4, American Medical Association and IMS Health.

has grown tremendously and in direct correlation to increased DTC advertising, according to Michael Dillon, Director of Pharmacy Services, Community Health Plan/Kaiser Permanente Northeast Division, Latham, New York.

And some disease categories are going to be aggressively promoted by the introduction of new drugs. One major pharmaceutical manufacturer is launching a new product for irritable bowel syndrome (IBS), a condition that is estimated to affect millions in the United States. However, it is usually not treated because there has been, up until now, no condition-specific drug and because it has often been seen as an "emotional" condition. The impact of a new IBS drug with a heavy DTC marketing component will be felt from the physician's office to the pharmacy benefits manager to the managed care organization.

The DTC phenomenon caused the pharmaceuticals to take notice. Consumer-directed advertising budgets began to grow, and there was a flurry of activity within the medical advertising agencies to establish consumer-oriented divisions. The revolution had begun. Net-directed DTC dollars gave the firms real value over their higher-cost counterparts, print and broadcast.

FROM "ASK YOUR PHYSICIAN" TO "TELL YOUR PHYSICIAN"

Pharmaceutical consulting firm Scott-Levin predicts that DTC advertising will top $5 billion in just two years, up over 1,000 percent. A significant portion of that will go toward Web-based advertising—reaching individual patients with specific diseases and generating the perceived need for certain drugs.

As Figure 14–2 shows, in the mid-1990s pharmaceutical companies began to spend enormous amounts of dollars on reaching and influencing consumers; from 1995, the spending increased dramatically. Still, the message was meant only to illuminate. For example: are your nails cracked and unsightly? Ask your physician about prescription medication for the condition. Do you frequently feel blue? You may be suffering from depression; ask your physician about medications that have helped millions. Did you know that certain medications might be right for your cardiac condition? Ask your physician if they might be right for you. The universal conclusion to DTC advertising at that time was "ask your physician." After all, the physician was the prescriber—the primary customer of the pharmaceutical company.

However, during this time, broadcast, specifically television, was opened up to the pharmaceutical companies as a legitimate advertising channel. While the FDA approved this new informational assault on the consumer, it made an embarrassing initial decision: it would not allow the pharmaceutical to link the product to the disease state. To its credit, after an outcry from consumers and a lot of ribbing from the media, the FDA quickly re-thought this and allowed pharmaceutical companies to link condition and product in broadcast.

The result of this DTC focus? Although pharmaceutical companies would continue marketing to physicians (Figure 14–3), never again would physicians be the only ones marketed to. Influencing and educating patients was improving sales. The stage was set for a full-scale strike on the consumer, and the marketing message began to change in a subtle but important way. As increased sales were linked to DTC advertising, what used to be "ask your physician" became "discuss with—*tell!*—your physician."

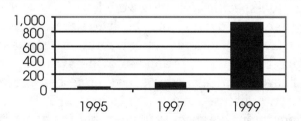

Figure 14–2 Spending Increases in DTC Advertising (in Millions). *Source:* Data from the National Managed Health Care Congress, 1999, Atlanta, Georgia.

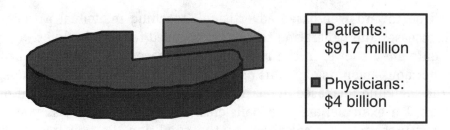

Figure 14–3 Advertising To Reach Patients and To Reach Physicians. *Source:* Data from the National Managed Health Care Congress, 1997, Atlanta, Georgia, Dr. Grant Lawless, V.P. Medical and Pharmacy Affairs/Corporate Medical Director, Highmark BlueCross BlueShield.

This change was only the beginning. The way pharmaceutical companies targeted consumers was about to change significantly. Where did pharmaceutical companies look next? The burgeoning world of real-time, user-specific information: the Net.

PHARMACEUTICAL COMPANIES GO ON LINE

The original DTC medium was print: newspapers, newsmagazines, and especially the so-called "women's magazines" (women heavily influence the purchase and use of both prescription and over-the-counter drugs). In print, the patient information (PI) was easy to provide; it usually ran on the page following the color ad for the pharmaceutical product. With the advent of broadcast, the PI became a problem. To overcome this, the FDA required a toll-free number to run in the televised spot, a number that the viewer could call to get all of the information on the drug. But the Web offered an even better solution: Launch a Web site that contains PI, and this site could contain even more influential advertising for the product. Plus, the cost of communicating in this medium was low (Figure 14–4). The drug-specific Web sites were born!

In 1999, there were well over 15,000 health-related Web sites—with more being created each day—that offered an extraordinary range of advice, education, and information to e-consumers and e-providers. Many of the most interactive are from the pharmaceuticals, which have large banks of substantive data about chronic and acute disease from which to draw. For the first time, the key elements of these enormous databases are available to the patient.

Based on an informal survey of *Med Ad News*, more than 80 of the top 100 pharmaceutical firms have Web sites. These sites introduce the firms to the

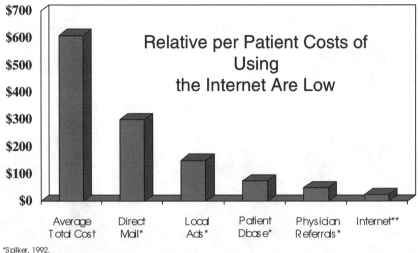

Figure 14–4 Per-Patient Recruitment Costs Are Low. *Source:* Data from Center Watch, Inc., and Spilker, 1992.

world, painting a picture of dedication to cures, research, and to substantive, positive involvement in the health care community. They provide the links that take providers and consumers to disease categories, health-related pages, product pages, disease-specific education, and usable tools to understand a disease or condition and engage in the care process. They are also used to inform investors and to list employment opportunities within the company.

The focus of each pharmaceutical company varies, but overarching goals are to educate consumers about product efficacy. It all adds up to one thing: the e-consumer is highly likely to ask for a prescription by name. Hoechst Marion Roussel (Figure 14–5) and Amgen (www.amgen.com) are good examples of companies that are reaching the e-consumer and e-patient under the umbrella of information and education.

Hoechst Marion Roussel offers brochures on topics such as diabetes. Physicians can download and distribute these brochures to patients. The brochures offer basic advice that reinforces what the physician may discuss with the patient during the medical interview. They strengthen the physician–patient relationship and help improve compliance.

Amgen offers a Reimbursement Hotline and a Safety Net® Program with toll-free numbers for patients and providers. The reimbursement program offers help

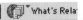

Netsite: http://www.hmri.com/onthehealthcareteam/

Hoechst Marion Roussel USA Home   Beyond Medicine to Health™

On the Health Care Team

information for health care professionals and executives

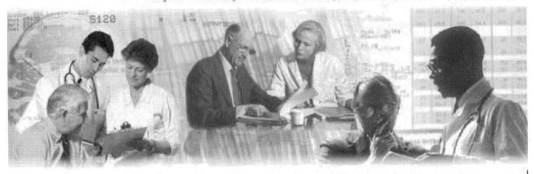

Figure 14–5 Hoechst Marion Roussel. *Source:* Reprinted with permission from www.hmri.com/onthehealthcare, © 1999, Hoechst Marion Roussel/USA.

in completing paperwork to get reimbursed for Neupogen® and Epogen®, two of Amgen's products that treat renal failure and end-stage renal disease. The Safety Net Program sets the wheels in motion to provide these two Amgen products free to indigent patients. Both of these programs, of course, help patients to use—and providers to request—Amgen products that may not be readily available. They not only promote the products but help build a stronger relationship between provider and patient, with each feeling that Amgen is looking out for their best interests. This type of low-cost program allows Amgen to build a relationship with not only the prescriber but the patient. The patient is very likely to request these products if he or she is in the position to do so. It is also an end run around the insurer, extending the influence of patients and prescribers by helping them to obtain reimbursement for off-formulary drugs more easily: Amgen is actually willing to give the product to patients who cannot afford them.

In addition to the Web sites that are specific to the manufacturer, some non-product-specific or non-company-specific sites are sponsored or underwritten by the manufacturers. These Web sites include items such as on-line health care magazines for providers. Between Rounds (Figure 14–6) is one example of this type of pharmaceutical company–sponsored site. It is an interactive magazine specifically for the managed care physician. The physician can interact with the "experts" at the on-line publication and get answers to specific questions and challenges—a feat impossible for print magazines to accomplish. It is this real-time aspect that gives the Web a distinct advantage.

Using the Web, pharmaceutical companies have an opportunity to create and re-create themselves in a medium that engages the user as an individual in a one-on-one interaction. The e-visitor understands the company from an intimate, personal perspective that was unlikely, even impossible, before the Internet. Pharmaceutical companies create an image that lingers after the informational or educational message has been forgotten. And, more than just image, the pharmaceutical sites offer information that is the result of research, substantive data, additional links, and evaluative tools.

The Internet is proactive. Traditional media are reactive. In an age when time poverty rather than economic prosperity is influencing Americans' shopping, purchasing, and other habits, the gold standard is the consumer who takes time

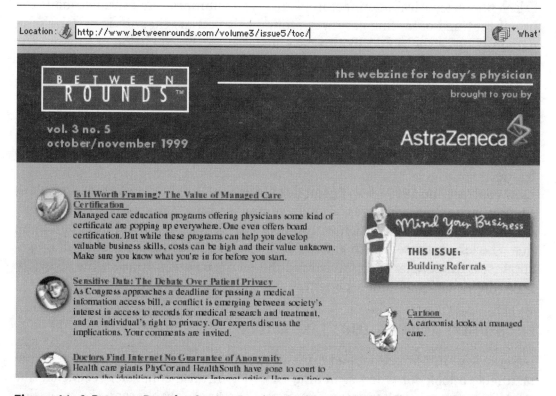

Figure 14–6 Between Rounds. *Source:* Reprinted with permission from www.betweenrounds. com, © 1999, Between Rounds.

to look for and purchase your product. Visitors to a Web site—e-consumers—seek out the site rather than merely coming across a message in a newspaper or viewing an ad on television. They have an agenda, and the pharmaceutical companies—masters of data capture—are rapidly accumulating e-consumer names and contact information, disease states, health concerns, and even buying habits.

What are they doing with that information? Right now, just a little. People are still learning about the Internet, much like they were just learning about managed care 20 years ago. How companies use and share the data captured is still influenced by consumers. In Baltimore, Maryland, in 1998 a supermarket chain and its in-house drugstores began to send disease-specific information to patients. They knew, from pharmacy data, which patients had which diseases, and decided to try to help those patients adapt to healthier lifestyles and to remember to fill and refill prescriptions. Recipients of this disease-specific information were outraged. They felt that the grocery chain was violating confidentiality by knowing who had what condition, even though it was the food chain's pharmacy that supplied the information.

The pharmaceutical manufacturers are being appropriately cautious about the use of captured data. One easy way around this barrier, though, is to ask the e-patient if he or she would like to have updates on the condition or product the manufacturers are investigating. A simple click of the mouse, and the pharmaceutical can send information and, not coincidentally, build a stronger relationship with someone who is likely sick.

Pharmaceutical companies consider their e-visitors to be potential e-customers. With new power to influence the prescription of drugs to treat their condition, these e-consumers or e-patients are fast becoming the e-prescribers of the future.

In contrast, in 1999, few hospitals, medical offices, or managed care plans even collect e-mail addresses. They have no idea how many patients are on line or how many they could reach with timely health and behavioral information on line. The longer these health and medical organizations wait to begin building e-databases, the further they fall behind the pharmaceutical firms in the ability to serve the e-consumer and e-patient.

E-CONSUMERS AND E-PATIENTS TAKE ACTION

Because of DTC broadcast and print advertising, consumers know which manufacturers to look for when searching the Web. If an e-consumer feels that she might have seasonal allergies, for instance, she has probably seen the television spots or read the print ads for Schering-Plough's Claritin® (Figure 14–7) and

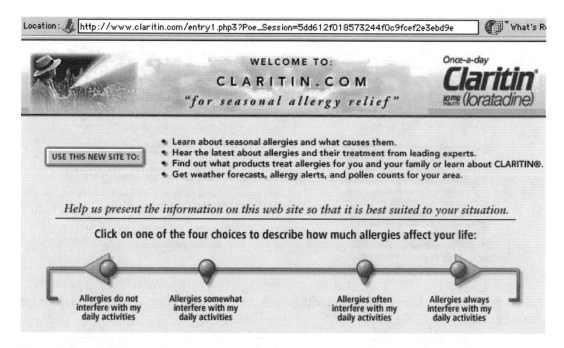

Figure 14–7 Claritin. *Source:* Reproduced with permission of Schering Corporation. All rights reserved.

Hoechst Marion Roussel's Allegra® (Figure 14–8). The likely next step—for about 38 percent of those who see the ad—is to investigate these companies on the Web, gathering information on seasonal allergies, but, more important to the manufacturer, gathering that information while also learning about the firm's product.

Schering-Plough's Claritin Web site allows visitors to interactively define how much allergies affect their lives; then it serves up information about what to do to manage daily life as an allergy sufferer. E-consumers set up a Personal Allergy Resource, and Schering-Plough collects demographic data. The customized page offers information based on the visitor's stated needs and interests, daily pollen counts, and a weekly giveaway. Visitors to Hoechst Marion Roussel's Allegra site can look up regional pollen forecasts, receive product coupons, and compare Allegra with other products.

This e-contact with the pharmaceutical company offers the e-consumer or e-patient a virtual lesson on seasonal allergies. From clinical explanations, to tools and strategies for avoiding allergens, the consumer gathers an amazing amount

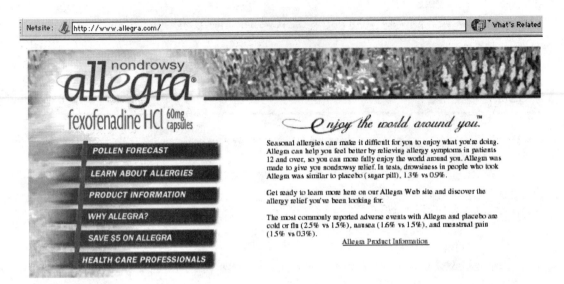

Figure 14–8 Allegra. *Source:* Reprinted with permission from www.allegra.com, © 1999, Hoechst Marion Roussel, Inc.

of information. The manufacturers provide both DTC advertising and scientific information. They recognize a responsive audience and are focusing, with laser accuracy, on the e-consumer.

GETTING TO REVOLUTION

Savvy e-patients ask for specific medical therapies and bring educational materials and information they downloaded from the Web right into the exam room. Why? According to a 1997 study by the Kaiser Family Foundation and Harvard University, 61 percent of consumers in heavily restricted health plans feel their managed care organization is more interested in the bottom line than in quality health care.[5] This sets the stage for supported self-care: patients (passive) morph into consumers (proactive) and look for the answers that they are convinced their health maintenance organization is not going to offer. And they take that information to the physician, requesting consideration for the viewpoint that they likely gained on a pharmaceutical or pharmaceutical-sponsored Web site. The e-consumer values the information on the pharmaceutical Web site. It is backed up by scientific fact, is well packaged, and tells e-consumers how to get what they want.

The major pharmaceutical companies have always lived in a world of data, trying to capture information to predict who will prescribe a drug, who will use it, and how it will benefit the patient. The Internet—itself a world of data—was a natural "e-home" for the pharmaceuticals. Here, they could tell their story as well as continue to capture data about both providers and patients. As Figure 14–9 shows, consumers access many types of information on the Web; when pharmaceuticals provide general and condition-specific health information not associated with their products on a Web site, consumers see pharmaceuticals more positively.

BUILDING RAPPORT: BECOMING THE E-CONSUMER'S FRIEND

Some pharmaceutical companies are continuing approaches they used before the Web existed, providing value-added services that do not promote products but build awareness. The Amgen pages for patients who suffer renal failure (see above) are a good example. Abbott Laboratories, which makes Norvir® for the human immunodeficiency virus (HIV), has a site (www.abbott.com/community/scienceofaids.htm) that takes the e-patient to science education programs on HIV and the acquired immune deficiency syndrome (AIDS). Visitors can take interactive quizzes to test their HIV knowledge and download a video tour of the Abbott-sponsored "AIDS: The War Within" exhibit at the Chicago Museum of Science and Industry. Abbott also features information on its long-term environmental and energy conservation programs, a philanthropic fund, and a program that contributes free pharmaceuticals in emergency situations such as natural disasters.

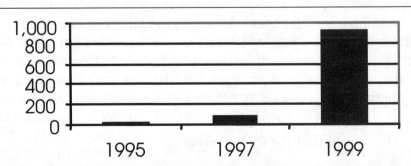

Figure 14–9 Top Five Topics by Those Seeking Health-Related Information on the Web. Data from Agency.com, Ltd., 1999.

Web sites such as Abbott's and Amgen's use the unique features of the Web to their best advantage, reaching consumers in a way impossible in print media. Imagine going from magazine to magazine, journal to journal, to find the multiple stories on what was offered at Abbott. On the Web, the e-consumer is always only a click away from more information.

One of the issues facing health care today is how providers are—or are not—using the Web. As e-patients become more involved in their own care, learning more about their condition and the therapies, they may very well be leaving the physician behind. Admittedly, physicians often do not have time to spend on the Net, finding out which are the most current therapies, where there are clinical trials in new medications, or which alternative therapies are being used by patients with a specific condition. But the medical profession must address this issue soon, perhaps making Net-based information available in sound bite style for providers serving patients in a particular plan. This is an e-opportunity. Smart pharmaceutical firms can establish a better relationship with physicians by giving them advance notice about what e-patients are likely to bring into their office.

PROVIDER? CONSUMER? BOTH?

Glaxo Wellcome's Healthy Lives page (Figure 14–10) provides information for e-consumers and e-providers, further blurring the traditional line between the two. Information is available on a variety of disease states and conditions, including asthma, chickenpox, depression, epilepsy, Lyme disease, HIV/AIDS, gastroesophageal reflux disease, and shingles. Each of the disease-specific areas offers information on symptoms, expected treatments, and health in general. In some cases, there is a glossary. The asthma area, for example, shows peak allergy periods and pollen counts on a map of the United States, "directing" the e-patient to the link between allergy and asthma. In the depression area, visitors can assess whether they are at risk for depression and learn about symptoms of depression and courses of treatment. The site offers links to two nonprofit organizations and other Glaxo-sponsored sites. Here, as in other locations, physicians can register and then tailor the information in printouts for distribution in the office. These customized printouts appear to have been produced by the physician, strengthening the relationship between the patient and the physician.

BUILDING SALES, BOOSTING E-COMMUNITIES

One of the magical things about the Web is its ability to connect people. Somehow, discussing a sensitive subject often becomes easier when consumers are in

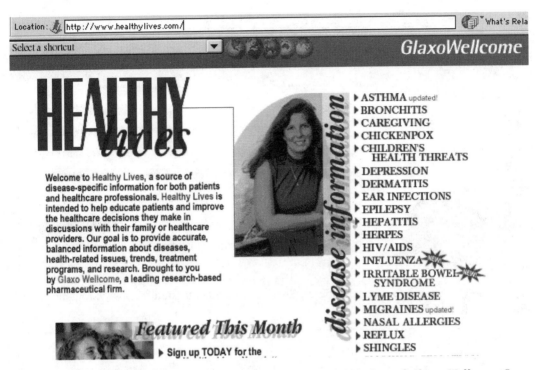

Figure 14–10 Healthy Lives. *Source:* Reproduced with permission of Glaxo Wellcome Inc., www.healthylives.com, © 1999.

cyberspace, not face-to-face. The Web has spawned a variety of health-related e-communities that range from bulletin board services to real-time chat rooms. It is in these cybercommunities that consumers share information with each other and learn that they are not the only ones suffering from what ails them.

For example, Pharmacia & Upjohn, maker of Rogaine™, offers a site to establish an e-community for those men and women (Figure 14–11) who are experiencing hair loss. Rogaine Online has two channels—one for men and one for women. In addition to education and information, visitors can exchange their own stories and issues, and, of course, enter an area for users of Rogaine to tell their success stories. Here, men and women can discuss the issue of hair loss and how it has impacted their lives without having to reveal their identity.

PROMOTING SELF-CARE: JUST GIVE 'EM THE PRODUCT

Self-care has taken on a new importance in health care as patients are encouraged to involve themselves in the care process, ask questions, comply with medi-

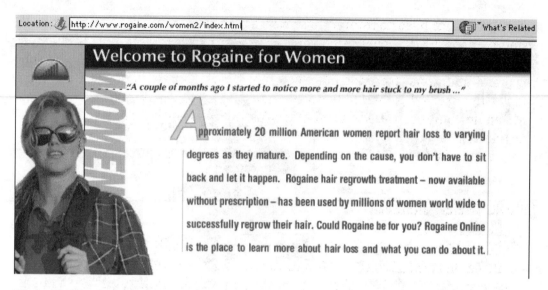

Figure 14–11 Rogaine for Women. *Source:* Reprinted with permission from www.rogaine.com, ©
1999, Pharmacia & Upjohn.

cal regimens and lifestyle modifications, and understand something about both
the illness and the consequences of noncompliance.

In an interesting twist on self-care through product sampling, Bristol-Myers
Squibb is using targeted on-line promotions to encourage site visitors to register
for free samples of Excedrin®, including a promotional spot on the TurboTax
page, touting relief from headaches during income tax time. Excedrin's Headache
Resource Center sends registered visitors a thank you note and a tin of 12
Excedrin in the mail during income tax filing time. When the visitor registers, he
or she receives information on headaches, a quarterly newsletter, and coupons
for products (for example, at the Excedrin Headache Resource Center at
www.excedrin.com). Bristol-Myers Squibb is not going to let the e-consumer forget the value of a relationship with this company. And it is playing nicely into
the fastest-growing aspect of health care: self-care.

There are consequences to self-care that the pharmaceutical firms need to
address, however. When selling a product for depression or cholesterol, it is not
just the pill that is being offered: the condition is being addressed as well. And
here, the manufacturers are not doing so well. According to the *Journal of Managed Care Pharmacy* (http://www.amcp.org), 28 percent of people do not know
the indications for depression. For high cholesterol, 79 percent do not know the
indications, and for migraine, 59 percent do not.[6] This indicates that the phar-

maceutical firms need to inform those who are the recipients of their DTC advertising perhaps a little more responsibly. Each of the sites listed in this chapter, and the many others out there, offer educational and informational tools, surveys, and additional methods of interaction for visitors. It is hoped that more people who use Web sites will learn the indications for the illness or condition.

Given how physician–patient relationships have suffered under managed care, the relationships being built between pharmaceutical manufacturers and patients are likely to have extraordinary implications in the process of care.

LURING THE E-CONSUMER

An age-old way to entice customers is to give something away. Pfizer has capitalized on this fact with a 150th Anniversary Sweepstakes, which was posted on the manufacturer's Web site in 1999. One hundred and fifty people had the chance to win $150 each if they could answer eight questions correctly—and all the answers were available within the Pfizer site. This sweepstakes may seem small, but relationships were being built. Pfizer accomplished two things: it got the site visitor to read all of the company's materials in search of the quiz answers, and it gathered data. Visitors entered the sweepstakes by keying their name, mailing address, and e-mail address. This e-database is worth more to Pfizer than the $22,500 sweepstakes payout.

Building an e-database is extremely important to a pharmaceutical company. Pfizer, for example, knows that the registered entrants looked at the Pfizer site for medical reasons because while they were searching for answers to health-related problems they happened upon the quiz. These people may be future users of Pfizer products.

The tone of the Pfizer site leaves most e-consumers thinking that Pfizer must be a consumer-friendly organization that invented good products and is willing to give away some of its money through a simple quiz. Most e-consumers who participated in the quiz probably did not realize that they traded information about themselves for the opportunity to win.

Interactivity—in the form of quizzes or assessments—is a significant part of a pharmaceutical Web site's value. Studies have shown that patients who are offered a method of participating in their own care tend to feel that they have a higher health-related quality of life and are more likely to comply with medical regimens and lifestyle modifications. Pharmaceutical companies get e-patients in the cyberdoor and give them what they want. They blur the line between provider knowledge and patient knowledge, creating consumers out of patients with—for the most part—well-designed, interactive sites that change perception at the same time as they maintain a level of control over that perception.

Make no mistake. Pharmaceutical companies are changing health care with their Web sites. They offer a previously unheard-of, though very controlled, look behind the doors of their organizations. At the same time, they gather information about visitors who have diseases and health-related conditions that may require use of the firm's products. Pharmaceutical manufacturers are leveraging the Net and going for the gold—the e-consumer motivated to practice self-care through e-care based Web sites.

DRUG REPRESENTATIVES REACH PRESCRIBERS IN AIR SPACE

Despite their focus on the e-consumer, pharmaceutical companies still employ significant sales forces (see Table 14–2) to reach physicians and other health care providers in real space. These efforts are combined with cyberspace strategies designed to get providers on line too.

The growth of pharmaceutical sales forces is due to multiple new products or line extensions as well as the fact that the population is aging and more drugs are being used. Managed care organizations, likewise, are adding drugs to their formularies. The Net is reaching the e-consumer, but the traditional prescriber is still very much on the radar screen.

Table 14–2 Top 10 Pharmaceuticals Ranked by Sales Force

Company	1998 Sales Force	Change in Sales Force between 1997 and 1998 (%)
Merck	4,700	+104.3
Bristol-Myers Squibb	4,200	+16.7
American Home Products	4,100	+4.3
Pfizer	4,100	−5.2
Glaxo Wellcome	3,400	+13.3
Schering-Plough	3,400	+70.0
Novartis	3,100	+3.3
SmithKline	2,900	+16.0
Johnson & Johnson	2,800	+36.1
Abbott	2,600	−52.7

Source: Data from Med Ad News, West Trenton, New Jersey and Salomon Smith Barney, New York.

Pharmaceutical manufacturers gaining access to prescribers is as common as the manufacture of pharmaceuticals themselves. Manufacturers have always approached physicians with clinical information about why their drug is better than another or why their drug is good in a specific medical situation. The traditional "door-to-door" drug sales representative still exists—at least for now. These representatives call on physician's offices, offering information, samples, and incentives. They fund local meetings and educational forums, entertain providers, and, in essence, make the wheels of the pharmaceutical industry run smoothly. The goal of the sales representative is and always has been to influence prescribers and thereby increase sales.

HITTING THE DETAILER BELOW THE MONEY BELT?

But how will these detailers be affected by DTC advertising and their own companies' creation of the e-consumer prescriber? A supply chain compression is likely, and DTC advertising may one day replace the drug representative. This may come to fruition slowly, however. In 1999, pharmaceutical manufacturers had an average sales force of 3,500, which was up from previous years. According to The Plymouth Group, a pharmaceutical consulting and analysis firm in Plymouth Meeting, PA, the future of the sales force is being driven by localization of the market, targeting of low-prescribing physicians, and more new product launches each year. Every new product accounts for about 100 new representatives. The sales representatives are, in fact, reinforcing what the e-patient is bringing into the physician's office and encouraging new prescriptions by stocking the office sample cabinet.

And DTC has not completely replaced advertising to providers. Pharmaceutical companies still spend $4 to reach providers for every $1 to reach consumers.[7] The focus on physicians should not be discounted; it is indicative of the fact that health care is evolving. While all participants in the health care system are furiously trying things on and discarding what they do not want, they are often keeping what they are simply afraid to throw away.

But the health care industry, and particularly the sales representatives, should look closely at what is happening and what can happen. Samples can be e-ordered for delivery at a specified time. Information can be sent directly to the office computer on not only a broad disease category but on the specific issues that the physician's patient faces. If the patient is an e-patient, the information can be forwarded to him or her as well. With the appropriate consent, even employers can be linked to this health continuum. Although sales positions will not disappear immediately, e-ordering and e-consumer advertising may change the sales landscape.

A WEB-ENABLED FOCUS ON DECISION MAKERS

As managed care reared its head in the early 1980s, the formulary was designed to standardize the care given to patients—including a reduction in the numbers of similar or "me too" drugs. Managed care organizations set out to save money. Savvy pharmaceutical firms began to approach formulary decision makers, attempting to influence this list of drugs. And the pharmaceuticals played the cost-savings game. At first.

Then new sales strategies came about, including the addition of value-added educational programs for plan members and prescribers, as part of the pharmaceuticals' approach to promoting product. Pharmaceutical companies quietly maintained lists of physicians who were friendly toward a particular product, who used it regularly for their patients, and who would, if necessary, go through the often arduous process of prescribing it if it were not on the formulary.

The Internet has now extended the reach of the pharmaceutical companies to the point where they can circumvent the formulary restrictions of managed care. Using Web-enabled technologies, pharmaceutical companies directly reach, teach, and influence the physicians that managed care hoped to isolate. And they promote the products that the managed care organizations hoped to eliminate. How did they accomplish this? They looked at what had always worked in real space, and using the power of the Net they promoted sponsorship of continuing medical education (CME) workshops and seminars on line.

The Web is well suited to reaching out to prescribers. In cyberspace, pharmaceutical companies can offer substantive clinical information to physicians and other providers. Secure Web sites, using physicians' licensing numbers or other data as passwords, offer an array of information. Included in this information is CME, important to physicians, who have to obtain an established number of credit hours per year to maintain their license.

Physicians frequently express the desire to obtain CME credits in settings other than workshops (Figure 14–12). They want to learn on their own time at their own pace. E-education is an excellent way for pharmaceutical companies to offer grants, even though physicians still express a preference for print. This is due in large part to the average age of a practicing physician, about 47. As the next generation of computer-literate physicians comes onto the scene, the story will

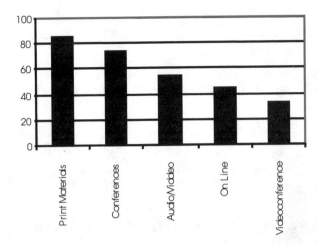

Figure 14–12 Settings (Other Than Workshops) in Which Physicians Would Like To Obtain CME. Data from Agency.com, Ltd., 1999.

change, and the most forward-thinking firms are ready. They understand the power of Net-based learning, and they will be ready when the physicians are.

Working with the traditional sponsors of CME—universities—pharmaceutical manufacturers have underwritten substantial numbers of e-CME programs. For instance, the University of Alabama at Birmingham, a leader in internationally oriented continuing education programs with a focus on Latin America, has taken a strong position in placing courses on the Internet. DuPont Pharmaceuticals, one underwriter of these programs, has sponsored University of Alabama programs on stroke (Figure 14–13).

Other organizations have sprung up to offer on-line continuing education units too. The Academy of Continuing Education Online (Figure 14–14) offers on-line courses for physicians. Procter & Gamble Pharmaceuticals has underwritten women's health programs for the Institute for Medical Studies (Figure 14–15), such as a CME course on urinary tract infection. The pharmaceutical companies, recognizing the value of using a variety of resources, have worked with these organizations just as they have with the more traditional venues. Each offers unrestricted educational grant money for continuing education and CME.

Providers other than physicians have access to Web continuing education, too. HELIX, sponsored by Glaxo Wellcome, is a meta–Web site that provides the P.L.A.N. database. This database allows users to search for all Academy of Con-

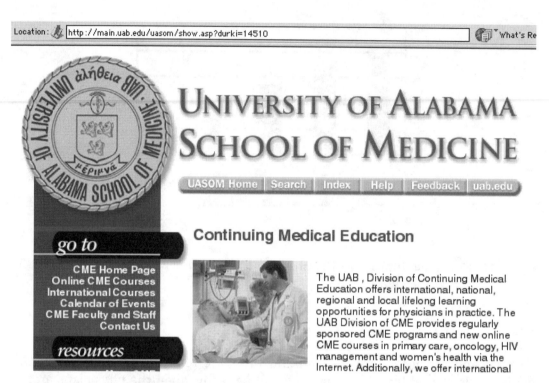

Figure 14–13 University of Alabama at Birmingham. *Source:* Reprinted with permission from www-cma.erep.uab.edu/onlineCourses/stroke/stroke.htm, © 1999, Continuing Medical Education, University of Alabama at Birmingham.

tinuing Pharmacy Education offerings. Glaxo also underwrites continuing education for the Physician Assistant AIDS Network on line (Figure 14–16).

Each of these sites uses the connective strength of the Web. The underwriter has access to physicians and allied providers as they interface with the continuing education site, gathers names and other important data, and can send the provider to other sites that it sponsors and influences. This is using the power of the Web, not merely residing in the neighborhood.

CLICK—YOU ARE IN OUR DATABASE, DOCTOR

Pharmaceutical companies are providing not only continuing education on line. In their ever-evolving push to provide non–drug products to providers, companies such as Hoescht Marion Roussel offer on-line brochure series. The company's Managing Your Health e-service, for example, offers physicians e-tools

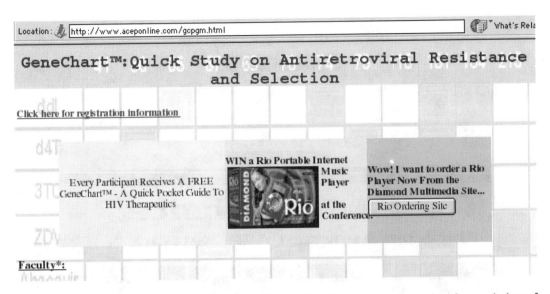

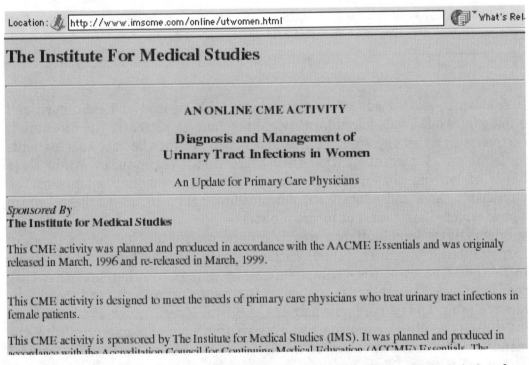

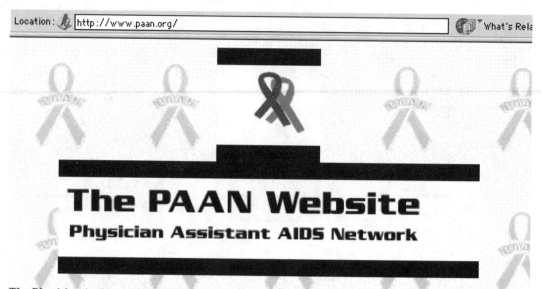

Location: http://www.paan.org/　　What's Rela

The PAAN Website
Physician Assistant AIDS Network

The Physician Assistant AIDS Network (PAAN) was formed to promote networking, continuing medical education, and symposia for PAs working in HIV/AIDS care. This webpage summarizes the most recent issue of our newsletter and reports recent advances in HIV/AIDS treatment.

Figure 14–16 The Physician Assistant AIDS Network. *Source:* Reprinted with permission from www.paan.org, © 1999, Physician Assistant AIDS Network.

that enhance patient education discussions. Click an icon and the physician's office prints out a valuable informational brochure to patients. The brochure is customized to the physician's office and makes up for the fact that patients forget about 75 percent of what they heard from the physician within three hours of leaving the office. In return, the drug company maintains the physician's name and educational downloading habits in its database—which allows targeted marketing of future products.

Bristol-Myers Squibb offers a weekly on-line newsletter that covers topics of current interest to primary care physicians (Figure 14–17). These link, of course, to the home pages of the pharmaceuticals as well as to other sites that they sponsor. Click. You are getting much of the information that was formerly offered in print, and you are now part of the Bristol-Myers Squibb database.

To attract health care providers who are visiting a nonpharmaceutical site, the manufacturers make themselves available with banners, tags, and "rooms" within other sites. Pfizer has a managed care news area in Physician's Online (www.pol.com). This area delivers feature articles, industry news, and business profiles from over 150 sources—one-stop information shopping for the busy professional.

CONCLUSION

This chapter examined the wide variety of ways that the pharmaceutical firms are harnessing the power of the Net and using the connective properties of the Web to guide e-patients through the maze of health and medical information. Is the pharmaceutical industry shaping a revolution, an irreversible new paradigm in health care? The answer is an unqualified yes.

Data captured by the pharmaceutical companies can benefit people in multiple ways. One may be transforming passive patients with chronic disease into active patients who participate in care or even in crucial clinical trials of new drugs (Figure 14–18).

The marriage of pharmaceutical companies and the Net is an excellent example of supply and demand at work—e-patients want exactly the kind of information that the pharmaceutical companies are delivering on line. The e-patient has a

Location: http://www.physweekly.com/  What's Rel.

Physician's Weekly

HIGHLIGHTS AND ANALYSIS OF MEDICAL NEWS

October 11, 1999 Vol. XVI, No. 38

IN THE NEWS

UNOS Imposes Liver Payback, Extinguishing a Prairie Fire

Data-Sharing May Spell Relief For Credentialing Process

GAO: Beware of the Overseers

POINT/COUNTERPOINT

THIS WEEK'S LEAD STORY

Merger on the Rocks
Financial stress threatens Stanford's two-year-old union with UC San Francisco

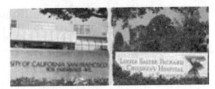

Figure 14–17 Physician's Weekly. *Source:* Reprinted with permission by Physician's Weekly © Copyright 1999 Physician's Weekly, Inc.

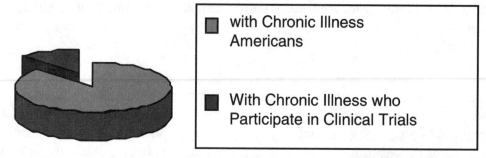

Figure 14–18 Incidence of Chronic Illness and Participation in Clinical Trials among 250 Million Americans. *Source:* Reprinted from U.S. Census Bureau, 1993.

consumerist bent that the pharmaceutical firms are responding to and encouraging. E-patients have become proactive participants in the continuum of care, and the pharmaceutical manufacturers, through product-specific and informational Web sites, are driving this new attitude. In contrast, physicians and managed care companies are woefully behind, often clinging to traditional, comfortable models of care.

It is likely that the pharmaceutical companies responded more to the medium than to the message. But the medium is the message. The Web presents a new e-communications, e-commerce, and e-care opportunity for an industry that was already comfortable with communication media. The efforts have been successful, and the pharmaceutical companies are funding this e-message to their own benefit. They understand who is on the Net and why. They are pushing the envelope in offering information to e-patients that formerly may have been offered only to their traditional customer base: prescribers.

The pharmaceutical industry is bringing the Net closer to provision of care than any other player in the health care industry. It is changing the way that e-patients—and often providers—understand their role in health care. The pharmaceutical manufacturers have set the stage: it is up to other major players to respond. Thinking "outside the box" has never been as important for those health care organizations that want to remain in the lead. And in business.

Undoubtedly, the pharmaceuticals will push the envelope further. With about 10 percent of physicians having a Web page in 1999, there is work that can be done to link with them. This is not so farfetched, nor as compromising as it might seem. The education that the e-patient is taking away from pharmaceutical Web sites and bringing to the physician is actually the first step in linking the two in the mind of the patient. Is it farfetched to consider a pharmaceutical link on a physician's Web site? No. Managed care organizations actively and aggressively promote the concept of self-care. Is it so difficult to imagine a day when people will visit an on-line physician, get a prescription, and take the cure? Absolutely not. And is it so difficult to think that a pharmaceutical rather than an insurer might sponsor that on-line physician? Maybe not. And is it so difficult to imagine a pharmaceutical firm offering a range of products through a pharmacy benefits management firm, at a deeply discounted price if e-patients buy health insurance through that company? Wait a few years and see.

The Net path for pharmaceutical companies is not all covered in roses, however. In 1999, some of the major firms actually began to pare down Net-based operations, scale back existing sites, or put new sites on hold. Why? Return on investment. Even the sophisticated pharmaceutical companies are having difficulty making the direct link between the amount they spend on the Web and prescription activity—even though the Web is one of the most cost-effective methods of reaching the consumer. It might be because the Net is new, it might be because the number crunchers trust other forms of DTC advertising more, but it is happening. Rest assured, however, those pharmaceutical companies dedicated to pushing information and products on line will find a way to justify the use of the medium. It is only a matter of time.

The Internet, with the ability to present information and e-service in an intimate, private setting—with astonishingly fast results, data aggregation, and interactive modalities—is having an enormous impact on the delivery of health care in the United States—and the prescribing habits and influence of physicians. Right now, it is the pharmaceutical industry that is truly harnessing the power of the Net, helping to create a new breed of e-patient, and offering what that e-patient wants.

What is your health care organization doing?

REFERENCES

1. R. Weissman, "But First, Call Your Drug Company," *American Demographics*, October 1998.

2. A. Holmer, "Direct-to-Consumer Prescription Drug Advertising Builds Bridges Between Patients and Physicians," *Journal of the American Medical Association*, Vol. 281, No. 4.

3. National Disease and Therapeutic Index (Plymouth Meeting, PA: IMS Health, 1996).

4. S. Engel, "The Golden Age," *Med Ad News*, Vol. 17, No. 9, 3–6.

5. M. James and T. Hoff, "Is There a Managed Care Backlash?" press release, Kaiser Foundation and Harvard University study, 5 November 1997.

6. M. Bloom, "Direct-to-Consumer Advertising Provides Challenge to Managed Care," *Journal of Managed Care Pharmacy*, Vol. 5, No. 2.

7. "IMS Reports Pharmaceutical Promotions Rose 16% in 1997," press release (Plymouth Meeting, PA: IMS Health, 1998).

CHAPTER 15

Searching for the Holy Grail: Integrated Electronic Medical Records and Beyond

Francis H. Rhie and Mark L. Braunstein

HEALTH CARE is an amazingly information-intensive industry. Physicians and other health care professionals spend more than 80 percent of their time collecting, processing, retrieving, and communicating information. Ironically, health care professionals typically do not see themselves as information gatherers and disseminators. As a result, when compared to other information-intensive industries, health care has been slow to capitalize on information technology. Most industries have allocated 10 percent of their capital budgets for information systems; health care providers have spent just under 2 percent.[1] Hospitals are higher spenders, but very little of that goes toward clinical systems. Physicians are minimal spenders, investing in virtually nothing beyond a billing and scheduling system for the office.

These technology spending lags have resulted in painfully slow implementation of both automated administrative functions and automated clinical records in the health care industry. Since physicians are the clear drivers of most clinical spending, it is not surprising that, many years after it became the "Holy Grail" of clinical computing, the computer-based patient record (CPR) has not become as pervasive as experts had predicted in the early 1990s.

The current health care delivery system provides ample incentives for the adoption of the CPR on a national scale. There is an ever greater need for clinical information for reimbursement, utilization management, risk-adjusted outcome research, and quality assessment. If the health care industry wants to successfully implement the CPR systemwide—which would rid the industry of many paper-intensive administrative functions, managed care hassles, and care delivery difficulties—it must understand why the CPR has taken so long to implement. Recognizing the barriers may help ensure quicker acceptance of the CPR by America's physicians and health systems.

AHEAD OF THE CURVE

Back in 1991, the Institute of Medicine (IOM) of the National Academy of Sciences issued a seminal report on the CPR. The IOM defined the CPR as "an electronic patient record that resides in a system specifically designed to support users by providing accessibility to complete and accurate data, alerts, reminders, clinical decision support systems, links to medical knowledge, and other aids."[2,p.11]

The IOM report, edited by Richard S. Dick and Elaine B. Steen, has provided guidance since its publication in 1991, but the bold vision remains just that—a vision.[3] The IOM saw a tremendous opportunity for the CPR to improve the quality of medical care and lower the cost of delivery by improving efficiency in the U.S. health care delivery system. But these ambitious thoughts were not widely accepted by the rest of the health care community. As a result, the 1999 adoption rate for the CPR is still no more than 5 percent—a percentage that has stayed almost the same since 1991.

In 1999, the predominant use of information technology in the health care delivery system is still financial—not clinical. Very few physicians use computer systems to even select diagnoses or procedure codes; most still rely on paper notes or dictation to document clinical encounters. The structured data collected are largely limited to encounter forms and information submitted on claim forms. Ironically, the need for reliable, consistent, and analyzable information is even more acute now than in 1991, when managed care was in its infancy and risk bearing by medical groups and health systems was rare.

The fact that physicians chose not to implement the CPR without clear standard or well-defined incentives should not surprise anyone. The impact of a new paradigm and the inherent behavioral changes necessary for physicians and other providers to use computer systems—with no economic incentive or assistance—were highly underestimated.

Much of this dilemma can be traced to the lack of a national consensus and standards for the CPR and a lack of economic benefit to the physicians who are required to make the investment to use it. Essentially, it was left to individual physicians and groups to invest in and implement this new technology, and that amounted to a sizeable sum. The potential beneficiaries of the electronically collected data (insurers and hospitals) did not offer to share the economic benefits with the collectors of the data (physicians).

Exactly what went wrong? Many of the answers can be found by looking back at events that happened during a decade that was supposed to see the implementation of the CPR on a national scale.

REIMBURSEMENT TAKES A DIVE

Our employer- or government-paid health insurance system has shielded consumers from the real cost of their health care. As a result, they have always demanded maximum health care benefits, regardless of cost. Over a period of years this led to a health care spending level, relative to gross domestic product (GDP), that was twice that of most other major industrialized countries. In 1998, health care accounted for more than $1.1 trillion a year, or 13.4 percent of GDP.[4]

Enter managed care, which began in the 1980s, became much more prevalent in the early 1990s, and continues today. Managed care left physicians and hospitals at the mercy of consolidated payers, who wielded tremendous bargaining power. Decreased reimbursement reduced capital budgets and lowered investment in long-term capital projects such as information systems and training.

Health maintenance organizations (HMOs) brought with them increased utilization management and "gatekeepers" that kept a tight control on access to specialists. Utilization management meant that medical practices and hospitals had more paperwork, longer waits on hold with insurance companies, and a need for additional staffing—which raised overhead at the same time that revenue streams declined. Because of this, a practice's or hospital's spending priorities, for the most part, were limited to dealing with the business side of managed care and contract management. Survival became the issue—not investment in new technology. A CPR typically was not even considered, despite the efficiencies and access to internal clinical databanks that could shift the balance of power to the provider at the managed care bargaining table.

INDEPENDENT PRACTICES FORM GROUPS

With the rapid growth of HMOs, many independent physicians organized themselves as independent practice associations (IPAs) in order to successfully contract. (An IPA is a loose organization of physicians whose only purpose is to manage risk-based contracts with managed care organizations.) Critical to an IPA's success were information management and connectivity. It was expected that the IPA would succeed in medical management through timely, high-quality clinical information.

Unfortunately, IPAs were often undercapitalized and lacked professional management expertise. Many did not even track incurred-but-not-yet-reported claims expenses and lost significant sums of money, which could have gone toward information technology. And since the IPA typically did not have the authority to demand that member physicians upgrade to new and standardized information systems, critical clinical and financial data stayed fragmented. For the most part, legacy systems with limited capability were left in place.

In the end, IPAs became an information flow bottleneck. They caused more redundant paperwork and operational inefficiency than existed before the IPA stepped in to "help." Most spent money only on financial systems for claims adjudication and administrative audits and reports; little was spent on clinical information systems or on linking providers electronically. Medical group or IPA competition was largely based on price, not quality, and health plans rarely reimbursed based on medical quality. So despite their lip service about quality, there was no clear message to physicians that a CPR or the tracking of clinical data was a priority.

WALL STREET BUYS PHYSICIANS

With the fragmentation of providers and undercapitalization of IPAs, there was a natural opportunity for entrepreneurs to step in and consolidate the provider market. Physician practice management companies (PPMCs) raised funds from the public market and acquired provider groups at a rapid clip. Providers sold an interest in their practice in hopes of gaining access to professional management and sorely needed capital to upgrade their inadequate information systems.

PPMCs and Wall Street were interested in efficiency gains from economies of scale, but they did not anticipate the drop in providers' productivity after they joined larger organizations and lost, to some degree, their entrepreneurial drive. There was no gain in efficiency when these diverse organizations were merged. And while there may have been some back office integration, there was rarely, if ever, any clinical integration.

Anyone who watches the news knows the fate of PPMCs: investors have reacted harshly to this failed strategy, and many front-runners have floundered, gone out of business, or divested themselves of the physician practice management market altogether.

HOSPITALS BUY PRACTICES

Hospitals led an effort to vertically integrate physicians and provide a continuum of care that could handle global risk capitation. Many figured that if this integrated delivery system (IDS) could streamline the continuum of care and reduce inefficiency and waste, the hospital could reap the benefit of lower costs and higher profits. To achieve full clinical integration, IDSs acquired multiple hospitals, physician practices, home care companies, rehabilitation units, and skilled nursing facilities.

IDSs created an environment with a tremendous need for information to manage complex clinical processes across the continuum of care. The next logical step: investment in a CPR to store clinical data in a single database and combine clinical and financial information.

Unlike PPMCs, hospitals at least had an appreciation for the potential impact of systems integration and standardization as well as the strategic role of clinical information systems. Like the PPMCs, however, many IDSs had great difficulty executing their information technology strategy. Many of the reasons were political. As mentioned earlier, hospitals have invested in information systems to a greater extent than most other segments of the health care industry. This seemingly positive attribute became a negative in an IDS when, ideally, one technology should have been used across the continuum of care. Battles over the "right" technology platform and the lack of vision within the IDS often led to stalemates—or at the very least, protracted decision making. With no real strategy, significant investments in cutting-edge technologies, such as the CPR, often got delayed.

Here again, physician practice purchases proved to be difficult to manage, and many IDSs lost money. Since most of the organizers of IDSs are hospitals with legacy information systems running their core businesses, they concentrated on replacing and upgrading mission-critical systems (and in 1999, Year 2000 issues drove investment and training priorities) rather than implementing new and innovative clinical systems. Medical groups that are part of IDSs have been the victims of this priority setting.

AN UNCERTAIN FUTURE

Physicians reacted to the uncertainties of managed care by signing en masse with many plans rather than proactively taking control or empowering themselves through the clever use of information systems. An uncertain future pushed some to cash out rather than invest for the long term. A provider market in flux and troubled PPMCs precluded the installation of clinical information systems. During consolidation and roll up, most resources were used to merge and acquire market share—not to invest in infrastructure.

Ironically, in 1999 physicians are right back where they started—fragmented and without clear direction. Perhaps the collective wisdom gained from what they went through can lead physicians to regroup and become active shapers of their own destiny.

THE DAWN OF A NEW MILLENNIUM

The time has come for a CPR that can be used universally across medical practices and health systems. According to practice management information system expert Vinson J. Hudson of Jewson Enterprise, Inc., CPR's market potential for 1997 was $7.6 billion and will grow to $8.4 billion in 2002. Hudson predicts a compounded annual growth rate (CAGR) of 2 percent thereafter.[5]

This CPR market analysis indicates that the actual CPR market will grow from $670.8 million in 1997 (9 percent of potential) to $1.5 billion in 2002 (18 percent of potential), a CAGR of 17.9 percent—a forecast of faster adoption over the next four to five years (Figure 15–1).

In the same report, Hudson lists factors that impede CPR implementation.

- Medical offices have placed a higher priority on contract management systems for managed care than on the CPR.
- Financial challenges and profitability pressures demand that systems with more immediate return on investment (ROI) be a higher priority than the CPR.
- The operational re-engineering required for CPR systems is complex. For these systems to succeed, workflow from every department has to change. This issue must be taken into account during the planning and implementation phases.

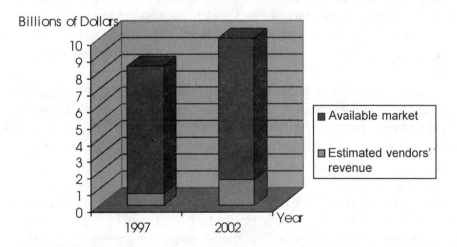

Figure 15–1 CPR Market in 1997 and 2002. *Source:* Adapted with permission from POMIS Knowledge Base, POMIS Report, © 1999, Jewson Enterprises, Inc.

- The cultural challenge among staff associated with automating the clinical aspects of medical practice delivery is underestimated. Implementation of a CPR system will require significant physician involvement at the front end.
- Although technology is ample, the human engineering required for the technology-averse clinician end-user is still lacking.[6]

We agree with Hudson but believe there are even more barriers to overcome if the CPR is to be successful.

TRANSCENDING BARRIERS

A more careful and detailed examination of the barriers to the implementation of the traditional CPR is essential to a real understanding of the problem.

First, the cost of purchase and implementation of the CPR is still formidable for most smaller physician offices. In 1998, about 136,000 physicians were in solo practice or two-physician groups, and about 229,000 were in medical groups of three or more.[7] Most of these practices use systems that are based on UNIX, DOS, or Windows. They utilize mini-computer or client/server architectures requiring on-site installation and support of powerful and complex computers, local area networks (LANs), wide area networks (WANs), and multiple ancillary devices such as printers, fax machines, and scanners. Replacing these legacy systems carries a high price tag.

The total cost of hardware and software is further increased by the high cost of training and the decrease in productivity during the early phases of introduction. Cost benefit analyses have been sporadic. Many physicians and health care executives feel there is not sufficient evidence that purchasing systems at this time will be cost-effective, particularly when there is no clear mandate to use the CPR.

Second, physicians are resistant to entering data. Having clinicians enter structured and standardized data at the point of care can benefit physicians and other secondary users of the medical record system. But to date, no standard format has emerged, and data entry continues to be more difficult with computers than with paper charts.

Most system designers and proponents of the CPR view direct entry of data by clinicians as one of the CPR's hallmarks. But even without direct data entry by physicians, there are significant benefits to be realized if documents and other information become available anytime, anywhere, across the continuum of care. Lack of physician data entry should not deter the implementation of a more limited CPR. For example, if progress notes, Current Procedural Terminology codes, and diagnosis codes are readily available to practices and secondary record users, the benefits will be substantial.

Data do not always have to be entered by the physician. Patient Care Technologies, Inc., has skilled nurses enter vital signs and monitor patient care (Figure 15–2).

Third, lack of clinical data standards impedes universal or nationwide implementation. This is not as much of a concern to individual or small practices. However, the issue has to be resolved at least at the enterprise level in order for enterprisewide implementation to be successful. Unfortunately, most of the current coding schemes are more focused on producing financial statistics than on solving clinical problems.

Fourth, to avoid significant redundancy of data entry, the CPR has to be integrated or interfaced with billing systems. Most popular billing software is based on legacy operating systems. It is difficult to adapt these legacy systems to the

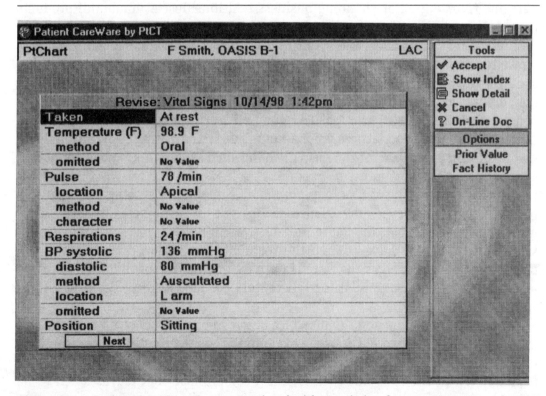

Figure 15–2 Patient CareWare. *Source:* Reprinted with permission from www.ptct.com, © 1999, Patient Care Technologies.

newer technologies typically used in the CPR. Further, Health Level 7, the evolving standard for information sharing and exchange among health care systems, deals only to a very limited degree with clinical information. So, once more, a lack of standards substantially complicates the widespread adoption of the CPR.

Fifth, multiple trading partners are difficult to connect universally. Even though physicians are often aligned with larger organizations, these are by no means exclusive arrangements. Even physicians aligned with well-established IDS networks still deal with multiple business partners—laboratories, radiology services, referring physicians, HMOs, preferred provider organizations, and IPAs. These trading partners are in different stages of technology adoption, which complicates communication with them. For example, some partners may communicate via fax or paper while others communicate electronically but on different vendor systems with different operating or database technologies.

Simplistic solutions will not work here since practices have to simultaneously deal with paper, fax, e-mail, Internet connection, and traditional electronic data interchange. To compound the problem, there is constant flux of trading partners due to emerging or changing business relationships. A number of products (integration engines, interface engines) strive to overcome this Tower of Babel problem. These systems, while often useful, add still more complexity and expense to the process.

Sixth, providers prefer to wait for newer technologies to mature. Physicians are bombarded with industry articles and vendor promotions about new and upcoming technology even though it is not necessarily ready for mass consumption. Among these products are voice recognition, handwriting recognition, integrated optical scanning for data entry, hand-held computers, and information appliances.

Rather than taking a technology plunge and upgrading systems as new technologies evolve, however, physicians tend to wait until the new, promised technology becomes stable and more widely available. This phenomenon is well known by those who have studied the technology adoption cycle. Most physicians would be classified as the "late majority" for adoption of computer technology even though they may be "early adopters" of new medical devices in their specialty field.

Seventh, form factors and the interface between people and computers are still major barriers. Keyboard entry in the examining room, laptop computers on wireless LANs, pen-based computers, and palm-top computers are available and have been applied to the CPR. But each is still a compromise that leaves much to be desired. Most software vendors have not put enough energy and research into the interface and into screen and workflow design. The tendency toward a universal approach to the "look and feel" of software, particularly within the Windows world, is not always good in an industry where the vast majority of potential end-users are technology novices. Familiarity with Windows and Internet Web browsers, however, has been a big plus in new user training.

Eighth, physicians and health care providers are mobile workers. Although this fact is obvious to those who work on the health care front lines, it is not often considered when discussing the use of technology. Think about it: for the most part, computers are still used while sitting down. This is equally true for notebook and desktop computers. The reasons are obvious and have to do with size, weight, the ergonomics of typing, and comfort.

But health care workers are classic mobile workers. They usually work while standing and move about during the day. Despite all the hype surrounding portable computers (beginning with the Apple Newton), they are still severely compromised by battery and screen limitations and by the absence of any truly good data entry paradigm for the smaller, hand-held devices.

Ninth, complex data requirements and obstruction of the physician–patient interaction have not been understood. Given the uniquely personal interaction between health care providers and patients, the providers are understandably leery about introducing obtrusive technology at the point of care. Moreover, the unusually complex data requirements within health care can strain the portable computer up to and beyond the breaking point. While portable computer devices have been well accepted in certain health care activities (mostly nursing and the allied professions), the much more complex data entry and retrieval requirements of the physician remain problematic for the most part.

Tenth, there is no consensus that "quality" pays. In industrial re-engineering, it is well established that quality will produce better products at a lower cost. In physician practices, product differentiation is largely done by price and not by quality. There is also the unsettled question of what constitutes quality and how to measure it. This is a catch-22. Payers will not pay for quality since they do not have reliable quality measures or information at the individual practice level. Providers are not really paid for quality, and therefore physicians feel that the CPR, which could go a long way toward providing the needed standards and data, is just one more added business cost that has no clear payback.

Eleventh, confidentiality and security are being discussed at the national level but are not firmly in place. The Health Insurance Portability and Accountability Act of 1996 mandates some standards and implementation guidelines and is slated for implementation in early 2002. In the heavily litigious health care environment, these concerns must be alleviated before widespread adoption of the CPR will occur.

Twelfth, state regulations vary. Absent federal regulation of the CPR, it falls to each state to define acceptable standards. For the most part, the states are very unsophisticated regulators of clinical information systems. As a result, very little is in place that governs truly paperless CPR systems. Absent this, even those providers who adopt a CPR may feel compelled to produce and store a redundant paper chart, further eroding the ability to cost-justify the CPR in the first place.

Thirteenth, the Food and Drug Administration (FDA) may soon join the fun. Clearly, FDA regulation of the pharmaceutical, instrumentation, and medical device industries creates major costs for those industries. Regulation of clinical software would likely raise the apparent cost of development but might, ironically, create the standards needed to spur more widespread adoption of the technologies.

Fourteenth, Year 2000 issues have taken attention away from the CPR. Even though CPR systems tend to be newly designed and avoid the Year 2000 bug, this has nevertheless been a barrier to purchase and installation of the systems. Further, many providers were preoccupied in 1999 with Year 2000 compliance and subsequently delayed or canceled new initiatives while they tried to replace or patch old legacy systems. This resulted in a significant decrease in spending on advanced products such as the CPR.

In 1991, the IOM estimated that, by the end of this decade, there would be nationwide CPR adaptation. Today's health care environment is more conducive to CPR adoption than was the case in 1991.

But the jig is up. It is time that these 14 barriers be addressed with new fervor. Given the current health care environment, consumer outrage with the status quo, and the pervasive use of the Web, a fundamental paradigm shift can and will take place in the health care system in the next several years.

CONSUMER OUTRAGE WILL FUEL CHANGE

In today's managed care environment, consumers feel they have lost control of their access to health care. Even before managed care, there was deep concern about health care quality. But now, consumers often feel like victims of cost-saving measures.

The e-healthcare revolution and the new e-consumerism allow consumers to regain this control and will reshape relationships between providers and patients. Since consumers will bear more and more of the financial burden of rising health care costs, it is likely that they will demand better services and more choices. They will also want access to quality data. The Web and rising e-consumer activism have led to much better educated consumers. Consumers want immediate access to their providers and want to communicate with their own providers about medical information they gathered through their on-line research.

E-consumers and e-patients are already playing a bigger role in their own care. In 1999, the trend was Web self-service—primarily accessing health information from Web services such as Intelihealth (www.intelihealth.com) or America's Health Network (www.ahn.com). But e-patients and e-consumers are fast wanting more. They want to e-communicate with their physicians or their physicians' staff. They want the ability to ask for appointments and check appointment status as well as obtain drug refills and laboratory notification on line.

They may, in effect, become the creator and warehouse of some or all of their own medical record. Medical record information may be deposited by the patient into a personal medical record folder that is stored in the patient's own secure Web site for this specific purpose. In order to accomplish this, e-mail and data transfer on a secure server will be essential.

FROM E-COMMUNICATIONS TO E-RECORDS

The 1991 IOM report listed technology barriers as minor impediments to the CPR. Major impediments listed were cultural, financial, and legal barriers. It may have been difficult to make that judgment without the benefit of foresight about the Internet. The explosion of Internet/Intranet and broadband WAN technologies will change the role and acceptance of information systems within health care delivery. Web applications have been adopted more quickly than any other new technologies. Tens of millions of health care consumers surf the Web, conducting business, shopping, receiving advice, and using e-mail. In greater numbers they seek health care information, e-services, and e-products as well.

The Internet is not just about high-bandwidth connectivity. It is a phenomenon that can deeply change cultural values. Broadband networking will enable e-connectivity for a whole new range of e-services; the .com revolution is much more than a larger pipe into the e-consumer's home-based personal computer (PC). The Web is revolutionizing how physicians and patients communicate. It confirmed that economies are now networked. Benefits of some technologies grow exponentially with the number of users of the same technology—evidence the telephone and fax machine.

E-communications, e-commerce, and the CPR have this same characteristic. Much larger benefits accrue as more patients and providers are networked. The

CPR used by only a few scattered groups of providers cannot provide the full economic benefit inherent in the technology. Since information sharing is the basis for much of the benefit (through reduction in error, waste, and duplication), CPR will realize its full potential only when there are numerous participants. Since the Internet provides this networking economically and universally, it must be an integral part of the CPR from now on. E-connectivity—between providers and e-consumers; e-consumers and providers; primary care providers and specialists; physicians and lab, pharmacy, and radiology services; and hospitals to each other and to community-based providers—is critical to success.

Any future CPR that does not take advantage of Internet integration will likely fail.

ENTER THE NEW HYBRID CPRs

With the Internet and increased e-consumer participation in health care delivery, health care information systems are experiencing a paradigm shift. The traditional model of isolated, remotely deployed systems that require multiple, intensive data entry at each location may not thrive. Data retrieval and transfer have to be seamless and inexpensive. The new CPR has to solve business problems that face today's practitioners by being connected to multiple trading partners. It has to create efficiencies and economic benefits for all participants who contribute data along the way. Primary users as well as secondary users of the medical record should benefit equally in this effort. New thinking must occur to accelerate widescale adoption of the CPR.

A centralized clinical and financial data center—available to a wide variety of participants through Web-enabled applications—offers the best hope for widespread adoption. The Internet pipeline can query and deliver administrative data such as eligibility, referral authorization, and formulary information. It can be used for claims submission and encounter reporting. It can deliver clinical data such as laboratory, radiology, and hospital discharge summaries. It can also deliver clinical reference data such as MEDLINE and on-line journals. In short, it is the preferred communication channel for delivering the CPR.

But the Web itself does not consolidate the physician's desktop. The Web may deliver data from multiple sources, but an integrated CPR that meets legal and medical record requirements is necessary to integrate data and images and store them either in local or remote servers connected to the Internet. A hybrid model that combines the Internet and distributed applications may be the answer—until more advanced technologies and very high-speed connections become less expensive and widely available.

OPTIMIZING THE EFFICIENCY OF CARE DELIVERY

Hybrid system CPRs with remote servers and a local, performance-enhancing cache can significantly improve the beleaguered workflow processes of medical offices and hospitals. Such systems offer CPR components, communication tools, office automation tools, practice management systems, and extensive reporting and query tools. The systems would include the following:

- *E-mail, voicemail, and faxing.* To enhance the usability and convenience of the system, there should be one in-box to unify all communication modalities available today. They are faxing and using voicemail and increasingly using e-mail. It should be easy to handle all three modes without getting out of the system and using disparate user interfaces. If the communication involves patient accounts, it should be automatically tagged and stored in the patient's file without human intervention.
- *Document scanning and management.* These tools are critical because there are multiple trading partners at various stages of technology adoption. Faxing and scanning of documents still offer a competitive advantage over monolithic system designs (such as a pure Internet implementation) in gaining early acceptance.
- *Clinical record components.* These include critical records such as problem lists, medication lists, allergy lists, and documentation of prior appointments and reasons for visits. They should be displayed visually and graphically alongside demographics, insurance information, and managed care affiliation. Their value would be greatly enhanced by secure access to this extensive clinical and administrative information anytime and anywhere, with proper authentication.
- *Office automation components.* Features such as pharmacy call-back for drug refills, scheduling, patient flow in the medical office, appointment reminders, telephone call-backs, and message handling should be integrated into the system.
- *Advanced clinical decision support systems.* Alerts and reminders for preventive care can help practices meet legal and population management mandates.

Hybrid CPR applications with these capabilities will improve efficiency tremendously.

- *Lower implementation and support costs.* The hybrid CPR lowers barriers to adoption by creating service options with lower capital outlay. The efficiencies of the Internet can lead to meaningfully lower total cost of ownership.

Thus, CPR and other business functions can be outsourced on the "rental" basis by monthly "subscription" through Internet application service providers. This has a strong potential to lower the barrier to entry for cash-strapped providers. New business models of Internet-based application service provider are starting up very rapidly.

- *Widespread, integrated practice management systems.* Since there will be no distinction made between financial and clinical transactions, they will be recognized as two sides of the same coin and will be recorded and managed as a single event. Moreover, to gain maximal benefits from the system, payers, consumers, and practitioners will want to analyze integrated clinical and financial statistics.
- *Networked systems that allow for easy outsourcing of noncore tasks.* Billing and collection and other nonclinical business functions, such as transcription or accounts payable, are likely candidates for outsourcing. The hybrid CPR makes outsourcing seamless.
- *Data-rich, accurate reporting.* The hybrid CPR is an excellent tool for collecting clinical data via ad hoc and preformatted reports and queries. Clinical analysis that aids in managing population- and disease-specific members will be an essential part of future disease management activities. This data management can be handled from a centralized data center, using benchmarking data from varied sources of information, which, up to this point, had not been available to independent physicians at an affordable cost.
- *Multiple data entry options.* Physicians have been concerned about slowing down their clinical encounters by being forced to use overly restrictive structured data entry. Allowing multiple modes of data entry, including old-fashioned paper entry and subsequent scanning, voice dictation, and structured data entry from a pick list, will enhance acceptance of new technology by physicians.

PHASING IN THE HYBRID CPR

Using any new technology—and most certainly the CPR—requires phased-in implementation. Even while practices phase in a CPR, they will see immediate information access benefits and the elimination of administrative hassles. Some of the sequential phases to be considered are as follows:

- Phase I: Control paper flow.
  - Scan paper documents into CPR.
  - Integrate computerized fax capability that handles incoming and outgoing faxes inside the CPR application.

–Initiate document routing and document review with electronic sign-off.
–Initiate paperless medical record (but not paperless office).
- Phase II: Connect with external business partners.
  –Connect with IPA or management services organization.
  –Connect with hospital.
  –Connect with laboratory.
  –Initiate two-way communication with e-patients.

Using Alteer.com (Figure 15–3), e-patients can e-mail their physician, keep track of their appointments, build a personal health profile, and request prescription refills.

- Phase III: Electronically document the care process.
  –Install templates for visits and letters.
  –Use a point-and-click process of documentation for structured data entry.
  –Employ a voice command or voice recognition program for visit documentation.

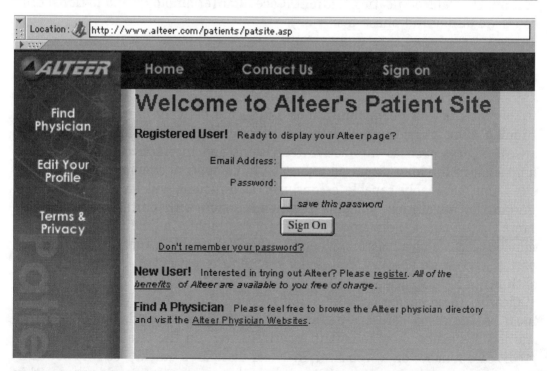

Figure 15–3 Alteer. *Source:* Reprinted with permission from www.alteer.com/corp/patients/about.html, © 1999, Alteer Corporation.

–Use hand-held computer devices for mobile documentation.

–Initiate order management, alerts, and reminders for follow-up care.

- Phase IV: Manage an internal data center.

–Review diagnosis and procedure statistics.

–Analyze utilization statistics for medications, laboratory procedures, and radiological procedures.

–Use outcome data for contract management.

–Benchmark data collection for comparison with outside organizations.

Although all of these improvements have merit, elimination of the paper medical record has the highest ROI because many of the inefficiencies in health care institutions are rooted in the paper record system. Whichever system is used to achieve these functions must be flexible and easy enough to include future plug and play components. A likely plug and play component is voice recognition or handwriting recognition technology that is adopted and improved with time; currently, these systems are not completely effective or reliable. Applications to assist providers with coding for International Classification of Diseases, Ninth Edition, Clinical Modification; Current Procedural Terminology; and national drug codes are also useful phase-ins.

E-OPPORTUNITIES AND E-CAVEATS

The potential of e-communications and e-care delivery grows even more intriguing when it is combined with the growing trend toward information appliances. Devices such as interactive televisions and interactive telephones may help achieve the long-promised reduction in computing complexity. As this occurs, any reasonably capable e-consumer or e-patient will be able to join the information revolution. Imagine e-patients armed with portable health assistants that monitor their progress and serve as highly individualized health reminders and health educators. When they are Web enabled, these devices become part of the e-care delivery process by keeping the patient in continual contact with his or her physician.

Clearly, these scenarios raise serious issues about security. Security issues must be addressed before e-patients will be fully connected. But laggards be warned. Remember how reluctant Americans were in the late 1990s to enter a credit card number on a Web site? That fear dissipated quickly, so it is not difficult to envision similar e-care delivery security concerns being addressed within a very short period of time.

When this radical shift takes place, Web-enabled systems will completely re-shape the landscape of e-care delivery. The traditional notion of data flow between the provider and the patient will change. Both will become comfortable with a more balanced two-way approach. The patient will become, in part, the source of medical insights or information. Weighty questions will flow both ways. Care decisions will become more of a partnership agreement—not strictly based on "doctor's orders."

Participants in the health care system may begin using a personal central data repository (CDR) of longitudinal medical records owned by patients and contributed to by both patients and providers. The Internet will replace the community health information network, and consumers will be a central part of the patient-centered CDR on the Internet.

Medical practices can no longer delay implementation of clinical systems to facilitate care delivery and improve customer service to patients. Selecting the right system will take some foresight. Web-enabled technology capable of meaningful e-connections to patients and the rest of the world is an essential first step.

EVALUATING YOUR HEALTH ORGANIZATION'S CPR FUTURE

Internet-Centric CPR Application Vendors

This section contains a list of companies that offer or might offer CPR applications in which the Web is central. These companies are discussed below, in alphabetical order. Remember that this industry is very dynamic. The list can become obsolete in a matter of months.

Abaton.com (www.abaton.com) is a Minneapolis-based company focused on developing Internet and Intranet technology that connects providers to laboratories, radiology services, IPAs, and pharmacies and capturing clinical information at the point of care. It is a venture-backed, privately owned company.

Alteer Corporation (Figure 15–4) is creating a new Internet-based physician office system using hybrid technology. The system is designed for providers as well as patients. Alteer products handle office functions such as scheduling, billing, document management, and e-connectivity to patients and other trading partners. Alteer Office® is designed as a paperless medical record system.

Confer Software (formerly Araxys; www.confersoftware.com) develops workflow engines based on Web technology platforms. The company is focused on practice guidelines and care flow integration.

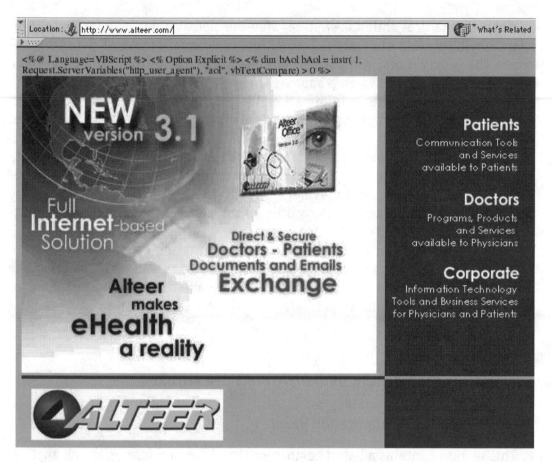

Figure 15–4 Alteer. *Source:* Reprinted with permission from www.alteer.com/corp/patients/ about.html, © 1999, Alteer Corporation.

E-physician (www.ephysician.com) is a start-up physician practice management system that is completely housed on a server accessible on the Web. Physicians and staff access e-Physician using hand-held computer devices.

Healtheon (www.healtheon.com) is a publicly traded company started by Jim Clark, founder of Silicon Graphics and Netscape. Healtheon develops Web-based systems that connect insurance companies and IPAs with physicians. Healtheon's goal is to connect physicians' offices to the Internet so that they may conduct business through Internet and Intranet technology.

iTrust (www.itrust.com) is located in San Francisco and is developing a CPR and office-based practice management system that is completely based on the Web.

Traditional CPR Vendors

There are several notable companies that provide "traditional" CPR products. It is likely that some of these companies are developing or will develop more Web-enabled products in the future.

Formerly called Visteon Corporation, Avio (www.avio.com) provides a suite of practice management, clinical records, and managed care products to large group practices and managed care organizations.

Epic Systems (Figure 15–5) is a successful private company with a MUMPS-based technology and a distinguished client list. Epic's customers have received Davies CPR Recognition Awards. EPIC has practice management software as well as a clinical electronic medical record (EMR).

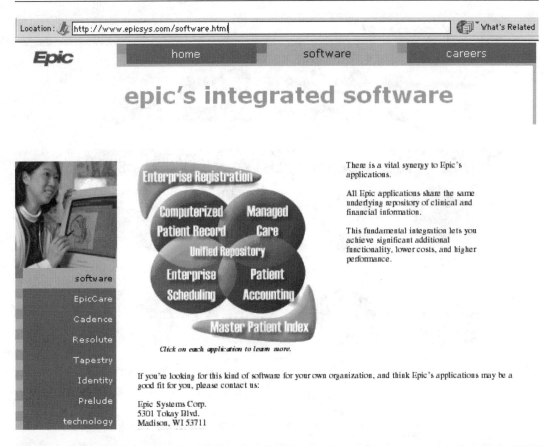

Figure 15–5 Epic Systems. *Source:* Reprinted with permission from www.epicsys.com, © 1999, Epic Systems Corporation.

MedicaLogic (www.medicalogic.com) is a pure EMR company targeting IDSs. Part of its overall solution is to partner with other vendors. The software has no practice management functions, but it interfaces with existing practice management software and IDS computer systems. MedicaLogic is developing a Web site that enables patients to review their history and perform certain tasks associated with managing their health care.

A market leader in home care EMR, Patient Care Technologies (Figure 15–6) offers hand-held point-of-care technology that emphasizes a structured approach to care delivery and documentation. A HITS award winner, Patient Care Technologies is actively developing Web-enabled direct care management applications.

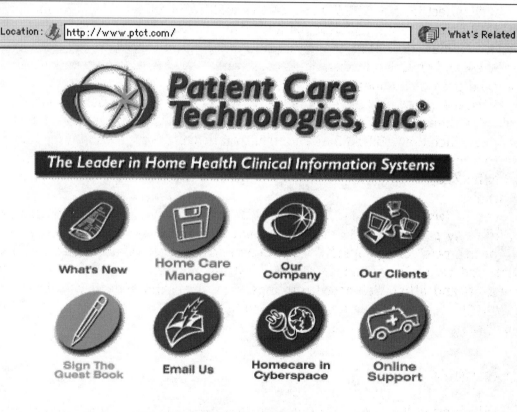

Figure 15–6 Patient Care Technologies. *Source:* Reprinted with permission from www.ptct.com, © 1999, Patient Care Technologies.

Aggregating Physician Desktops

The following companies use Web applications to offer services and information to physicians. Each of the companies allows for cost reduction via on-line transactions and push technology. These companies have achieved a very high profile on Wall Street as part of the general Internet phenomenon. Some of them are making deals with major media companies and other large corporations. They may, in time, help realize the hybrid CPR model by facilitating communications with physicians and adopting the Internet as the basis for a hybrid CPR tool.

Medcast (www.medcast.com) has a unique hybrid approach using in-office, PC-based software as well as software running on a robust office computer. Physicians can receive news and information and use applications that encompass disease management, patient concerns, and practice management. Medcast is a fee-based service.

MedConnect (Figure 15–7), a free service with advertiser sponsorship, provides medical information to physicians and other health care professionals. Other services include free MEDLINE access and access to board review articles, news updates, and on-line journals. The company is creating six on-line journals to be sent via push technology.

Medscape (www.medscape.com), a free service with advertiser sponsorship, provides thousands of articles for on-line browsing plus a variety of other free services, including MEDLINE. They recently hired Dr. George Lundburg, former editor of *JAMA,* and subsequently started Medscape General Medicine (MedGenMed), a fully electronic, comprehensive peer-reviewed general medical journal.

WebMD (www.webmd.com), a fee-based site, connects physicians, hospitals, third-party payers, and consumers to medical information, tools, and services. A "health care portal," WebMD is a single point of access to insurance verification and referrals, enhanced communications services, branded health care content, and other Web-based offerings. Healtheon and WebMD will merge in late 1999 with unprecedented market capitalization for health care information companies.

CONCLUSION

CPR adoption has been painfully slow over the years due to multiple barriers. These barriers have often been underestimated by manufacturers and businesspeople who have tried to automate clinical recordkeeping. But as an industry largely focused on information collection, analysis, and dissemination,

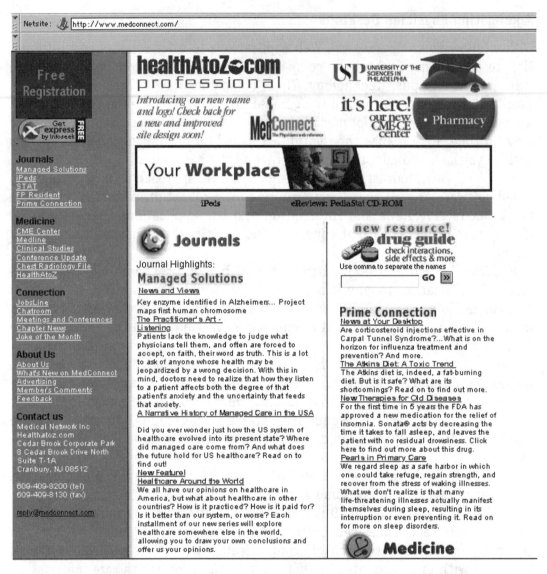

Figure 15–7 MedConnect. *Source:* Reprinted with permission from www.medconnect.com, ©
1999, Medical Network, Inc., also known as HealthAtoZ.com.

health care cannot ignore the importance of building the infrastructure to manage clinical information much longer. Because health care is being pressured as
never before to re-engineer itself and become more cost-effective, the CPR is an
e-tool whose time has come. And with the Medicare risk-adjusted capitated pay-

ment scheme based on ambulatory diagnoses expected to take effect in the next three to four years, it will be even more imperative to work with other provider partners to collect physicians' clinical information.

As patients are asked to accept an increasing share of health care costs, they will continue to be a significant driver in this transformation. The pervasive use of Web applications in many Americans' everyday lives provides renewed hope that clinicians and patients alike will adopt clinical information technology. An e-patient-centered CPR can automate the collection of relevant clinical information and present it in a way that is helpful to e-patients as they manage their own care. Patient self-care will continue to be an area of intense product development as new point-of-care technologies enable more extensive direct patient involvement in the management of chronic diseases. Such automation also stands to lower the overall cost of health care delivery.

Well-funded companies are rushing to build an infrastructure that connects providers, payers, employers, and patients using the Internet. Many companies want to build a portal to providers and patients by offering free medical content along with e-commerce products such as pharmacy and alternatives to traditional medical care. Innovative companies are developing applications and services that will eliminate administrative hassles and lower costs for providers and patients. We believe that, given the current state of technology, the most successful CPR will be a hybrid of Web-enabled technology and plug and play software for the physician's office.

Many issues remain before the CPR will be widely used. Among them are structured data entry, human–computer interface and form factors, and financial incentives to providers to acquire clinical information systems. When providers are compensated for quality (and better documentation is necessary to prove that quality), there will be a rush by providers to acquire clinical information systems. Until then, providers will be hesitant to acquire and assimilate information systems without clear economic payback. For the short term, it is likely that information systems that manage administrative and financial business processes will continue to be more common than CPR systems.

The impetus is clear. The Web stands to be the biggest catalyst for change that the health care industry has ever seen. And with both patients and providers on line in one virtual health care enterprise, the Web may finally help people benefit from a networked community that truly improves the health of the nation.

Where To Go for More

As you can imagine, the information about Web-enabled CPRs changes nearly daily. To keep your practice or health care organization up to date, visit the

Location: http://www.medrecinst.com/index.shtml   What's Related

MEDICAL REC🌐RDS INSTITUTE
shaping the world of electronic health records

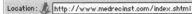

Home

Who We Are

What We Do

Press Center

Publications

Survey Results

▶ The Caregiver and Provider

▶ System Integrators and Component Vendors

▶ You and Your Health Information

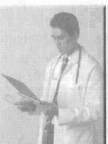

The Caregiver and Provider

From the small office physician to the largest metropolitan hospital, the electronic health record will change the way you provide care. Click here to learn about the technology behind the EHR and the legislative acts and standards that are driving the industry. Tap into our 16 years of resources and experience and stay in the forefront of the EHR movement.

System Integrators and Component Vendors

Click here for updates on the standards and legislative acts that are defining your marketplace. Learn about our excellent marketing and promotional opportunities at our national and international conferences.

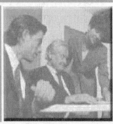

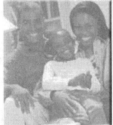

You and Your Health Information

Electronic Health Records affect everyone. Click here to learn more about your rights concerning your health record and hear opinions on who owns your record.

Figure 15–8 Medical Records Institute. *Source:* Reprinted with permission from www.medrecinst.com/Index.html, © 1999, Medical Records Institute.

following information sources regularly. Sign up for their e-newsletters and stay abreast of trends in medical recordkeeping.

The Computer-Based Patient Record Institute (www.cpri.com) was the result of the IOM report on CPR. It serves as a neutral forum to promote CPR and works closely with private vendors and government agencies.

The mission of the Medical Records Institute (Figure 15-8) is to promote the creation and implementation of the electronic patient record. It holds an annual meeting called Toward an Electronic Patient Record every May.

The Health Care Financing Administration (Figure 15-9) is a definitive source on health care services, policies, and costs.

Healthcare Informatics (www.healthcare-informatics.com) is an excellent resource for CPR and up-to-date information in the health care informatics area. It publishes annual CPR reviews with vendor updates. The last update was in May 1998.

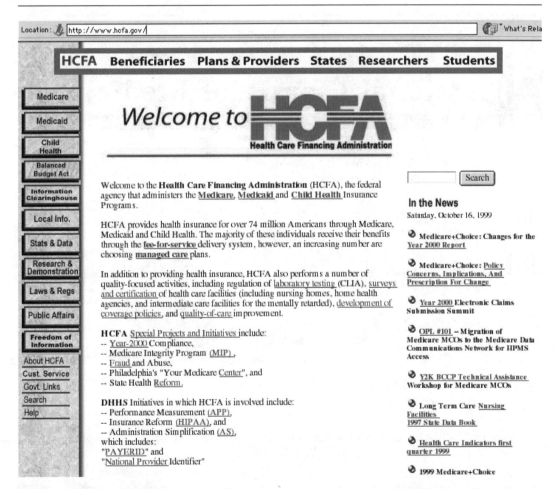

Figure 15-9 The Health Care Financing Administration. *Source:* Reprinted from www.hcfa.gov, 1999, Health Care Financing Administration.

The American Medical Informatics Association (www.amia.org) is dedicated to the development and application of medical informatics in the support of patient care, teaching, research, and health care administration.

The Healthcare Information and Management Systems Society (HIMSS; www.himss.org) is a nonprofit organization representing information and management systems professionals in health care. The annual HIMSS trade show is the industry's largest annual gathering.

The National Library of Medicine (Figure 15–10), a component of the National Institutes of Health, is a major sponsor of research in clinical computing and

Location: http://www.nlm.nih.gov/

UNITED STATES
National Library of Medicine

Site Index | Search Our Web Site

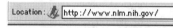

HEALTH INFORMATION
MEDLINE, MEDLINE*plus*, and other resources

LIBRARY SERVICES
Catalog, Databases, Publications, Training, Grants

RESEARCH PROGRAMS
Computational Molecular Biology, Medical Informatics

NEW & NOTEWORTHY
Announcements, Exhibits, New on this Site, Hot Topics

GENERAL INFORMATION
Visiting the Library, FAQs, Directories, Jobs

Welcome to the world's largest medical library and creator of MEDLINE.

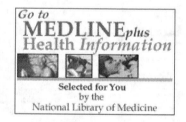
Go to
MEDLINE*plus*
Health *Information*
Selected for You
by the
National Library of Medicine

U.S. National Library of Medicine, 8600 Rockville Pike, Bethesda, MD 20894
National Institutes of Health
Department of Health & Human Services
Copyright and Privacy Policy

Figure 15–10 Medline. *Source:* Reprinted from www.nlm.nih.gov, 1999, National Library of Medicine.

provides Medline, the leading on-line index to peer-reviewed journals of all kinds.

REFERENCES

1. C. Clark, "Healthcare Info Systems," *Value Line Report,* 7 April, 1995, 679, quoted in M.L. Millenson, *Demanding Medical Excellence* (Chicago: University of Chicago Press, 1997), 91.
2. R.S. Dick and E.B. Steen, eds., *The Computer-Based Patient Record—An Essential Technology for Healthcare* (Washington, DC: National Academy Press, 1991), 11.
3. C. Marietti, *Healthcare Informatics* (May 1998), 77.
4. V. Hudson, *The POMIS Report 1999,* Vol. 1, 5–7.
5. Hudson, *The POMIS Report 1999,* 8–30.
6. Hudson, *The POMIS Report 1999,* 8–20.
7. Hudson, *The POMIS Report 1999,* 3–31.

CHAPTER 16

e-Health and the Law

Laura J. Oberbroeckling

$\mathbf{F}$OR YEARS, health care providers have employed various technologies to improve diagnostic capabilities, expand treatment options, and treat chronic conditions. Whether it be through imaging technology, the development of new drug therapies, or the advent of laser surgery, technology has always been key to our nation's health care system. Until recently, however, technology had not realized its full potential as a means of reducing health care costs. Ironically, instead of cutting costs, technology has helped drive up health care costs (Figure 16–1).

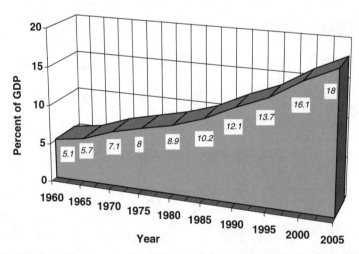

Figure 16–1 Health Care Costs as a Percentage of Gross Domestic Product (GDP). *Source:* Reprinted from aspe.hhs.gov/96gb/cappend.txt, 1999, U.S. Department of Health and Human Services.

Acknowledgments: Special thanks to Valerie E. Hurt for her assistance in researching and drafting this chapter.

- Consumer-oriented health care
- Professionals as information sources for patients choosing self-care options
- Focus on preventive care
- Electronic communications between providers as well as patients and providers

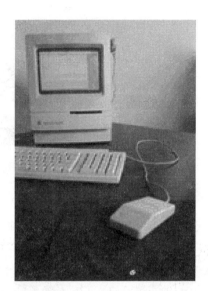

Figure 16–2 Health Care Trends

The advent of the Internet and the Web, however, has the potential to reshape the health care delivery system by improving quality of care and increasing efficiency—while at the same time helping to control or curb the ever-rising cost of providing health care. The Web has this potential because, unlike any other technology available today, it can help control costs associated with both the demand for and supply of health care services. Figure 16–2 lists some of the trends currently shaping health care.

From the e-patient's perspective, the Net is an information pipeline that extends the health care system into the home—which ultimately decreases the need for expensive visits to the emergency department or physician's office. It also empowers e-consumers and e-patients with the knowledge necessary to help select their own treatment options, including self-care. From a physician's or other health care provider's perspective, the Web can contribute significantly to cost containment through e-commerce solutions that improve information, e-communications, and e-care delivery. The Web also presents an opportunity to get a piece of the health care dollar (Figure 16–3), e-health care having been described as "the trillion-dollar opportunity."[1] But physicians, health care providers, and e-patients have concerns about how technology will affect access, quality, and patient confidentiality. Although the benefits of using Internet-based applications to improve the delivery of health care to patients are enormous, the legal issues surrounding implementation of a Web-enabled application

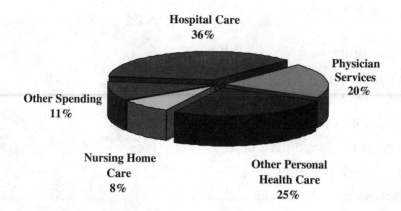

Figure 16–3 Allocation of Health Care Dollars. *Source:* Data from hsriv.kee.aetc.af.mil/market/healthexp.html, 1999.

are complex. Health care organizations need to understand the issues and take steps to minimize the risks of legal liability.

Recognizing the practical use of e-communication, e-communities, e-commerce, and e-care delivery, this chapter discusses their legal ramifications in the health care industry and provides guidance on how to establish Web-enabled applications in compliance with applicable laws and regulations. The chapter is divided into two parts, each of which is designed to provide basic information necessary to understand the legal implications of implementing an e-strategy in your health care organization. The first part provides information regarding laws and regulations generally applicable to any business using the Internet—laws concerning privacy and confidentiality, trade practices, copyright, and e-commerce. The second part discusses legal concerns for health care providers specifically—some of which apply whether or not the provider is using the Web, and others that apply specifically to the use of the Net. Privacy and confidentiality of medical record information, licensure and accreditation, malpractice liability, and Food and Drug Administration (FDA) regulation of drugs and devices are covered in this second part.

CAVEAT: LEGAL "E'S" ARE MOVING TARGETS

One of the challenges associated with writing this chapter is the rapid pace of change in the health care industry and the extraordinary pace of change in communications technology. In the 105th Congress alone, approximately 350 bills were introduced concerning privacy protections—about 50 of which concerned protections for medical record information, and nearly 25 of which concerned electronic privacy.

Therefore, rather than focusing on the latest legislative proposals or regulatory developments, this chapter concentrates on legal trends and the importance of developing a framework for understanding the myriad legal issues relevant to the use of Web applications in health care. By the end of the chapter, you should feel more comfortable about introducing Web-based strategies into your health care organization and taking advantage of the enormous potential to improve quality of care and save money—without running afoul of the law.

THE GENERAL LAW OF THE INTERNET

It is no secret that e-commerce is growing rapidly. Businesses in virtually every sector of the economy, including health care, are beginning to use the Web to cut the cost of purchasing, manage supplier relationships, streamline logistics and inventory, plan production, and reach new and existing customers more effectively.[2] In the midst of the economic benefits associated with this growth, the federal government has called for a "non-regulatory, market-oriented approach to electronic commerce," based on the theory that unnecessary government regulation will stifle future growth and, thus, the well-being of our increasingly wired economy.[3] Despite this stated hands-off approach to regulating e-commerce, however, there have been numerous federal and state efforts to regulate e-commerce. In addition, e-commerce is not exempt from the usual laws and regulations governing commerce generally. Figure 16–4 and the paragraphs below give a brief overview of some of the laws of general application that are of special concern for companies conducting business over the Internet, with special focus on those laws specifically tailored for e-commerce.

Regulating e-Commerce

Laws and regulations governing e-commerce encompass a crazy quilt of international, federal, and state laws and regulations. Legal issues that previously concerned only a small number of international businesses, such as jurisdiction across state and national borders, are receiving a great deal of attention now that a small business in Dubuque, Iowa, can have global reach over the World Wide Web.

International jurisdictional issues aside, the fact that business is conducted in cyberspace does not exempt the business from the usual laws and regulations

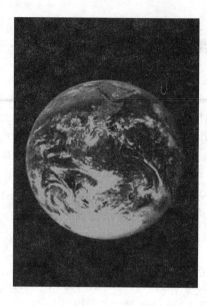

- Contract laws
- Copyright
- Trademark
- Domain name registration and use
- Consumer protection
- Licensure and accreditation of professionals
- Professional liability

Figure 16–4 Global Legal Issues

affecting commerce. Every state in the United States, for example, has adopted some version of the Uniform Commercial Code (UCC), a collection of laws governing commercial relationships. For several years now the National Conference of Commissioners of Uniform State Laws (NCCUSL) and the American Law Institute (the bodies responsible for drafting revisions to the model UCC) have been working to adapt the UCC to e-commerce.[4]

If adopted by the states, the proposed model statute, the Uniform Electronic Transactions Act, would revise existing general contract law to create uniform guidelines for the use of e-communications and recordkeeping in contractual transactions. In addition, separate work is proceeding on drafting an electronic contracting and records act for e-transactions not covered by the UCC. This second model act, originally proposed as a new article 2B of the UCC,[5] concerns transactions involving information that can be copyrighted—including transactions involving software, e-commerce information, and licenses for data, text, and similar materials.

After considerable controversy and discussion about the proposed article 2B, in early 1999 the NCCUSL announced that it would promulgate the draft article 2B as a separate uniform act (the Uniform Computer Information Transactions Act), to be finalized and sent to the states by the end of 1999.[6] Internationally, the United Nations Commission on International Trade Law has drafted a model law supporting the use of international contracts in e-commerce.[7] This model law establishes rules and norms that validate and recognize electronic contracts and defines the characteristics of a valid e-contract.

Consistent with these national and international efforts, almost every state in the United States has considered or enacted laws or regulations requiring some method to authenticate individual authorization for e-commerce and e-business.[8] Because most states have a statute of frauds that operates to deny enforcement of certain unwritten contracts (such as those in operation for one year or more), authentication laws are critical to validate e-contracts. In order to give e-documents the same indicia of reliability as signed, written documents, authentication laws require the use of letters, characters, or symbols presented in electronic form to authenticate a writing, or other methods to ensure that the document received is an authentic copy of the document sent.[9] The laws vary from state to state, but the trend appears to be toward a recognition of the validity of e-documents.

Whatever the final result of these legal developments at the international, federal, and state levels, lawmakers at all levels have attempted to adhere to the same general principles:

- *Draft provisions using technologically neutral language.* New laws and regulations, to the extent possible, are drafted with technologically neutral language so that they will not become outdated or require substantial revision with the next generation of technological development.
- *Facilitate continued growth of e-commerce.* New rules are designed to facilitate e-commerce, rather than restrict its development with onerous administrative and regulatory barriers.
- *Recognize and accept electronic communications.* Laws and regulations encourage the recognition and acceptance of e-communications.
- *Promote consistency and certainty.* Efforts are aimed at creating a seamless web of regulation so that companies utilizing electronic communications can operate under one general guiding principle.

Assuming that lawmakers continue to adhere to these guiding principles, e-commerce should continue to grow and thrive despite increased regulatory interest in an increasingly paperless world. In the meantime, e-health companies transacting business in cyberspace should ensure that business transacted on line is in compliance with all requirements in the jurisdictions in which they operate, so that all agreements entered into are enforceable. Figure 16–5 outlines some important issues with paperless contracts. This is particularly impor-

- E-negotiations save time and expense.
- There is a growing legal recognition and acceptance of e-communications.
- E-contracts may be validated through the use of keys and codes.

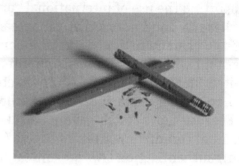

Figure 16–5 The Paperless Contract

---

tant for those contracts that fall under the jurisdiction of the statute of frauds and, thus, require a signed writing to be effective.

Making Your Mark with an e-Trademark

Federal and state trademark law protects any word, name, symbol, or device intended to be used in commerce to identify or distinguish goods or services.[10] Traditionally, trademark law protected a mark from use by a person or entity in competition with the owner of the mark (i.e., protecting BandAid® from use by a competing plastic strip bandage company) or from use that would likely cause confusion, mistake, or deception, even if the infringer is not in direct competition with the owner (i.e., use of the name Jeep Cherokee® by a clothing manufacturer). Since 1996, however, the Lanham Act has also protected against trademark dilution by providing a right of action to an owner of a *famous* mark against another person's commercial use of the mark.[11] An example of dilution but not necessarily infringement would be "[t]he use of DuPont shoes, Buick aspirin, and Kodak pianos."[12]

In short, federal trademark law protects brand names such as Kaiser Permanente or WebMD from unauthorized reproduction. Federal law does not require the registration of a brand name in order to obtain this protection; certain common law rights arise from actual use of a mark. However, there are benefits to registering a mark, including notice to the public of a claim of ownership for the mark, which is a legal presumption of nationwide ownership. The first to use a mark in commerce or file an intent to use application with the Patent and Trademark Office (PTO) has the ultimate right to use and registration. In order to determine whether a mark has been registered already, the PTO's files may be searched. Searches can be conducted at the PTO offices in Arlington, Virginia, or on the Web at www.uspto.gov/tmdb/index.html.

For a company whose primary interest is doing business on the Web, the most important trademark is not necessarily the company's name (such as Columbia/ HCA, Inc.) or the name of one of the company's key product lines (such as Claritin). In e-commerce, the most important trademark is the company's Web address or domain name, such as askadoc.com (Figure 16–6). Ask a Doc's "Who we are" Web page notes its relationship with PTC International, Inc., yet the domain name, not PTC International, is the key trademark. A domain name is critical to an e-commerce company because it provides a unique identity to communicate to customers and the market.

Until recently, Network Solutions, Inc. (NSI) was the exclusive registrar for all domain names using .com, .org, and .net. NSI also had some responsibility for registration for more than 240 country codes, such as .uk. In 1997, however, the Department of Commerce began moving away from its exclusive agreement with NSI and toward a competitive, market-oriented registration process. Pursuant to this initiative, the Department of Commerce turned over much of the responsibility for managing the domain name system to a nonprofit California-based company, the Internet Corporation for Assigned Names and Numbers (ICANN).[13] On April 21, 1999, ICANN announced that it had selected five new companies to participate in domain name registration on a test basis from April 26 through June 24, 1999. Following the conclusion of this test period, the registration for .com, .net, and .org domains will be opened on equal terms to all companies that meet ICANN's standards for accreditation.

It is important to note that although registration of a domain name is necessary to use a name on the Internet, it is not the equivalent of registering a trademark and vice versa. Registration of a domain name does not entitle the registrant to trademark rights, and registration of a trademark does not reserve the domain name. Because of this seemingly two-track system for registration and protection of an e-company's most important identifier—its domain name— conflicts have arisen where parties have registered Internet domain names that are the same as, or substantially similar to, registered or common law trademarks. To date, most conflicts between owners of trademarks and domain names have been resolved through negotiation, but increasingly the parties have been forced to litigate these matters.[14] These negotiated and litigated disputes have not resolved the underlying confusion between domain name registration and

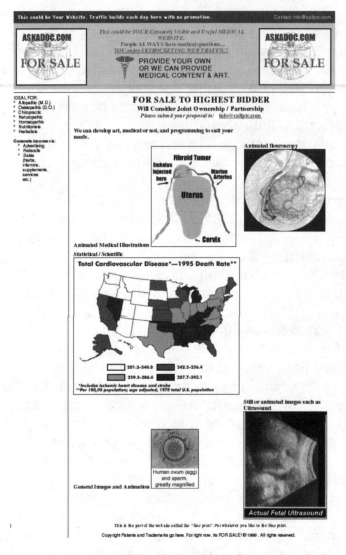

Figure 16–6 Ask a Doc. *Source:* Reprinted with permission from www.askadoc.com, © 1999, PTC International, Inc.

trademark laws. Therefore, there remains a great deal of tension between domain name registration requirements and trademark laws.

Keeping this tension in mind, any company considering using and registering a domain name should consider the trademark implications of using a domain name. It should also ensure that its domain name is not another company's trademark and that it registers its domain name, as Figure 16–7 notes, as a trademark to obtain the protections afforded under the Lanham Act. Consideration of the trademark implications of a domain name is good practice, especially in light of the trademark dilution provisions of the Lanham Act. In addition, in order to register a name with NSI, for example, an applicant must certify that the proposed use does not interfere or infringe on any trademark rights. If the name is rightfully owned by someone other than the applicant, NSI may revoke the right to use a particular domain name and may assign the applicant a new domain name and put the disputed name on hold pending resolution of the dispute.

Understanding e-Copyrights

Federal copyright law secures legal ownership rights for the author of a creative expression, such as a book, work of art, or Web page.[15] The owner of the creative expression, or intellectual property, can sell or license the rights to the property or otherwise control other people's use of the property by granting or denying others the privilege of using the work, making copies, and controlling the manner of making copies, or derivative works.

It is important to keep in mind that copyright protects expression, not facts or ideas. Only a creative work existing in some tangible form can be copyrighted. An idea in someone's head or the expression of that idea through a conversation

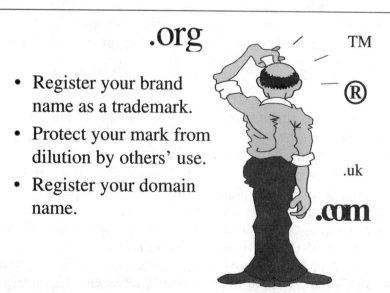

Figure 16–7 Protecting Your Good Name

with a friend is not tangible—it has to be fixed in some form, whether it be in electronic form or on disk, paper, canvas, or the like. But the fact that an idea is fixed in tangible form does not alone make it copyrightable. The expression must also be creative and not merely factual.

A recitation of statistical information regarding the symptoms of a disease posted on the Web or sent via e-mail, for example, while fixed in tangible form, is not copyrightable standing alone. Factual information can be used freely—there are no ownership rights in facts or ideas. The *expression* of these facts, on the other hand, is a creative work that is protectable by copyright even if the underlying facts and ideas are not. Therefore, the recitation of information concerning angina in an on-line medical textbook is copyrightable as a creative expression because of the organization and presentation of the underlying facts. For example, a page on the www.emedicine.com Web site shows an emergency medicine textbook on angina.

Although copyright law protects creative expression fixed in tangible form, it does not offer absolute protection from use of expression ad infinitum. Since 1978, federal law has provided copyright protection for works for the life of the author plus 50 years. In addition, under some circumstances otherwise copyrightable works may be used by another person or company without the permission of the copyright owner as long as the use does not unreasonably prejudice the legitimate interests of the author (e.g., "fair use").[16] The unauthorized use of a copyrighted work not protected by the fair use doctrine can subject the person using the work to possible criminal and civil liability.

Generally, if a person or company copies a protected work for its own use by, for example, copying an answer provided by askadoc.com (www.askadoc.com) or a list of recommended physicians from findadoc.com and reprinting it on another e-health Web page without permission or attribution, it is considered direct infringement. In the on-line context, however, an increasing number of claims have been brought under theories of contributory and vicarious liability.

Under these theories, the sponsor of the Web site on which the infringing material was posted would be liable directly, and the on-line service provider (OSP) or Internet service provider (ISP) enabling the Web site to be viewed might be liable indirectly. Courts have held that merely providing the site and facilities for known infringing activity is sufficient to establish contributory infringement.[17] Not surprisingly, OSPs have opposed vigorously theories of vicarious and contributory liability for such activities, arguing that it is difficult to police the overwhelming amount of information on their services. As a result of this outcry and the growing number of copyright issues created by the expansion of e-commerce, Congress enacted the Digital Millennium Copyright Act of 1998, signed into law by President Clinton on October 28, 1998.[18]

In an attempt to limit ISP and OSP liability, the Digital Millennium Copyright Act provides safe harbors for ISPs and OSPs for infringement by transient transmissions (such as e-mails) passing through their computers. It allows these same providers to escape liability for more permanent transmissions (such as Web pages) if they promptly remove infringing material upon request. Finally, the act also prohibits the falsification of identifying information accompanying copyrighted works.[19]

Because of the vital role that the expression of ideas plays in e-commerce, any e-health company must take steps to ensure that its intellectual property is protected to the fullest extent possible under the law. Some of these steps include the following:

- Register copyrights, when feasible, to take full advantage of the copyright protections afforded under the law.
- Notify all users of the copyright protection in a work your company has produced.
- Establish clear written policies and procedures governing Web links and the permissions to copy and use copyrighted material.

Equally important to protecting your own company's intellectual property is the need to take steps that ensure your company does not infringe on any other person's copyright. As Figure 16–8 discusses, one way to do this is to require that any hyperlinks on your company's Web site are posted with full disclosure to, and permission of, the owner of the Web site.

Consumer Protection, Spam, and Unfair Trade Practices

Both the federal and state governments—through the Federal Trade Commission (FTC) and the state attorney general offices—have authority to regulate e-commerce to protect e-consumers from unfair trade practices. The FTC has authority over all products that travel in interstate commerce (encompassing virtually all e-commerce transactions), and the states have limited authority to deal with commerce that affects their particular jurisdictions.[20] Both the federal government and the states have adapted laws generally applicable to trade practices—such as those mandating "truth in advertising"—to e-commerce and have enacted laws and regulations specifically addressing e-commerce-related concerns.

On the federal level, the FTC has brought enforcement actions against companies found to be engaging in unfair or deceptive trade practices over the

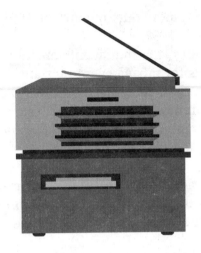

- Register copyrights.
- Notify users of copyright protection.
- Adopt and implement permissions policy.
- Obtain permission before hyperlinking or copying others' works.

Figure 16–8 Copyright Compliance

Internet.[21] On the state level, unfair and deceptive trade practice prosecutions have proceeded for similar reasons.[22] Most of these cases involved old marketing scams recycled on the Internet. The companies behind these scams were held in violation of existing laws and regulations, but the FTC has also taken action against unsolicited commercial e-mail and schemes unique to the Internet.[23]

For example, on August 13, 1998, the FTC and GeoCities, an ISP and Web site proprietor based in Santa Monica, California, agreed to settle charges that GeoCities "misrepresented the purpose for which it was collecting personal identifying information from children and adults."[24] Applying its existing rules and regulations to the on-line context, the FTC required GeoCities to cease misrepresenting the purpose for which it collected and used consumer personal identifying information and to provide full disclosure regarding, among other things, the dissemination of personal identifying information. In addition, the FTC required GeoCities to post on its site a clear and prominent privacy notice explaining to consumers what information is being collected, why it is being collected, to whom it will be disclosed, and how consumers can access and remove the information.

Because of the appearance of Web-based fraudulent schemes and other violations of trade practice laws in cyberspace, the FTC has considered promulgating a separate policy concerning the applicability of its current rules to e-commerce.[25]

Such a policy statement would clarify how existing FTC rules and regulations apply to any information or activity communicated through electronic media. In addition, the FTC has been developing new regulations that respond to concerns related to the collection of information about, and targeting of product sales to, children.[26]

A key area likely to be addressed by the FTC, either through independent action or at the direction of Congress, is unsolicited bulk commercial e-mail, or "spam." The federal government and the states are exploring ways to limit spam through legislation. Nevada, for example, banned unsolicited e-mail advertisements unless the message is "clearly and conspicuously" identified as an advertisement and imposed fines of $10 per e-mail message or actual damages for violations.[27] Other states, especially those with economies closely tied to high-tech industries, have enacted even broader legislation.

California regulates the content of unsolicited commercial e-mail and imposes criminal penalties on senders who violate its requirements.[28] California requires anyone who sends an e-mail that "promotes directly or indirectly, the sale or distribution of goods or services" to a party with whom the sender does not have an "existing business or personal relationship" to include in the subject line of the e-mail the term "ADV:" to designate the message as an advertisement. This requirement identifies the message as spam prior to reading and enables software filters to discard the message automatically. In addition, senders must include in the message a valid e-mail address for replies and clear instructions on how the recipient can request to be removed from the distribution list. Violation of these requirements is punishable by a fine of up to $1,000 and up to six months in prison.

The state of Virginia adopted restrictions on spam in 1999. As part of comprehensive legislation aimed to facilitate e-commerce and Internet growth, the Virginia legislation did the following:

- It criminalized the transmission of a false or forged e-mail message sent in connection with unsolicited bulk e-mail.
- It criminalized the sale, distribution, or possession of software whose principal purpose is to facilitate such e-mail.
- It expanded the state's long-arm statute ensuring that personal jurisdiction could be exerted over anyone that uses a computer or computer network located in Virginia.
- It provided penalties of up to $25,000 per day to be collected by people and e-mail providers injured by unsolicited bulk e-mail.[29]

The Virginia law also allows ISPs to limit the activities of advertisers who send unsolicited commercial e-mail. This provision is especially important given the fact that America Online's headquarters are located in Virginia.

Whether in Nevada, California, Virginia, or any other state with spam restrictions, it is important to keep in mind there is a trend toward criminalizing spam, providing individuals the right to collect civil penalties and giving ISPs immunity from prosecution or civil liability if they adopt policies limiting or prohibiting spam transmission.

Even absent federal or state consumer protection statutes or regulations governing the Internet, courts increasingly are finding ways to apply existing laws to regulate the excesses of e-commerce, especially with regard to spam. In 1997, for example, a federal court in Ohio enjoined an ISP, Cyber Promotions, from sending unsolicited e-mails to CompuServe subscribers, on the ground that such solicitation constitutes trespass.[30] The plaintiff in the case, CompuServe, was granted injunctive relief to protect its property, namely its proprietary nationwide computer network. Given these judicial restrictions, as well as the increasing number of federal and state laws affecting e-commerce and e-advertising, your health care organization must adopt trade policies simultaneous with the launch of an e-business on the Web. The following steps are recommended:

- Comply with federal and state trade practice laws and regulations, including "truth in advertising" laws and restrictions.
- Monitor legislative and regulatory developments.
- Use special caution when using bulk e-mails or other forms of unsolicited communications with consumers or potential consumers.
- Use extra caution when dealing with children or products or advertising that may be targeted to children or be of special interest for children.

Addressing e-Patient and e-Provider Confidentiality and Privacy Concerns

One of the greatest challenges facing e-commerce is balancing the need to maintain and protect the privacy of e-consumers and the confidentiality of data transmitted over the Internet against the need for access to data. In health care, this subject becomes extremely dicey, given the fact that patient medical records deserve a high level of confidentiality.

In general, privacy protections are a function of state law and are enforced either through consumer protection statutes, like those governing spam, or common law tort actions—intrusion, appropriation, public disclosure of private facts, false light, and so on. There are, however, several federal statutes that specifically govern on-line privacy. For example, there are provisions designed to protect children and disclosure of government information.[31] Federal laws of more general application, such as the Electronic Communication Privacy Act of 1986 (ECPA), also merit attention.[32]

Congress adopted ECPA in 1986 to update the federal wiretapping statute and to contemplate electronic messaging technology long before the potential of the Internet was realized. ECPA broadens the wiretap laws to prohibit unauthorized persons from intercepting e-communications in transmission or disclosing or using any intercepted communications.[33] The catch is, ECPA applies only to electronic communications using "common carrier" facilities available to the general public, such as private telephone systems and branch exchanges. Therefore, interception and divulgence of an internal company e-mail to a third party does not violate ECPA if the company is not a provider of an electronic communication service to the public, even if the company's system allows communication to third parties over the Internet.[34]

Considering the myriad of federal and state laws governing on-line privacy, as well as the heightened interest in this topic by legislators at the national and state level, it is safe to conclude that privacy concerns will continue to drive legislation affecting e-commerce. Given the proliferation of federal and state efforts to protect consumer privacy, anyone conducting business on line should carefully monitor legal developments to ensure compliance. Any health care organization that conducts e-business should adopt and implement a "fair information practices" policy that specifically addresses the concerns in Figure 16–9, described in detail below.

- *Privacy.* A fair information practices policy should describe the means by which the company collects, maintains, uses, distributes, and protects data; consumer or user rights with respect to personal data; and procedures for allowing consumers or users to make choices with respect to how their data will be used. A good privacy policy details policies and procedures for limiting access to personal identifying information to only those persons to whom access is required.
- *Security.* Hand in hand with a privacy policy is a security policy to ensure the physical integrity of the data. Unless precautions are taken to protect data from loss, theft, misuse, alteration, or destruction, no amount of restrictions on access to data will be effective. A security policy also must ensure that, consistent with the law and privacy policy, if data are shared with any third

- Privacy
    - —limiting access to and use of patient-identifiable data
- Security
    - —safeguard physical integrity of data
- Integrity
    - —ensuring data are accurate, complete, and current
- Training and continuous quality improvement/quality assessment— educating and monitoring staff on compliance with policies
- Enforcement

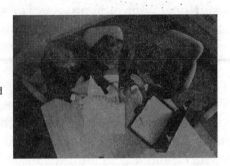

Figure 16–9 Elements of a Fair Information Practices Policy

party, that third party has similar security measures in place so the data remain secure upon transmission.

- *Integrity.* An integrity policy ensures that any information collected and stored in a secure environment is accurate, complete, and current. In order for the data to have any value or relevancy, the integrity must be safeguarded through intake and input procedures. The most foolproof privacy and security measures amount to little if the data being protected have little use or value because of poor intake or input procedures.
- *Enforcement.* Any good policy must include compliance mechanisms. The best and most detailed policies are of little value if there is no recourse for any violation.

Revise and update your organization's fair information practices policy regularly, to take into account changes in the law.

HEALTH CARE LAWS AND REGULATIONS

The first part of this chapter discussed the legal issues related to e-commerce generally. This part of the chapter will take a look at how laws and regulations governing health care providers play out—or could play out—in the e-health industry.

Protecting the e-Patient Record

For many years, medical record information has been maintained in paper charts in a physician's office, and/or in a file folder at a patient's insurance company. In the computer age, however, medical records are moving away from being paper based and increasingly are maintained in electronic format. Maintaining electronic records and large databases means patient information can be accessed by health care professionals and organizations anywhere in the world. The benefits to this are many: e-records are easier to store, more comprehensive, and arguably more accessible to providers, payers, and other interested parties.

While computerization of medical records is more cost-effective and convenient, the fact that so much data are collected together in one location and can be accessed by so many people poses new security concerns. Just as with paper records, providers are legally required to protect the confidentiality of electronic records from unauthorized access. If your health care organization plans a Web-enabled strategy that includes personal e-patient records, or any health information that is personal, accessible to both patients and providers within an Extranet, be prepared to address the privacy and confidentiality issues that come along with this strategy.

Because of the highly personal nature of medical record information, state and federal governments have become increasingly concerned about protecting the confidentiality of electronic health data. This heightened concern has resulted in an explosion of interest in safeguarding access to, and dissemination of, electronically stored health data. Because a new legislative or regulatory proposal is suggested almost daily, it is virtually impossible to provide an up-to-the-minute account of state and federal law in this area. However, because traditional confidentiality laws provide the basis for, and extend to, health data protection, they provide a framework for developing a sound confidentiality policy.

State law provisions generally permit medical records to be created and maintained electronically so long as security measures to prevent unauthorized access are in place. The Health Insurance Portability and Accountability Act of 1996 (HIPAA)[35] requires Congress to enact legislation adopting standards with respect to the privacy of personal identifying health information, and it is the first federal law to address electronic medical records.[36] HIPAA mandates that health care entities adopt reasonable and appropriate administrative, technical, and physical safeguards to protect the integrity and confidentiality of medical information.[37] For example, HIPAA requires the development of unique health identifiers for each individual, employer, health plan, and health provider. Developing procedures for the electronic transmission and authentication of signatures for use in financial and administrative transactions is another goal. And special regulations for health care clearinghouses will require that where a clearinghouse is part of a larger entity, it must isolate its activities to prevent the larger organization from having unauthorized access to the records.

Medical privacy laws have traditionally developed through case law or state statute.[38] Generally speaking, patients have the right to access their treatment records and maintain some proprietary interests over them, but the physical records themselves belong to the health care provider.[39] Though the records are "owned" by the health care provider, a patient's record is still subject to the patient's privacy rights and must be kept confidential from unauthorized parties. Common law confidentiality requirements often supplement statutory confidentiality requirements, and a breach of health care record information can result in lawsuits for breach of duty of confidentiality, breach of contract, invasion of privacy, negligence, intentional infliction of emotional distress, and defamation. Furthermore, a health care provider who willfully misrepresents health information practices or fails to tell patients about the uses and disclosures of health information may be liable for fraud, consumer fraud, or fraudulent or deceptive trade practices.

Confidentiality of health care information is not absolute; there are numerous exceptions that allow the disclosure of confidential information with or without patient consent.[40] In most states, patients have access to their medical records and may also grant permission to third parties to have access to their records, which may take the form of a release.[41] To be valid, a release must be within the limits of the patient's authorization and should be preferably in writing. Patient consent is generally unnecessary when giving authorized health care personnel access to hospital medical records.[42] There are also exceptions for disclosure to employees and agents, for disclosure to other providers, in an emergency, to obtain payment, to carry out peer or medical review, for communicable disease reporting, or for some types of research.

But disclosure without patient consent does not apply to highly sensitive health information. Federal and state statutes and regulations impose stringent confidentiality requirements for defined records and sensitive information, including alcohol and drug abuse patient records,[43] mental health records,[44] records containing human immunodeficiency virus (HIV) test results or information relating to an acquired immune deficiency syndrome (AIDS) diagnosis,[45] and, increasingly, information concerning genetic screening and testing results.[46] Stiff penalties accompany the unauthorized disclosure of these types of records. For example, Virginia imposes civil penalties of up to $5,000 for anyone who discloses that a patient is HIV-positive, and in California the unauthorized disclosure of HIV test results can subject the violator to penalties of up to $10,000 and/or imprisonment.[47] As a rule of thumb, health care providers should have tighter safeguards in place to protect the confidentiality of these more sensitive records.

Although confidentiality of health record information traditionally has been an area of concern for state legislators and regulations, a growing number of federal laws and regulations also address the privacy and confidentiality of health care medical records. The Health Care Financing Administration's (HCFA's) Rules on Medical Records Services require that hospitals have a procedure to ensure the confidentiality of medical records to qualify for Medicare funds.[48] The hospital may release medical records only pursuant to state and federal laws, court orders, or subpoenas and must prevent unauthorized people from gaining access to or altering the medical records.[49]

Federal law also provides privacy protection for the records of patients in federally assisted drug and alcohol treatment facilities.[50] Patient consent is required (with limited exceptions) before the contents of the treatment records may be disclosed. Privacy of research subjects also is protected by federal law.[51] The failure to abide by relevant federal or state laws can lead to criminal penalties,[52] civil penalties, private rights of action and damages, attorney's fees and costs, and licensure sanctions.

Pursuant to HIPAA's requirements, a number of bills related to medical records privacy have been introduced, but no legislation has yet been enacted. If Congress fails to enact legislation enforcing the privacy standards by August 1999, HIPAA requires that the secretary of Health and Human Services promulgate final regulations with confidentiality standards by February 2000. One way or another, new standards for privacy of personal identifying medical information will be in place by February 21, 2000. More than likely, these federal regulations will preempt all contrary state law except those state requirements that are more stringent than the federal legislation. Thus, some state laws would remain in effect.

Once HIPAA's federal health information privacy and security standards become effective, providers will need to fully comply with all technical requirements in order to avoid severe criminal penalties for wrongful disclosure. Wrongful disclosure of personal identifying health information results in a fine of up to $50,000, imprisonment for one year, or both.[53] If the disclosure is malicious or for pecuniary gain, the penalties can go as high as a fine of $100,000 and/or five years in prison. Plainly, health information confidentiality and security are critical compliance issues for e-health companies.

No question about it—complying with the hodgepodge of overlapping state and federal laws addressing medical privacy and confidentiality can be confusing. This is particularly true for providers venturing into the e-health arena; they must comply with the confidentiality requirements of the jurisdictions at both ends of each e-communication and must develop policies and techniques for storing, managing, retrieving, searching, safeguarding, and encrypting computerized medical information. Below are some tips to get you started:

- *Check the applicable laws and regulations in each state where you serve patients or otherwise conduct business.* Do not forget to check laws and regulations governing electronic transmissions generally, as well as medical records generally, and laws governing specific types of information such as information about HIV, mental health, or substance abuse. Monitor developments at the state and local level.
- *Monitor federal laws and regulations.* Consider participating in the legislative and rule-making process through lobbying and commenting on proposed regulations.
- *Develop written confidentiality policies that delineate exactly who may have access to what information.* Define the circumstances under which information may be disclosed and set forth penalties for the unauthorized use or release of confidential information.
- *Establish monitoring practices and enforcement procedures for violations of the confidentiality policy.* Some providers may wish to consider using employee and contract agreements to ensure confidentiality.
- *Implement technological safeguards such as personal identification and verification techniques, access control software, and audit controls.* Access can be controlled by passwords, key cards, or access codes that may not be disclosed or shared with other users. And users' access should be limited to only what they need to do their duties; systems can be programmed to lock out users who attempt to access information that is outside their authority.
- *Conduct employee education and training programs.* Make sure that employees understand the confidentiality program in effect and the critical importance of the policy to the viability of the company.

The bottom line: health care providers are obliged to use reasonable precautions to preserve the confidentiality and freedom from unauthorized access of confidential medical information and records.[54] This requires good computer and data security as well as appropriate training and monitoring of staff. As technology constantly evolves, the reasonableness of security measures for e-records is likely to be judged relative to current systems security technology and security practice.

Because extra protections are required for sensitive health care information such as HIV test results and substance abuse records, as a practical matter, physicians and health care organizations should take the strict standards required to maintain the confidentiality for HIV test results and substance abuse records and apply those for all health care records. Besides avoiding the complexities of having two confidentiality policies, this provides the broadest protection possible for all records and reduces the likelihood of an unauthorized disclosure.

"How Do I Code for That?"

Although the federal government provides reimbursement for e-health services, reimbursement has been limited to certain special circumstances. For example, for several years, Medicare has reimbursed for teleconsultation services involving specialists as part of demonstration projects in 57 facilities in Georgia, North Carolina, West Virginia, and Iowa.[55] The federal government also has authorized state Medicaid programs to provide reimbursement for telemedicine services on a state-by-state basis.[56]

More recently, the federal payment programs have expanded their reimbursement for e-health services beyond demonstration or experimental projects. Driven, in part, by lower costs,[57] improving technologies,[58] congressional interest,[59] and increased acceptance of payment for e-health services by the states[60] and private payers,[61] HCFA has expanded its recognition of reimbursable e-health services.

For example, effective January 1, 1999, HCFA began providing Medicare reimbursement for services rendered to individuals located in rural health personnel shortage areas.[62] Reimbursement under this program is limited to real-time or interactive video consultations between certain categories of providers, including physicians, physician assistants, nurse practitioners, clinical nurse specialists, and nurse-midwives. Consultations with clinical psychologists, clinical social workers, certified nurse anesthetists, and anesthesiologist assistants are excluded, as are consultations with other providers referred by nurse anesthetists and anesthesiologist assistants.

Under this rule, HCFA recognizes only live audio and video transmissions, thereby excluding telephone, fax, and e-mail services or other services using store-forward technology,[63] although these services may be reimbursable under other provisions of the Medicare Act. The Medicare Carriers Manual, for example, indicates that some forms of diagnostic testing that do not require face-to-face consultations are reimbursable.[64] These services are outlined in Table 16–1. Despite these limitations, e-health providers should expect increasing acceptance of e-consultations by government and private payers alike. Several states already have adopted nondiscrimination statutes prohibiting insurers from denying payment for e-health services if the services would be reimbursable if provided in a traditional setting.[65] Reimbursement for electronic physician-to-patient interactions is likely to gain acceptance by payers as e-providers demonstrate their ability to reach rural, elderly, or otherwise vulnerable patient populations, thereby expanding access to health care services.

e-Licensure for Physicians and Other Health Professionals

States typically require that physicians, pharmacists, nurses, and other providers obtain a license that authorizes them to practice their profession within their state. State licensure laws generally require licensed practitioners to have a certain level of education and training and to have passed an entrance exam in order to obtain the privilege of practicing their profession. State licensure requirements make the performance of certain services within that state illegal if the practitioner is not properly licensed.[66]

To offer e-advice or e-consultation on its Web site or Extranet, health care organizations' practitioners must be properly licensed. After all, a radiologist viewing an X-ray through a Web site or Extranet is practicing medicine, just as a nurse sending an e-mailed response to an e-patient question about a child's fever is practicing nursing. The fact that there has been no face-to face contact between the referring physician and specialist, or the nurse and patient, does not alter the fact that the practitioners are providing health services that require a

Table 16–1 1997 Medicare Telemedicine Coverage

Code	Service	Payment ($)	Number of Services
93012	Transmission of electrocardiogram (ECG)	651,500	10,578
93014	Report on transmitted ECG	1,939,900	89,084
93733	Telephone analysis, pacemaker (dual)	20,111,700	871,429
93736	Telephone analysis, pacemaker (single)	18,477,500	908,360
G0004	ECG transmission physician review and interpretation	4,443,300	21,652
G0006	ECG transmission and analysis	8,445,600	48,785
TOTAL		54,069,500	1,949,888

Source: Data from 1997 Medicare Telemedicine Coverage, 1998, ATA News Update at 2, American Telemedicine Association.

- Use only licensed professionals to dispense advice and counsel.
- Ensure that professionals are licensed in the jurisdiction where the advice is being rendered (location of patient).
- Limit responsibilities and advice provided to scope of license.
- Document licensure status of employees.
- Work with licensing bodies and associations to clarify law.

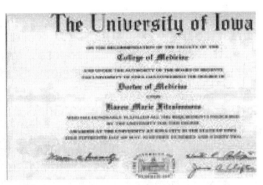

Figure 16–10 Steps to Ensuring That Practitioners Are Properly Licensed

license. Figure 16–10 describes the steps necessary to ensure that your organization's providers are properly licensed.

The requirement for state licensure poses a unique problem for practitioners who offer medical services or practice medicine on the Web. Claims of licensure violations or the unauthorized practice of a licensed profession may arise either because staff are providing advice in a field in which they are not licensed or because licensed staff are providing advice in a state where they are not licensed to practice.

Failure to comply with state licensure laws can result in severe sanctions. For example, if a Web-based medical consultation service is held to have violated state laws governing physician licensure or the practice of medicine, it and the individuals working for it could be subject to civil or criminal penalties, including the payment of fines or incarceration.[67] In addition, any licensed physician who assists a Web-based medical consultation service in the unauthorized practice of medicine may be subject to license revocation and be unable to practice medicine again.[68]

Some states have addressed this problem in the context of specific telemedicine services, such as radiology.[69] Other states require by law that individuals who provide diagnostic or therapeutic services via electronic means be licensed in the state where the patient is located.[70] Oklahoma, for example, requires licensure in Oklahoma for "performance by a person outside of this state, through an ongoing regular arrangement, of diagnostic or treatment services though electronic communications for any patient whose condition is being diagnosed or treated within this state."[71] Regulations in some states, usually adopted by the state medical board, also require full licensure for telemedicine consultations by out-of-state physicians.[72] Frequently, however, state licensure requirements may contain exemptions for occasional, or "consulting" physicians.[73] In addition, there are numerous proposals to circumvent repetitive state licensure requirements in the context of telemedicine or Web-based health care services (see below).

Efforts to require interstate providers of medicine to be fully licensed in each state are underway in many states, including Arizona, Arkansas, Connecticut, Georgia, Hawaii, Illinois, Indiana, Iowa, Kansas, Maine, Massachusetts, New York, North Carolina, Oklahoma, and Pennsylvania.[74] To counteract the efforts to require that practitioners be licensed in multiple states, several associations have drafted interstate telemedicine licensure and mutual recognition proposals. Among the organizations making these proposals are the Federation of State Medical Boards (FSMB), the National Conference of State Boards of Nursing (NCSBN), and the Association of Telemedicine Service Providers (ATSP).

The FSMB's Model Act to Regulate the Practice of Telemedicine was adopted as policy by the Federation in April 1996.[75] The FSMB Model Act requires physicians seeking to practice medicine across state lines to obtain a special license from each state medical board. Practicing medicine across state lines in this context is limited to "any medical act that occurs when the patient is physically located within the state and the physician is located outside the state."[76] The special license would be limited to such practice and would not allow a physician to enter a state for the purposes of practicing medicine. Several states, including Alabama and Texas, adopted legislation based on the FSMB's Model Act.[77]

The NCSBN's proposal for an Interstate Compact on Mutual Recognition for Nursing Regulation (Nurse Licensure Compact) was adopted by the NCSBN in December 1997.[78] The Nurse Licensure Compact permits nurses licensed in one state to practice in other states that are signatories to the compact, much like people licensed to drive in one state may be permitted to drive in other states. Utah became the first, and to date the only, state to adopt the proposal in March 1998. Utah Senate Bill 146, the Nursing Regulation–Interstate Compact bill, will be effective January 1, 2000.[79] In accord with its efforts to promote interstate licensure, the NCSBN entered into contracts with five technology companies to develop a national system to verify and report nurse licensure information in July 1998.[80]

ATSP also developed a draft interstate telemedicine licensure compact.[81] The ATSP compact, like the NCSBN's Nursing Licensure Compact, would permit practitioners fully licensed in one state to practice in other states, though it would limit their practice to telemedicine. To date, no states have passed legislation based on the ATSP compact.

Given the endorsement of these proposals by the regulators themselves, e-health providers should not expect significant opposition to practicing e-health services across state lines. Until proposals become law, however, e-health professionals should be licensed in all jurisdictions where their patients are being served. In the meantime, e-health providers should work with state regulators and legislators to bring about regulatory and legislative change to allow e-health professionals to realize the full potential of Web-enabled applications.

e-Fraud and Abuse

E-health ventures that involve federal payment programs, such as Medicare or Medicaid, must consider compliance with federal and state antifraud and abuse laws that restrict certain referrals and other business practices that, outside of the health care arena, may be commonly accepted and widely utilized. There are a wide variety of criminal and civil statutes—both federal and state—that hold health care providers liable for fraud and abuse, including the False Claims Act,[82] the antikickback statute,[83] and self-referral statutes, known as "Stark" at the federal level.[84] Any e-health provider giving or receiving remuneration of any kind to induce referrals of patients covered by federal programs, any provider seeking reimbursement from Medicare or Medicaid, and any physician group or organization providing e-health services that enters into a joint venture with a hospital or other institutional provider should pay close attention to the fraud and abuse laws.

Consider, for example, an e-health provider that contracts with physician groups to operate a Web-enabled advice service targeted to health concerns for the elderly. This service would be staffed by nurses available around the clock. Consumers logging into the system would likely be Medicare eligible or contacting the service on behalf of their Medicare-eligible mother or father. If a consumer has a problem that merits medical attention, the e-health provider would then recommend a physician associated with one of the physician groups with which it has a contractual agreement. The physician groups would in turn pay the e-health provider a flat fee for each new patient referred through the Web service. This type of arrangement could constitute an illegal kickback resulting in criminal prosecution.

As e-health services continue to grow, so will the fraud and abuse implications of providing e-health services. Any e-health provider participating in federal programs or considering participating in federal programs should invest the necessary resources into developing and implementing a fraud and abuse compliance program to ensure that the business is conducted within the bounds of the law.

This is especially true with regard to those e-health ventures that are owned by physicians who deliver e-health services and refer patients to those who do not provide e-health services.

Quality of e-Care Delivery—e-Providers Beware

Health care professionals practicing medicine, pharmacy, or nursing over the Web are not exempt from laws and regulations governing patient rights and quality of care. Therefore, any health care professional practicing e-health can be held accountable for advice under common law malpractice theories. Although there have not been any reported malpractice cases involving Web-based health services, there are a few reported cases involving call centers, and these cases indicate several trends for e-health liability. Because call centers, like Web-based providers, provide services to patients using communication lines and without face-to-face interaction, the call center cases are applicable to e-health providers generally.

First, e-health providers do have a duty to provide consumers with quality care consistent with the governing standard of care.[85] The fact that there is no face-to-face interaction between the patient and professional does not eliminate or diminish the duty owed the patient. Second, e-health providers are considered specialists whose care should be judged by the standard of care applicable to that specialist community.[86] This trend is significant because it means, for example, that e-pediatricians who do not see their patients do not owe a duty to exercise the degree of care and skill exercised by ordinary pediatricians in the same or similar locality who have the ability to see and examine their patients. Third, corporations can be held liable for the negligence of professionals providing e-health services through the corporation.[87]

In addition to providing a window into the future of e-health liability litigation, the call center cases highlight some of the key areas of concern for e-health providers interested in avoiding or minimizing liability. In each of the most publicized cases, one of the driving forces in the litigation was the fact that the provider appeared to place a premium on cost savings at the expense of quality of care. For example, in one well-publicized case a call center nurse advised the mother of a six-month-old infant to take him to a distant hospital under contract with Kaiser instead of a closer hospital.[88] While driving to the recommended hospital, the child suffered from a cardiac arrest and respiratory failure. Three days later, the child's limbs turned black, and he later had to have parts of his hands and legs amputated.[89]

More recently, a court in Pennsylvania gave the plaintiff a green light to proceed against a health plan's call center because its staff encouraged a pregnant woman to seek hospitalization services at an in-plan hospital at some distance from her home.[90] In another publicized case, a West Coast health maintenance organization's after-hours call center received a telephone call from a mother of a sick child. After hearing the details of the child's condition, the nurse advised the mother to bring her child to the emergency department but warned her that her insurance would not cover the visit if it was not deemed an emergency.[91] The mother consequently decided not to bring her child to the emergency department, and the child died before the physician's office reopened the next morning.[92]

With respect to documentation, the facts as described by the court in the Pennsylvania case, *Shannon,* seem to indicate that the patient's previous calls were not documented so that when the patient called for a second or third time, the nurse did not have important information about the patient's calling history that could have helped the nurse evaluate the urgency of the situation presented by the caller. Whether or not these were the facts of the case, the importance of documentation and having systems and procedures in place cannot be overemphasized.

Although any health care provider understands that there is no sure way to avoid the risk of malpractice liability, e-health providers can take several steps to avoid or minimize their potential liability. E-health providers should keep the following principles, listed in Figure 16–11 and detailed below, in mind when implementing a risk management program.

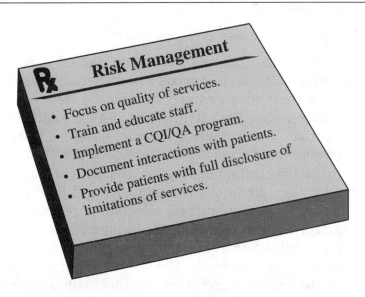

Figure 16–11 Risk Management

- *Focus on the quality of the services provided.* The best risk management plan is the provision of quality services.
- *Hire highly qualified staff and train and educate staff to stay abreast of the latest care-related developments.* Staff also should be trained to deal with crisis situations resulting from a patient interaction or a breakdown in the system.
- *Develop systems and procedures that ensure that staff treat similarly situated patients similarly.* Advice-oriented services should be providing consistent advice and counsel.
- *Implement a comprehensive continuous quality improvement/quality assessment (CQI/QA) program that continuously evaluates the quality of services being provided as well as identifies any "weak links" in the system.*
- *Document interactions with patients and retain records of interactions.* Records of interactions should be audited as part of the CQI/QA program and can be used for education and training of staff. Records also can be used to defend any criticisms of advice provided.

Finally, an effective risk management program should ensure that the representation of the services provided does not create inflated expectations. E-health providers should not create expectations of physician care if advice is provided by nurses only. E-health providers should make full disclosures to patients utilizing the e-health services of the scope of services being provided and any limitations of the services provided.

Regulation of Drugs, Devices, and e-Pharmacies

The federal FDA, under its authority to regulate medical devices,[93] has taken the position that it is authorized to regulate computer-based diagnostic software programs.[94] Many of these programs may be used by Web-based providers of medical consultation services. The extent of the FDA's regulation of these types of programs is uncertain, but in general, software governed by the Food, Drug, and Cosmetic Act must be cleared for marketing by the FDA, have clear and accurate labels, and satisfy certain quality controls. Although the responsibility to ensure that a software product is properly approved lies squarely with the manufacturer, the cost of doing business using these products may change if regulation increases. Therefore, e-health providers should be aware that the software they use may be subject to a regulation now and/or in the future.

In addition to regulating devices, the FDA has jurisdiction over the marketing of drugs. Although the number of companies offering to fill prescriptions over the Internet is increasing, there are significant questions about how drug transactions can be regulated over the Internet, resulting in numerous calls for regulation of the dispensing of drugs over the Internet.[95] Concerns about patient safety and potential fraud in the absence of face-to-face encounters between patients and pharmacists are the primary drivers of this call for action. The FDA has discussed this issue but has not yet taken any formal steps to restrict on-line pharmacies or the sale and dispensing of drugs on line. Given the heightened concern about consumer safety, however, the FDA is likely to examine this issue in some detail and, at the very least, make some recommendations with respect to "best practices," if not adopt regulations specifically governing on-line drug sales.

Of even greater concern to lawmakers and consumers, however, is the proliferation of prescription services on line. These services circumvent the traditional physician–patient relationship and allow a patient to obtain a prescription drug on line without ever having a face-to-face interaction with a physician. Although increasingly common, this practice is prohibited by some state laws that require an examination prior to a prescription drug sale and is considered an ethical violation by the American Medical Association (AMA).[96] The California physician licensure statute, for example, provides that it is unprofessional conduct for a physician, surgeon, or podiatrist to prescribe, dispense, or furnish drugs without a good faith prior examination.[97] This California statute was enacted before e-health services were contemplated, but given lawmakers' concerns and the AMA's position on physician prescriptions over the Internet, it is not likely to be amended to allow physicians to prescribe over the Internet.

CONCLUSION

Combining technological innovation with quality care has enormous potential to improve access to health care services and control the costs associated with providing those services. But in order to realize the full potential of increased access and cost savings, e-health providers must develop strategies and plans that maximize their compliance with the myriad of laws and regulations that govern their business, as well as minimize their exposure to legal liability. In this regard, it is important to recognize that e-health providers are subject to the same laws and regulations as other health care providers—licensure requirements, reimbursement rules, fraud and abuse restrictions, and malpractice liability. In addition, e-health providers must comply with laws and regulations governing commerce generally and e-commerce specifically, whether it be confidentiality and privacy restrictions, intellectual property concerns, or fair trade practices laws.

Exhibit 16–1 e-Health Compliance Strategies

- Make legal compliance a top business priority.
- Focus on quality patient services.
- Monitor federal, state, and local developments.
- Educate and train staff on legal issues.
- Maintain comprehensive documentation.

Once e-health providers incorporate a legal compliance program into their business plans, they will begin to see cost savings and improved quality of care. The following "prescription" can help physicians and health care executives avoid some of the legal pitfalls that are inherent in Web-based technologies (see Exhibit 16–1):

- Make legal compliance an integral part of your business plan. An effective compliance plan should ensure compliance with intellectual property laws, consumer protection provisions, privacy and confidentiality restrictions, and licensure statutes, as well as any other applicable laws and regulations.
- Focus on providing high-quality services using highly skilled and licensed professionals.
- Monitor international, federal, state, and local developments, and draft and implement a compliance plan tailored to the most restrictive applicable legal requirements.
- Educate and train staff on legal issues and underscore the importance of compliance.
- Maintain complete, accurate, and comprehensive documentation on patient interactions.

REFERENCES

1. *See Taking the Internet Cure: Health and Medicine Online*, THE INDUSTRY STANDARD, April 5, 1999, at 30.

2. *See generally Secretariat for Electronic Commerce, U.S. Department of Commerce, The Emerging Digital Economy (1998)* <http://www.ecommerce.gov/emerging.htm>.

3. *See generally The White House, A Framework for Global Electronic Commerce (1997)* <http://www.ecommerce.gov/framewrk.htm#BACKGROUND>.

4. NCCUSL, *Draft of Uniform Electronic Transactions Act (1998)* <http://www.law.upenn.edu/library/ulc/uecicta/98am.htm>.

5. NCCUSL, *Draft of Uniform Commercial Code Article 2B (1997)* <http://www.law.uh.edu/ucc2b/031098/031098.htm>.

6. *See NCCUSL To Promulgate Freestanding Uniform Computer Information Transactions Act* (last modified April 7, 1999) <http://www.nccusl.org/pressrel/2brel.html>.

7. UNCITRAL MODEL LAW ON ELECTRONIC COMMERCE, reprinted in BENJAMIN WRIGHT, JANE K. WINN, THE LAW OF ELECTRONIC COMMERCE, Appendix E (1999).

8. *See generally*, Internet Law and Policy Forum, *UPDATE: Survey of State Electronic & Digital Signature Legislative Initiatives* <http://www.ilpf.org/digsig/digrep.htm> (Appendices A through C describe state electronic authentication laws and legislation).

9. Authentication technologies can include voice recognition and fingerprints. *See, e.g.*, Rob Fixmer, *Tiny New Chip Could Pit Protection of Property against Right of Privacy*, N.Y. TIMES, Sept. 28, 1998, at F6 (describing computer chip that transmits a unique serial number over computer networks, including the Internet, to authenticate a computer processor).

10. The Lanham Act, 15 U.S.C. § 1125, *et seq.* (act protects against misappropriation, passing off, trademark infringement, invasion of right of publicity, false advertising, likelihood of causing consumer confusion, and unauthorized commercial endorsements).

11. *See* The Federal Trademark Dilution Act of 1996, 15 U.S.C. § 1125(c).

12. H.R. REP. No. 104-374, at 3 (1995), reprinted in 1996 U.S.C.C.A.N. 1029, 1030.

13. For more information, *see* ICANN's Web site at <http://icann.org>.

14. *See generally* Victoria Slind-Flor, *The Domain Name Game Is Heating Up the Internet*, NAT. L.J., June 3, 1996, at B1.

15. *See* 17 U.S.C. § 101, *et seq.*

16. *See* 17 U.S.C. § 107.

17. *See, e.g.*, Fonovisa, Inc. v. Cherry Auction, Inc., 76 F.3d 259, 264 (9th Cir. 1996) (holding that a trademark holder adequately stated a claim for contributory trademark infringement by alleging that operators of a swap meet were supplying a necessary marketplace for the sale of substantial quantities of counterfeit recordings by independent vendors).

18. Pub. L. No. 105-304, 112 Stat. 2860 (1998) (codified as amended in scattered sections of 17 U.S.C.).

19. Congress recently enacted additional copyright provisions strengthening the criminal enforcement of the Copyright Act. *See* The No Electronic Theft Act (NET Act), Pub. L. No. 105-147, 111 Stat. 2678 (1997) (amending Copyright Act to include additional criminal enforcement provisions).

20. *See* The Federal Trade Commission Act, 15 U.S.C. § 41, *et seq. See, e.g.*, Nevada Unfair Trade Practices Act, Nev. Rev. Stat. § 598A.

21. *See, e.g.*, Global World Media Corp., No. C-3772 (Oct. 9, 1997), reprinted in 5 Trade Reg. Rep. (CCH) ¶ 24,306 (alleging false claims about herbal supplement advertised over the Internet); FTC v. Fortuna Alliance, L.L.C., Civ. No. C96-799M (W.D. Wash., filed May 23, 1996), reprinted in 1997 Trade Reg. Rep. Transfer Binder (CCH) ¶ 24,039 (alleging illegal pyramid scheme marketed over the Internet); FTC v. Brandzel, 98C 1440 (N.D. Ill., filed Mar. 14, 1996), reprinted in 1997 Trade Reg. Rep. Transfer Binder (CCH) ¶ 23,999, ¶ 24,112 (alleging violation of FTC Act and Mail or Telephone Merchandise Rule for computer products paid for on Internet but not delivered).

22. *See, e.g.*, New York v. Lipsitz, 663 N.Y.S. 2d 468 (N.Y. Sup. Ct. 1997) (finding sufficient jurisdiction in New York to enjoin Internet magazine subscription sales when advertising included fictitious testimonial messages).

23. FTC v. Thomas Maher, et al., Civ. No. WMN-98-495 (D. Md., filed Mar. 4, 1998), reprinted in 5 Trade Reg. Rep. (CCH) ¶ 24,397.

24. *See* GeoCities: Analysis To Aid Public Comment, 63 Fed. Reg. 44,624 (1998).

25. Interpretation of Rules and Guides for Electronic Media: Request for Comment, 63 Fed. Reg. 24,996 (1998); Announcement of Date of Public Workshop on the Interpretation of Rules and Guides for Elec-

tronic Media, Procedures for Requesting To Participate, and Request for Submission of Advertisements, 64 Fed. Reg. 14,156 (1999).

26. *See, e.g.,* Children's Online Privacy Protection Rule, 64 Fed. Reg. 22,750 (1999) (proposing regulations to prohibit unfair and deceptive acts in connection with the collection and use of personal information from and about children over the Internet).

27. Nev. Rev. Stat. § 41.730(1)(c).

28. Cal. Bus. & Prof. Code §§ 17538.4, 17538.45; Cal. Penal Code § 502.

29. Va. Code Ann. §§ 8.01-328.1, 18.2-152.2, 18.2-152.4, 18.2-152.12 (1999).

30. *CompuServe v. Cyber Promotions*, 962 F. Supp. 1015, 1017 (S.D. Ohio 1997). Cyber Promotions suffered a similar setback in 1998 when it settled a lawsuit brought by Earthlink for $2 million. *See* Amy Harman, *Biggest Sender of Junk Mail on Internet Agrees To Stop*, N.Y. Times, March 29, 1998, Sec. 1 at 23.

31. Industry self-regulation is also used to enforce consumer protection standards. For a summary of the policy debate surrounding acceptance of such third-party review, see Nadya Aswad, *Industry Hopes Seal-of-Approval Programs Will Meet Privacy Self-Regulation Challenge*, Daily Rep. for Executives (BNA), No. 248, at C-1 (December 29, 1998).

32. Electronic Communications Privacy Act of 1986, Pub. L. No. 99-508, 100 Stat. 1848 (1986) (codified at scattered subsections of 18 U.S.C.).

33. 18 U.S.C. § 2510, *et seq.*

34. *See* Andersen Consulting v. UOP, 991 F. Supp. 1041 (N.D. Ill. 1998) (holding that contractor's divulgence of internal e-mail to newspaper did not violate ECPA because Andersen was not a provider of electronic communication services to the public, notwithstanding the company's Internet capabilities).

35. *See* Pub. L. No. 104-191, 110 Stat. 1936 (codified at scattered sections of 18, 26, 29, and 42 U.S.C.) (hereinafter referred to as HIPAA); *see also* H.R. Rep. 104-496 (1996), reprinted in 1996 U.S.C.C.A.N. 1865 (providing legislative history of HIPAA).

36. *See* Pub. L. No. 104-191, § 264(c), 110 Stat. 2033 (codified at 42 U.S.C. § 1320d-2).

37. *See* 42 U.S.C. §1320d-6.

38. *See, e.g.,* De May v. Roberts, 9 N.W. 146 (Mich. 1881) (physician liable for damages for bringing a friend to witness a childbirth without patient's consent).

39. *See* McGarry v. J.A. Mercier Co., 262 N.W. 296, 297 (Mich. 1935) (medical records are the property of the physician because the records are "practically meaningless to the ordinary layman"). *See, e.g.,* Calif. Code Regs. Tit. 22, § 70751(b).

40. *See* Whalen v. Roe, 429 U.S. 589, 602 (1977) (holding that disclosures of private medical information to physicians, to hospital personnel, to insurance companies, and to public health agencies do not automatically amount to an impermissible invasion of privacy).

41. *See, e.g.,* Mass. Gen. Laws Ann. ch. 111, § 70(E).

42. *See* Ind. Code Ann. § 34-6-2-15 (granting access to hospital medical records to physicians or other professionals in a hospital; patient consent is not required for this purpose).

43. *See, e.g.,* Colo. Rev. Stat. § 25-1-1108(1); N.Y. CLS Men. Hyg. § 23.05, *et seq.*; Ohio Rev. Code Ann. § 3793.13.

44. *See, e.g.,* Cal. Welf. & Inst. Code § 5328; Colo. Rev. Stat. § 27-10-120; Fla. Stat. § 394.455; Iowa Code § 228.1, *et seq.*; Md. Code Ann., Health-Gen. § 4-307; Tenn. Code Ann. § 33-3-101, *et seq.*

45. *See, e.g.,* Fla. Stat. § 381.004; Iowa Code Ann. § 141.21, *et seq.*; Md. Code Ann. Health-Gen. § 18-336; N.Y. CLS Pub. Health § 2782; Ohio Rev. Code Ann. § 3701.243, *et seq.*

46. *See, e.g.,* Cal. Health & Safety Code § 124980; Md. Code Ann. Health-Gen. § 13-109; Or. Rev. Stat. § 659.700, *et seq.*

47. *See* Cal. Health & Safety Code § 120980.

48. *See* 42 C.F.R. § 482.24(b)(3) (1997).

49. *See, e.g.,* Alaska Stat. § 13.23.100; *see also* Cal. Health & Safety Code § 123149(g) (requiring a provider that chooses to use an electronic recordkeeping system to develop and implement policies to include safeguards for confidentiality and unauthorized access to electronically stored patient records, authentication by electronic signature keys, and systems maintenance). Other states, such as Illinois, Utah, and Washington, have more comprehensive requirements and detail minimum procedures for the authentication of electronically stored medical records.

50. *See* 42 U.S.C. § 290dd-2; 42 C.F.R. pt. 2.

51. *See, e.g.,* 42 U.S.C. § 241(d) ("The Secretary may authorize persons engaged in biomedical, behavioral, clinical, or other research (including research on mental health . . .) to protect the privacy of individuals who are the subject of such research by withholding . . . identifying characteristics of such individuals"); 21 C.F.R. § 20.63(a) (requiring patient-identifying information in medical files of controlled-drug research subjects to be deleted before such files are made public).

52. *See, e.g.,* Me. Rev. Stat. Ann. Tit. 5, § 19206 (liability for actual damages and civil penalties from $1,000 to $5,000 for unauthorized disclosure of HIV test results).

53. *See* Pub. L. No. 104-191, § 262(a), 110 Stat. 2029 (codified at 42 U.S.C. § 1320d-6).

54. *See, e.g.,* Estate of Behringer v. Medical Center of Princeton, 592 A.2d 1251 (N.J. 1991). The court found that although Medical Center policies limited access to electronically maintained medical records to persons having patient care responsibility, in practical terms, the charts were available to any physician or nurse and to other hospital personnel. Because the Medical Center failed to take reasonable precautions to limit access to the plaintiff's chart where the impact of easy accessibility of the chart was clearly foreseeable, this constituted negligence.

55. *See For the Record,* MODERN HEALTHCARE, Dec. 2, 1996, at 34 (describing HCFA's approval of a three-year demonstration project to reimburse providers for telemedicine services).

56. As of January 1998, those states were Arkansas, California, Georgia, Iowa, Montana, North Dakota, South Dakota, Virginia, and West Virginia. *See* D. Ward Pimley, *Technological Changes May Prompt Growth of Telemedicine in Near Future,* 7 Health Law Rep. (BNA) 51, 52 (Jan. 8, 1998) (describing how some Medicaid programs reimburse for telemedicine services).

57. As part of its implementation of the Telecommunications Act of 1996, 47 U.S.C. § 254(h), the Federal Communications Commission has authorized expenditures of $400 million per year to support telecommunications services for nonprofit health care providers in rural areas. *See* Statement on the FCC's plan for Implementing Universal Services before the Senate Subcommittee on Communications, Committee on Commerce, Science, and Transportation (statement of Reed E. Hundt, Chairman, FCC) (June 3, 1997). The FCC also has directed the administration of the universal service program in such a way to enable rural health care providers to obtain lower, urban rates for telecommunications services.

58. *See, e.g.,* Pimley, *Technological Changes,* at 51 (describing existing technology and innovations applicable to the health care setting).

59. *See, e.g.,* Balanced Budget Act of 1997, Pub. L. No. 105-33, 111 Stat. 251 (codified at 42 U.S.C. § 332(a)(1)(A)) (Congress required Medicare to reimburse for some teleconsultation services starting in fiscal year 1999 for rural areas designated as suffering from a shortage of providers).

60. *See* Cal. Bus. & Prof. Code § 2290.5(c) (requiring health service plans to pay for "services appropriately provided through telemedicine"); Cal. Health & Safety Code § 1374.13(c) (requiring that health care services plans issued, amended, or renewed after January 1, 1997, may not require face-to-face contact as a prerequisite for payment on services that are appropriate for delivery by telemedicine).

61. *See* Pimley, *Technological Changes,* at 52 (describing how, for example, BCBS of Kansas provides for reimbursement and BCBS of North Dakota reimburses for telemedicine consultations).

62. *See* HCFA, Final Rule, Medicare Program: Revisions to Payment Policies and Adjustments to the Relative Value Units under the Physician Fee Schedule for Calendar Year 1999, 63 Fed. Reg. 58,879 (1998). A list of eligible rural HPSAs can be found at <http://158.72.105.163/databases/ppsa/hpsa.cfm>.

63. This limited construction of what services will be reimbursed has caused some debate in Congress and may be revised in the future by legislation. *See* Rural Health Improvement Act of 1997, S. 415, 105th Cong.; Comprehensive Telehealth Act of 1999, S. 770, 106th Cong.; *see also* ATSP, *Advocacy Alert: November 4, 1998, Medicare Reimbursement for the Practice of Telemedicine in Rural America* <http://www.atsp.org> (describing proposed legislation).

64. Medicare Carriers Manual ("MCM") § 2020(A).

65. *See, e.g.*, Cal. Ins. Code § 10123.13 (referring to Cal. Bus. & Prof. Code § 2290.5 defining telemedicine as "the practice of health care delivery, diagnosis, consultation, treatment, transfer of medical data, and education using interactive audio, video, or data communications"); La. Rev. Stat. Ann. § 22:657; *see also* Leslie A. Sandberg, *Telemedicine Continues To Wrestle Wicked Problems: Reimbursement, Licensure, and Bandwidth Rules or Is It Compliance?* 20 HEALTH MGMT. TECH. 134 (Feb. 1, 1999) (discussing states adopting nondiscrimination provisions).

66. *See generally* American Health Lawyers Association, HEALTH LAW PRACTICE GUIDE § 1:34, *et seq.* (general discussion of state licensure of individual practitioners).

67. *See, e.g.*, Cal. Bus. & Prof. Code § 2052 (classifying the practice of medicine without a license as a misdemeanor); Fla. Stat. § 921.0012 (classifying the unlicensed practice of medicine as a felony).

68. *See, e.g.*, Cal. Bus. & Prof. Code § 2264 (classifying the employment of or the aiding or abetting of any unlicensed person to practice medicine as unprofessional conduct that under § 2221 may result in revocation or suspension of license).

69. Conn. Gen. Stat. Ann. § 20-9 (1998).

70. Ind. Code § 25-22.5-1.-1(4); K.A.R. § 100-26-1; Nev. Rev. Stat. § 630.020(3); Okla. Stat. Tit. 59, § 492(3)(b); Tex. Admin. Code §174.1; Conn. Gen. Stat. Ann. § 20-9(d); Fla. Stat. Ann. § 458.355.

71. Okl. Stat. Ann. § 492(C)(3)(b).

72. Kan. Admin. Reg. § 100-26-1, 1997; Mass Board of Registration in Medicine general counsel opinion letter; JOINT WORKING GROUP ON TELEMEDICINE, TELEMEDICINE REPORT TO CONGRESS, January 31, 1997, at 47 ("JWGT Report") (*citing to* Letter from Pennsylvania Board of Medicine to Teleimaging Chartered (March 29, 1996)), available at http://www.nha.doc.gov/reports/telemed/legal.htm.

73. Exemption for consulting: Ariz. Rev. Stat. § 32-1421(B) (emergencies); Ind. Code Ann. § 25-22.5-1-2(a)(4); Idaho Code § 54-1804(1)(b); Fla. Stat. Ann. § 458.303 (exempt from licensure when meeting with licensed Florida physicians for consultation purposes); N.H. Stat. Ann. § 329:21(II); N.C. Gen. State § 90-18(11) (regular or frequent consultation may eliminate the exemption of out-of-state physician consultation); Ohio Rev. Code § 4731.01; Penn. Stat. § 63-6-204; Utah Code Ann. § 58-12-30(2) (emergencies); Ark. Code. Ann. § 17-95-203(2) (exemption from licensing requirement for physician who has no hospital connections or office in state and who sees patients only "occasionally"); Conn. Gen. Stat. Ann. § 20-9(b)(4); Kan. Stat. Ann. § 65-2872(j).

74. *See Interstate Licensure for the Practice of Telemedicine* <http://208.129.51/InterstateLicensure.html>.

75. *See* <http://www.fsmb.org/telemed.htm>.

76. Federation of State Medical Boards of the United States, Inc., *An Act to Regulate the Practice of Medicine Across State Lines* <http://www.fsmb.org/telemed.htm>.

77. Ala. Code § 34-24-500 to -508; 22 Tex. Ad. Code § 174.1-174.14.

78. *See* Multi-State Regulation Task Force, BOARDS OF NURSING APPROVE PROPOSED LANGUAGE FOR AN INTERSTATE COMPACT FOR A MUTUAL RECOGNITION MODEL FOR NURSING REGULATION, April 1998, 1, 4.

79. S.B. 146, 52d Leg., 1998 Gen. Sess. (Utah 1998).

80. *See* Multi-State Regulation Task Force, How Does the Interstate Compact for Mutual Recognition Work? July 1998, 3.

81. *See* <http://www.atsp.org>.

82. Civil liability for filing false claims arises under 31 U.S.C. §§ 3729-3731. Criminal liability lies under 18 U.S.C. § 287.

83. *See* 42 U.S.C. § 1320a-7b(b). Many states have similar antikickback provisions. *See, e.g.,* N.Y. Code R. & Regs., tit. VIII, § 29.1(b)(3); Md. Code Ann., Health Occ. § 12-313(b)(11).

84. *See* 42 U.S.C. § 1395nn.

85. *See* Bienz v. Central Suffolk Hosp., 557 N.Y.S.2d 139 (2d Dep't 1990) (recognizing that a telephone call to a physician's office for the purpose of initiating treatment could be sufficient to create a physician-patient relationship); *see also* Starkey v. St. Rita's Medical Center, 1997 Ohio App. LEXIS 137 (Ohio Ct. App. Jan. 8, 1997) (concerning malpractice liability of hospital-sponsored call center; case discussion centers on causation and duty appears to have been conceded by the call center); Shannon v. McNulty, 718 A.2d 828 (Pa. Super. 1998). *See generally* James L. Rigelhaupt, Jr., J.D. Annotation, *What Constitutes Physician–Patient Relationship for Malpractice Purposes*, 17 A.L.R. 4th 132 (1981).

86. *Shannon*, 718 A.2d at 832.

87. *Shannon*, 718 A.2d at 835–836.

88. Adams v. Kaiser Found. Health Plan of Ga., 93-VS-79895E (Fulton Co. Ga. Feb. 2, 1995) (jury awarded plaintiff $45.54 million; the case was later resolved for an undisclosed amount under a confidential settlement agreement). *See Settlements,* Nat. L.J., Feb. 5, 1996, at C14.

89. In 1996, Kaiser also ran into difficulties with regulators concerning the operation of their call center in California. Officials at the California Department of Corporations found "widespread shortcomings in the quality of services" performed by Kaiser Permanente, including with the operations of the telephone advice line. The report issued by the state expressed concern that the nurses staffing the line did not give advice "free of cost-cutting pressures." *See Kaiser Permanente: Under Fire from California Regulators,* Health Line, Aug. 29, 1996.

90. *Shannon*, 718 A.2d at 832.

91. The advice given about payment also might raise concerns under prudent layperson provisions applicable under some federal programs, adopted in many states, and proposed in many more jurisdictions. Under prudent layperson provisions, insurers must cover and make reasonable payment for emergency services if a person is suffering from symptoms that would reasonably suggest to a prudent layperson an emergency medical condition.

92. Deborah Grandinetti, *Patient Phone Calls Driving You Crazy? Here's Relief,* Med. Econ., June 24, 1996.

93. *See* 21 U.S.C. § 321, *et seq.*

94. Radiology Devices; Proposed Classifications for Five Medical Image Management Devices, 61 Fed. Reg. 63,769 (Dec. 2, 1996).

95. *See, e.g.,* Charles Marwick, *Several Groups Attempting Regulation of Internet Rx,* 281 JAMA 975 (1999).

96. *Internet-Based Pharmacies Raising Regulatory Questions,* Med. Industry Today (Apr. 7, 1999).

97. Cal Bus. & Prof. Code § 2242.

e-Services: Planning Process for e-Business Development

Douglas E. Goldstein and Michael Stull

IF YOU ARE a physician or health care executive who recognizes the significance of the health care e-revolution and have begun to envision the future, then the question is "how" to guide change in your organization. Perhaps the preceding chapters have helped you see the need to energize and fortify your business using enterprisewide, Web-enabled e-commerce solutions. But what are the e-business processes that enable you to "do it better...on line"? Take the e-plunge and initiate the e-business action planning process in this chapter; there is no better time than the present.

Understand at the outset, however, that to achieve e-service success, you must recognize the pervasive impact of this decision. For example, as administrative costs fall due to the low cost of moving data through "e" technology and the Internet, there will be a dramatic reallocation and reorganization of company resources and staff. Also, the various supply chains will shorten and decompress, taking with it employees and long-term relationships with certain suppliers. And customer service relationships will shift from telephone-based centers to real-time multimedia customer service centers—there will be much more of a focus on the e-consumer and e-patient. These changes will not be easy for everyone in the organization to accept, and that fact needs to be recognized before you begin. It is also critical to realize that true e-service means doing service on the Net. It is not a passive content Web site!

PLANNING CHALLENGES

As the saying goes, if you do not know where you are going, any road will take you there (see Figure 17–1). The same holds true with planning and implementing your organization's e-strategy and e-action plan. Without clear e-business objectives, the implementation of e-commerce and e-care and related e-services

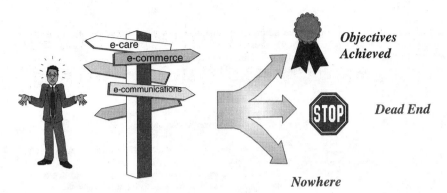

Figure 17–1 Selecting the Correct Path. *Source:* Copyright © 1999, Douglas Goldstein and Michael Stull.

could take an unintended fork in the road. Because true e-services and e-commerce will pervade the very fabric of an organization, there are a number of key challenges to assess for successful planning, development, and implementation of e-care, e-commerce, and e-communications. Articulating this brave new e-care world, enterprisewide (or in the future "interprisewide"), is critical for your e-service plan to be sustainable, manageable, and upgradeable. Each challenge is listed in Figure 17–2 and further highlighted below.

Defining e-Business Objectives

Saying that your organization will use e-service solutions to "increase shareholder value" is not a clear enough company objective. As is the case with good diagnosis coding, specificity counts. Do you want to increase sales or reduce operating costs—and to what degree? Does the organization need to improve operational efficiencies such as claims submission, eligibility verification, referral authorization, or customer support? Do you want to increase sales volume and the organization's e-customer base—for example, sell more policies or products? Perhaps your desire is to increase access to services or products for current e-customers as well as expand market share or increase gross margins. Each business objective must be translated into an e-process and measurable e-business objective. In 1999, Dell Computer was selling millions of dollars in computers a day, and this fact allowed them to keep operating costs low despite adding thousands of new staff. The objective scope may be *product specific,* such as putting a product catalog on the Web; *companywide,* for example, putting all products on the Web, or linking your supply chain electronically; or *function specific,* such as putting customer service on line. After determining the scope, it is necessary to

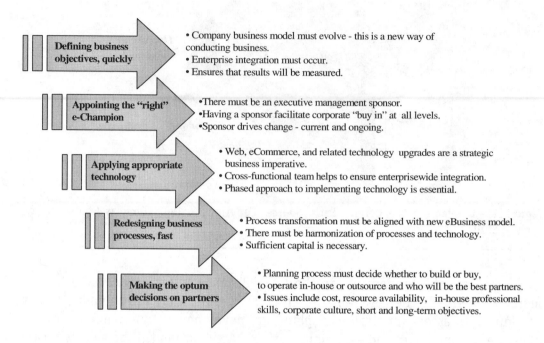

Figure 17–2 Key Challenges in the e-Service Planning and Development Process. *Source:* Copyright © 1999, Douglas Goldstein and Michael Stull.

project the impact of a new e-business process in specific percentage increases or decreases.

Appointing an e-Champion

Active executive leadership and sponsorship are crucial to achieving e-service business objectives. Without an e-champion leading the change effort, your organization will experience serious bumps in the e-commerce road. Without direction and vision, it is difficult to achieve critical mass and sustained change is virtually impossible. Just as there has never been a Super Bowl winner without a strong, visionary coach, the implementation of e-services cannot be achieved without solid leadership and defined e-service job accountabilities.

The corporate e-champion participates in the development of the e-service delivery framework and oversees execution from an enterprise perspective. Remember, implementing true e-communications, e-commerce, and e-care impacts the very foundation of each major business function and operating unit within the organization. A senior company executive with both the perceived and the real power to effect change is critical to your e-team. Many organizations are finding that establishing a new position such as senior vice president of e-services—or starting an entirely new .com company to exploit the on-line opportunities—is absolutely essential.

Applying e-Technology Wisely

Internet and information technology is evolving very rapidly. Be sure to align the changes in "e" technologies that create new capabilities and opportunities with stated e-business objectives, and be careful not to fall into the "latest and greatest" product trap. E-services are not dependent on a particular technology, product, or platform—despite what a Microsoft, Netscape, or IBM salesperson might tell you. What is critical is elevating the technology function within your company from a support group that is buried under a line manager to a strategic business unit that is on the same level with your sales and marketing, finance, and operations teams. It most frequently requires a detailed analysis and comparison of how processes are completed before and after "e" service.

Web-enabled solutions for a truly Web-centric enterprise that operates at lower costs and higher efficiencies requires:

- front-end Web servers and applications servers, customer relationship software, Intranets for sharing company information and collaborating locally and remotely
- Extranets for linking to key customers, virtual private networks to establish an integrated, secure network infrastructure supporting geographically dispersed organizations, e-commerce software, sales and marketing software, procurement
- order processing/management applications designed for e-services
- integration with back-end systems (accounting, finance, inventory management, etc.) to develop a truly Web-centric enterprise that operates at lower costs and higher efficiencies

Redesigning Business Processes with "e" in Mind

For years, health care organizations have had the luxury to run inefficiently and still stay in business. E-commerce, however, forces medical offices, hospitals, and insurance companies to re-think their labor-intensive procedures and hierarchical processes. Health care organizations can develop Internet-supported processes and organizations that work more effectively and give better customer service through integrated telephone and Web real-time call centers and processes. (See Chapter 8 for more information.)

In the twenty-first century, the rapid advancement of new "e" software and hardware and technology product introductions force business processes to change at a pace that is faster than ever. Introducing new "e" technology without a corresponding transformation of business processes is like trying to fit a V8 engine into a four-cylinder compartment—it does not work. Mobile computing, ubiquitous wireless connectivity, high-speed transaction processing systems, knowledge management solutions, and related technology improvements drive business process change, and they must evolve together. Do not make the mistake of leaving your business process transformation and re-engineering initiatives behind the introduction of new "e" technologies and Web-based services. The Web front end must be tied into your legacy systems or a complete 100 percent Net process must be in place for true e-services. If you do redesign processes as you implement e-technology, return on technology and Net investments will pleasantly surprise you.

Determining the Shortest Path to Implementation

Trying to be all things to all e-consumers all at once can end in disaster. Pick your priorities and focus on the most important opportunities for your organization—plan the e-service delivery model using "build it or buy it" analyses, and remember that one size does not fit all. As you consider your build/buy, outsourcing, and cosourcing options for Internet solutions, be sure to review available technical and design staff resources. Consider the other current corporate initiatives and the skill set of your technical staff. How well do they understand Java, hypertext markup language, XML, secure sockets layers, and other standards of Web and e-commerce? And as you consider outsourcing, think about your organization's corporate culture. Some companies have not been able to successfully outsource systems development and operations because they have always handled them in-house. In cases like this, outsourcing may be difficult because it requires relinquishing some control and relying on a new generation of Net-based technology companies.

In the new Web world, it could make sense to cosource the development and operation of new e-services with a partner organization. A good example of this is the HealthOnline.com network of on-line health and medical channels. In this case, Health Online, Inc., operates this private-label solution as an interactive media management company through a business model that lowers all the operating costs for members of the network. One key element of this approach is a cost center of hosting Web services, which was converted into a revenue-generating business model with leading health systems.

As you begin to develop and implement an effective e-service plan, the preceding five issues will get you from your own 20-yard line across midfield. At that point, you can ensure that the results achieved meet your newly defined e-business objectives and that the process can be adapted as market conditions evolve.

Successful organizations have something very important in common—the ability to plan for, respond to, and manage change. IBM, Microsoft, GE, McDonald's, America Online, and other successful companies have dynamic rapid response planning processes in place that enable them to respond to changing market conditions. To effectively launch Net-based and other e-service solutions, health care organizations must develop and restructure their product and service offerings and support environment in a rapid response manner.

E-SERVICE DEVELOPMENT FRAMEWORK

There is an action-oriented approach to planning for the development of e-services—the "e-service development framework," illustrated in Figure 17–3. The authors developed this approach over a number of years, as a result of many engagements with leading health care companies nationwide. The approach and key steps to the e-service success pipeline are outlined below.

First, Formalize e-Business Function and Priorities

A carefully developed, formalized e-business function—with dedicated senior executive time and support—is the overriding priority under any circumstance

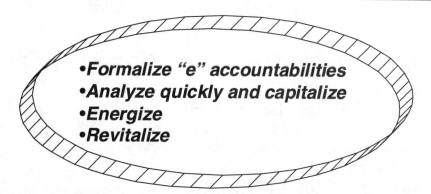

Figure 17–3 e-Service Development Framework. *Source:* Copyright © 1999, Douglas Goldstein and Michael Stull.

when developing a successful Web-centric, e-service business environment. One element involves establishing a new position such as chief "e" development officer who is responsible for inventorying, cross-fertilizing, focusing, and coordinating all the Internet, Extranet, and Intranet activities going on across the organization. The e-actions that are described below will guide the way to success and achievement of e-goals.

- *e-Action #1: Articulate the e-Services Concept and Strategy Over and Over.* No matter which tools or methodologies are used to develop an e-service infrastructure, there is one overriding principle that must be promulgated throughout the company: e-service delivery through e-commerce and e-care systems is a fundamental change in the way health care organizations do business. It affects all areas of the organization, from the front line to the board room. A commitment must be made from the executive level to implement, manage, and continuously evolve the corporate focus on e-services. This message of priority and e-action must become part of the culture. Anything less will result in a suboptimal return on Net investment and a reduction in long-term benefits from these activities.

A corporate memo, a meeting, or an e-mail message sent companywide describing the company's commitment to e-service delivery will not do. What is needed is a comprehensive, structured, ongoing new, dynamic "e" process to move an organization into the world of e-service opportunity.

- *e-Action #2: Hire a High-Level "e" Executive, Create a Cross-Functional e-Team, and Enact the e-Service Strategy.* Successful e-service implementation must be planned for and managed by an internal team comprising the "e" executive, corporate e-champion, key business unit and support managers, key front-line staff, and potentially, the involvement of key customers. After your organization has set the e-priority, it is challenged to:

- Articulate the company vision and define objectives for e-commerce and e-care
- Guide the development process and ensure speed to market
- Determine the best organizational structure (such as an owned e-business unit or a separate .com e-company that is initially wholly owned but uses external capital to grow and disseminate e-services and products)
- Assign development actions to e-team members
- Prioritize e-service development in Internet, Extranet, and Intranet initiatives
- Educate and support all team members with appropriate capital resources

- Review and benchmark results
- Manage ongoing change and process/technology upgrades based on competitive market forces

The "e" executive must take the lead in organizing, motivating, and managing the efforts of the e-team.

Figure 17–4 illustrates the composition of the e-teams, which is responsible for leading, articulating, developing, and managing e-services across the enterprise. The total number of people in the e-group is less important than their ability to articulate strategy, get their peers and associates to implement actions, and otherwise contribute to the process. That said, for large organizations, three or four representatives is not a big enough e-team, 8 to 15 people is manageable, and more than 20 is too large. The e-team is the nexus of the infrastructure.

The e-team is critical in motivating change, sponsoring e-technology education, delivering capital and resources, encouraging creative "e" thinking, and, most important, developing speed to market tactics. Remember, in less than four years, Yahoo.com went from a list of Web sites to a leading Net search engine, to a leading media company, to one of the world's most recognized brands! The e-team should not get hung up on excessive analysis. It supports implementation and learning during initial operations, as the groundwork is laid for the next version of your e-service or e-product.

Second, Analyze Quickly and Capitalize

Once you have articulated the organization's e-business objectives, *analyze* each activity that supports e-implementation. The planning activities and corre-

---

Executive e-Team Action Group
- Executive sponsors
- Dedicated Chief e-Development Officer
- Key corporate managers
- Key corporate staff
- Multidisciplinary team

Figure 17–4 e-Group Members. *Source:* Copyright © 1999, Douglas Goldstein and Michael Stull.

sponding e-actions are listed in Exhibit 17–1 and described below. An organization must aggressively analyze its corporate strategy, practices, technologies, partnerships, industry and competition, and *capitalize* e-solutions that provide a competitive advantage in key business areas. In achieving success in retail, the mantra is "location, location, location." In providing e-services, the guiding motto is "fast and right!"

• *e-Action #1: Review Existing Technology Systems.* Many major corporations cannot accurately estimate the number and type of technologies, products, and solutions they use. Without taking inventory and creating this baseline, an e-service framework using Web-enabled systems will experience integration troubles and cost run-ups—and support requirements will miss the mark.

• *e-Action #2: Evaluate Industry "Best e-Practices."* Review and analyze both your competitors' approach to e-based service delivery and industry best e-practices. Are your competitors offering only marketing information, or are e-consumers and e-patients able to buy products or register for local workshops? Do medical office or hospital staff have e-commerce solutions—such as eligibility verification or on-line supply ordering—on their desktops? Visit powerhouse e-commerce companies such as Amazon (www.amazon.com), Dell (www.dell.com), CDNow (www.cdnow.com), and Cisco Systems (www.cisco.com) to see what they are doing and how they personalize and energize their services for e-customers.

Exhibit 17–1 The "Analyze Quickly and Capitalize" e-List

- Review existing technology systems.
- Evaluate industry "best e-practices."
- Analyze e-service technologies and solutions.
- Visit informative Web sites.
- Review industry trade information.
- Attend industry conferences on e-health care.
- Be a beta site for e-solutions.
- Learn from industry analysts.
- Put yourself in your customer's shoes.
- Transform business processes.

Source: Copyright © 1999, Douglas Goldstein and Michael Stull.

The e-service requirements of most organizations can be met by adopting industry solutions and best practices that already exist and partnering with innovative e-solutions that enhance a core platform.

- *e-Action #3: Analyze e-Service Technologies and Solutions.* Analyze leading e-products, technologies, and systems within the industry and across industries. These include Web and applications servers, application software (customer relationship, sales and marketing, procurement and order processing and e-commerce), company Intranets, Extranets for interface with key clients, and so forth.

- *e-Action #4: Visit Informative Web Sites.* It is important to visit Web sites that offer credible and current information about e-business trends. Some good choices include www.cnet.com, www.cyberatlas.com, www.thestandard.com, and a whole host of technology Web sites. Join their e-newsletters, and visit the sites frequently based on need.

- *e-Action #5: Review Industry Trade Information.* *Modern Healthcare* covers aspects of e-business in the health care industry, while magazines like *Managed Care Interface* have regular monthly Internet columns and articles. Plus a new generation of print and e-newsletters like "Medicine on the Net" are dedicated to e-healthcare and growing rapidly. *Inter@ctive Week, Internet Week,* and *Network Computing* will keep you up to date with the Internet industry in general.

- *e-Action #6: Attend Industry Conferences on e-Healthcare.* The Healthcare Information and Management Systems Society (www.himss.org), INTEROP, Internet World, and ComNet (examples of industry technology conferences and trade shows) are leading organizations that hold informative meetings on a regular basis. Recently, a conference called eHealthcare World (www.ehealthcare-world) has been held twice a year. Network with other members and attendees to find out what has worked for them.

- *e-Action #7: Be a Beta Site for e-Solutions.* Consider partnering with an emerging Net solutions company in a beta site effort. Test new Net-based software, hardware, and tools. Work with technology vendors and offer to be a demonstration site for their Web-enabled products and solutions at a reduced cost, of course. Many health care providers—integrated delivery networks, regional health systems, large hospital groups, physician groups, and so on—already work closely with technology and services vendors such as Microsoft, IBM, Netscape, Oracle, WebMD, SMS, and McKesson HBOC, evaluating new releases of applications and software. This provides familiarity with the products and facilitates trust and a better working relationship with vendor partners.

• *e-Action #8: Learn from Industry Analysts.* Savvy health care organizations subscribe to research services provided by the Gartner Group (www.gartner.com), Forrester Research (www.forrester.com), and the Yankee Group (www.yankeegroup.com). Gaining access to these companies' information libraries and industry analysts is an excellent way to learn about industry dynamics and leading technology and product companies by industry and by capability. It also helps to position e-products, focus research, and achieve speed to market.

• *e-Action #9: Continually Put Yourself in Your Customers' Shoes.* "Customer value" is a buzzword in today's marketplace, but the idea needs to be integrated into your organization, not just discussed. Understand what your customers need and want, why they remain loyal, and how the organization could better respond to their needs through cheaper, better, faster e-solutions.

To address these issues, schedule focus groups and get user feedback through on-line interactive surveys. Get a clear understanding of e-customers' perception of the company and the value its products and services deliver. Do e-customers think of your company as a progressive, high-quality organization with a customer-centric view? Is your organization helping their pocketbooks, their health, their wardrobes, their psyche? What are customers doing on line today, and what do they want to do on line with you. If you can accurately answer these questions, your e-service strategy will be much more likely to achieve prescribed company e-objectives.

• *e-Action #10: Go to Digital Processes.* Do not waste valuable time and resources trying to fit current business processes to the e-business environment. Begin breaking down each existing process, and think about how to reassemble it in an e-commerce environment now. Everything—from work flow, management oversight, and staff roles and responsibilities to customer interaction and supply chain management—must undergo some level of re-engineering or transformation in order for e-business processes to work. Often, the choices are to integrate with legacy systems through detailed processes or to just start from scratch with an entirely new e-business system.

Do yourself a favor—go for the biggest bang for the buck. Start by re-tooling those business processes that benefit from e-commerce the most, with the least amount of implementation difficulty. Hospital organizations may want to start by allowing e-customers to register prior to an admission and pay for it on line. Medical offices may choose to do new patient registrations on line and direct e-consumers to access it on line prior to their arrival to save patient time and staff effort.

Third, Energize

Step three in the infrastructure development process requires *energizing* the organization for e-action and rapid evolution. Listed in Exhibit 17–2, energizing activities are those that help your organization plan a successful implementation of the desired e-result. E-actions for the energizing process are described below.

- *__e-Action #1__: Deliver Capital That Supports e-Business Initiatives.* The capital expenditure will be related to the organization's telecommunications center, customer service center, or data and e-commerce center, the staffing required for new work flows, business processes, and responsibilities. It will be based on e-business plans and financial projections.

- *__e-Action #2__: Continually Evolve the e-Plan.* Once you have already successfully articulated the e-service vision, created a functional e-group, and analyzed existing technologies, competitors, and opportunities and begun implementation, it is essential to constantly revise the strategic e-Plan. This plan must address e-service objectives, the activities necessary to achieve these objectives, the capital and operating costs associated with required activities, and the time horizon estimated to reach identified objectives. In this regard, the company's e-strategy plan addresses the activities listed in Exhibit 17–3.

E-business initiatives should be factored into all major corporate business activities, and a detailed e-service project plan must be developed—by business unit, line of business, regional unit, and product unit. Charge specific operating

---

Exhibit 17–2 "Energize" Activities

- Plan for facilities that support e-business initiatives.
- Update the company's strategic plan so that it includes e-commerce, e-operations, and e-care delivery.
- Schedule pilot programs before you roll out e-solutions enterprisewide.

Source: Copyright © 1999, Douglas Goldstein and Michael Stull.

Exhibit 17–3 Corporate e-Strategy Plan Activities

Affected Business Areas and Corporate Infrastructure	Strategic Plan Activity
Organization structure and staffing	Redefine company organization, lines of responsibility, reporting, and so forth to support e-service delivery. Plan for increase in staffing in certain areas and reduction in others. Plan for reorienting responsibilities of managers and key business unit and support staff.
Major business services and related processes, including • patient care • physician services • member services, including benefits and enrollment • hospital and facility services • customer service, including call center operations • finance and accounting, including payer relationships • sales and marketing • human resources • technology infrastructure, including integration of legal systems	Define high-level, strategic e-objectives companywide and by operating unit and support organization. Describe high-level process change due to e-service implementation and based on interrelationships of key corporate functions, including sales, purchasing, inventory management, fulfillment, and customer service.
Budgeting/forecasting	Develop the overall corporate budget to plan, implement, and operate/manage the new e-business environment above and beyond current planned estimates. Describe the overall increase in corporate value and return on investment based on implementing e-services.
Facilities	Describe general facility changes necessary to accommodate the digitally focused e-business model.
E-security	Describe an overall security framework with defined objectives enterprisewide.

Source: Copyright © 1999, Douglas Goldstein and Michael Stull.

and support departments with the development of the tactics and objectives for implementation. For example, if the purchasing department is charged with the ownership of a Web-based storefront for suppliers to purchase standard, recurring items electronically to reduce time, cost, and error, the managers and staff in that department, working in conjunction with corporate information technology specialists (or an information technology vendor) should outline the key activities required to support this e-commerce solution. Use Exhibit 17–4, the e-activity checklist, as part of this evaluation.

- *__e-Action #3__: Schedule Pilot Programs before You Roll Out e-Solutions Enterprisewide.* On-line project planning is critical to ensuring that when e-systems, e-services, e-products, and e-solutions are developed, they are accurately tested and measured against identified requirements and commitments. Fully functional on-line Intranet servers are essential tools to support necessary activities. This is especially important when the e-service involves multiple entities such as e-customers or suppliers. Test the key, high-visibility programs with influential customers to obtain buy-in and input prior to the formal rollout.

Fourth, Revitalize and Evolve

The e-service implementation is not complete until a revitalization and evolution system is in place. This evolution system makes "e" an essential part of the organization. It must come alive! Net years are measured in months; an action or

---

Exhibit 17–4 e-Activity Checklist

- Does our current staff have the skills required to support this initiative?
- Which automated tools and technologies are needed to implement the service?
- In what time frame will the e-services be rolled out?
- Should internal technology staff build interfaces with existing databases—or is outsourcing this development a better strategy?
- What risks are associated with implementation?
- Who will operate the new system?
- Who will provide training to internal staff and key customers, suppliers, and others?
- How will our business processes change based on Web-enabled service delivery?

Source: Copyright © 1999, Douglas Goldstein and Michael Stull.

enterprise education effort about the digital "e" revolution is necessary. Measurement dimensions include:

- *Short-term success.* This is measured by budget versus actual costs, resource expenditures, and adherence to schedule.
- *Long-term success.* This is measured in relation to specific business objectives (e.g., increased sales opportunities, increased sales to current customers, decreased call center or medical office call volume, and improved ratings on patient satisfaction or e-customer surveys).
- *Intangible success.* This is measured by overall increase in corporate value, brand building, and customer perception.

Be sure to delegate responsibility and accountability to upgrade and continuously develop e-services based on results, changing market conditions, competition, corporate focus, and overall company strength. Changes to Net e-services must be on the fly. It is much better to launch the initial 1.0 version of the Internet, Intranet, or Extranet service in three months and add features as you go, then wait a year to launch e-service and miss the market. Every Net effort is a work in progress. Evolution is rapid and the best proving ground is with the customers on line!

KEY E-HEALTHCARE METHODOLOGIES

E-Healthcare methodologies are supported by e-vision, e-management, and constantly evolving plans that will lead to success. Outlined in Table 17–1 and described below, these methodologies support e-objectives being implemented on time and within budget. These methodologies are critical to energizing change within the organization.

- *e-Methodology #1: Ongoing e-Team Success Sharing Sessions.* These sessions must be regular, planned events with attendance by all e-team members. Meeting objectives include

  - sharing of lessons learned, key success, and strategies to improve
  - reporting, by business area, the planning milestones, status, and project problems
  - development of action items, with assigned responsibilities and due dates
  - continued feedback on overall e-progress

Table 17–1 Methodologies To Implement e-Initiatives

Methodology Component	Key Factors
Executive oversight e-council meetings	Held at regular intervals—weekly, biweekly, or monthly. Ensures assignment of action items and reporting on progress achieved on assigned activities.
Interactive workshops	Among and between executive e-council, key managers, key corporate staff, key business partners, customers, and suppliers. Held during the planning process as well as during periodic status reviews.
Companywide correspondence	Top-down, continuous, of a constant theme, with updated messages—Intranet and Extranet enabled.
Facilitator	May require an outside expert to help facilitate the planning process.

Source: Copyright © 1999, Douglas Goldstein and Michael Stull.

Critical to the success of these meetings is strong leadership from the corporate e-champion. A clear, written agenda should be distributed prior to each meeting. Assign responsibility for action items throughout each meeting, and discuss progress status reports and updates. A positive energy of confidence, excitement, and learning should pervade all meetings and communications.

• *e-Methodology #2: Ongoing "e" Workshops.* E-team leaders must demonstrate by example "excitement." Facilitated by various e-team members, on-line workshops are designed to share extensive information about the market, players, e-opportunities, and e-strategy options and to assess internal sales, service, and operational aspects of the company. The workshops include members of operating business units, administrative support units, other executive management staff, and—depending on circumstance and relationship—a key customer, supplier, or business partner. If properly executed, these workshops build the foundation for e-services and recommendations and will lead to the overall corporate e-strategy and specific actions by business unit.

• *e-Methodology #3: Set Up Project Intranet and e-Casting Channels.* All existing corporate communication channels (e-newsletters, etc.) must be partnered with new media like broadcast Internet e-mail daily and weekly updates and an e-services project Intranet. A continuous stream of relevant, current information related to e-service efforts must be sent throughout via the Intranet, print, etc. Beginning in the executive offices, the messages and content should be clear, concise, upbeat, and generally available enterprisewide—without giving away trade secrets to potential competitors. The company's corporate Intranet should establish a special information repository to support daily work and, depending on the strength of external relationships, an Extranet may be extended to key suppliers, customers, or partners, allowing them to participate in the e-service effort through a secure channel.

• *__e-Methodology #4__: Engage an Experienced Health Care Expert and Facilitator.* It is often helpful to engage an outside consultant to assist in e-service development. Your organization may never have undertaken such a large technology or change project; an expert can help facilitate project planning sessions and get the organization farther, faster. Or, as is the case in many health care organizations, there may be no in-house e-business expertise that can support the company's e-initiatives. A skilled e-expert can be very useful in guiding the organization and help your organization avoid the mistakes encountered by others. Finally, outside experts can cut through the corporate politics that often rear their head during critical planning, development, and implementation phases.

If your e-team has planned and effectively executed the methodologies, you are on the way to achieving e-business goals—such as improving patient care, lowering costs, etc. There is little magic in planning for e-service delivery; but, it takes commitment, vision, hard work, and the pressing desire to stay ahead of the competition. If your organization follows our formula for e-business services, outcomes can include

- clear e-business objectives related to e-solutions that cut costs and improve sales
- companywide enthusiasm for the new e-world
- a dynamic e-business plan that includes all priority opportunities
- tactical development and operations plans that focus on e-services and the actions required to achieve success
- pilot e-services to market, test, improve, and expand
- detailed Net security plan that enables e-business initiatives to protect confidentiality
- an e-infrastructure that constantly introduces e-products, e-services, and e-solutions to beat the competition

CONCLUSION—E-BUSINESS PLAN

Integrating e-Services Success with MedStrategy Matrix

Are your organization's Internet and "e" efforts considered a:

A. *"Tactic" to lower costs or source new business*
B. *Key "strategy" to achieve a competitive advantage*
C. *Vital "element," integral to the fabric of our organization, as it seeks to transform itself from a 1990 information/industrial company to 2010 knowledge and e-services organization?*

Success depends on taking the mental position reflected in "c." This is the correct path to prosperity in the next millennium.

A change in thought and attitude is needed before you guide revolutionary "e" change within your health care organization. Internet e-commerce and e-care are fundamentally shifting "bricks and mortar" business models into "clicks and mortar" e-businesses. As bandwidth to homes and businesses expands exponentially, the depth and breadth of what can be done on line will continue to increase dramatically. Yesterday, the Net moved text and graphics. Today it is moving real-time audio and video.

There is a new saying in .com companies: *"if it is not broken, break it!"* The Washington Post is a great example of how to break and reinvent a business model. The Post has been a consistent investor in on-line initiatives for the past five years. Some efforts—such as its proprietary on-line service—have not fared well, but the Web-based version of the Washington Post newspaper (www.washingtonpost.com) has been a huge success. In the latter half of 1999, the Washington Post was one of the first on-line newspapers to launch 24-hour, on-line news. Post leaders learned from past mistakes, and came out stronger and more knowledgeable the next time around.

The beginning of this chapter outlined four major elements to the e-services development framework:

1. Formalize "e" Business Priorities.
2. Analyze Quickly and Capitalize.
3. Energize.
4. Revitalize and Evolve.

Throughout this chapter a series of action steps and recommendations for the planning and development of your e-commerce and e-care efforts have been discussed. It is essential to visualize these four areas as part of an integrated e-

Exhibit 17–5 e-Business Plan Development Process

e-Business Plan Elements	Development Actions
Formalize Priorities:	
• e-Leadership	Corporate executive must "sponsor" and actively coach and drive e-initiatives.
• e-Vision	Company leaders must live the "e-vision" enterprisewide.
• e-Team	An e-Leadership Council and management team must support the e-vision and action plan.
• e-Customer (involvement)	Affected key customers should be involved in the e-business change.
Analyze and Capitalize:	A strategic plan and detailed tactics must:
• Action Plan	• define e-strategies required to achieve articulated business objectives
– e-Strategy	
– e-Budget	• develop budgets necessary to support e-initiatives
– e-Service	• define e-service related to support e-commerce and e-care activities
– e-Sales	
– e-Timing	• develop project plans that define the planning and implementation cycle for e-actions
Energize and Revitalize:	Change core business processes to support e-service delivery and e-solutions.
• e-Process Transformation	
• e-Legacy Integration and Web Systems	Current legacy systems must be integrated into deployed e-based solutions where it makes business sense or completely new Web-based systems put into place.
• Speed of Development	Move into the e-action now, target our e-opportunities, develop key pilot projects, and "get the ship moving."

Source: Copyright © 1999, Douglas Goldstein and Michael Stull.

Business Planning and Development Matrix as illustrated in Exhibit 17–5. This matrix is a template for an e-Business Plan. It highlights an e-Services development framework, lists an e-Business Planning Element, and delivers a summary of key Development Actions within each row. When implemented carefully, it can deliver a competitive advantage in the highly competitive, e-healthcare marketplace.

"Formalizing 'e' Business Priorities" involves leadership, vision, teamwork, and customer involvement around the "e" initiative. The President and CEO must set the tone and direction. The entire management of the health care enterprise must truly understand that the wise applications of "e" products and services through the Internet, Intranets, and Extranets is the key to better service, lower costs, and future success. Achieving this depends on multimedia communication and education throughout the organization and the use of Internet technology in vital internal and external areas. One example of this is Sentara Health System, which made no-interest loans for employee to purchase home computers. Setting priorities depends on having an effective inventory of internal and external use of Internet technology to sell more, cut costs, improve service, and achieve other benefits.

Various rating and selection systems can be used relative to the organization's strategic near- and long-term goals to select the greatest market opportunities to invest capital and human energy. Your e-Team, coupled with experienced outside consultants, can support the analysis, selection, development, prototyping, and implementation efforts of the highest priority e-commerce or e-care projects.

"Analyzing Quickly and Capitalizing" means getting the e-business Action Plan drafted with focused strategies, budgets, e-services, sales forecasts, sales tactics, and timing imperatives. Draft this plan within 30 to 90 days or less. The speed of Internet time is so fast that not acting quickly could render your organization's strategies and e-services out of touch with the market on the day they are launched. All Net initiatives are a work in process. It is much better to get a version 1.0 e-service up and running and evolve it over time than to wait until it is "perfect." But be careful to balance this rate of development speed with "right." Moving through the process "right" means addressing the internal needs of key stakeholders and external customers, so that when the e-business plan is in place there is extensive buy-in across the organization.

Laggards beware. One of the major issues facing large existing health care organizations is whether the bureaucratic structures and leadership vision (or lack of vision) hinders the ability to respond to a rapidly changing e-business environment. The loss of Borders' market share—both on line and off line—to Amazon.com, is a classic example of this. At least one CEO (Borders, Inc. in 1999) lost his job because of slow and poor on-line e-commerce development. One option to speed development is to set up a .com subsidiary that has the freedom and flexibility to move quickly. Initial funding comes from the parent health care organization, but capital strategies that leverage other financial investments (from institutional, strategic, or venture investors) help to brand and implement new e-commerce services.

Getting "energized" demands dynamic enthusiasm and leaders to guide the entire e-team and the whole organization. Comprehensive process transformation is essential to achieve true e-services, e-commerce, and e-care. Simply putting up a Web site that promotes a product but does not deliver on-line ordering, on-line support, or "better, cheaper, faster" is not a competitive advantage to your organization.

In 1999, drugstore.com, PlanetRX.com, and others had pharmacists on line 24 hours a day, 7 days a week to answer consumer questions. AmericasDoctor.com has doctors on line round the clock as well. Some of these health information services answer questions by e-mail, on-line chat, and real-time interactive video. *To effectively compete in the twenty-first century, health care organizations must implement robust health and medical e-services.* This means creating services that are effectively and seamlessly integrated with legacy systems and offer better customer service at lower costs. The other option is to define and implement an entirely different Web-based customer e-service function built on new technology that bypasses and replaces legacy systems.

When BankOne, one of the largest bank holding companies in the country, decided to move quickly into the on-line banking e-world, it created an entirely new company—Wingspan Bank (www.wingspan.com). Wingspan Bank's mission was to establish a beachhead in cyberspace that attracted new, cybercustomers and delivered on-line lessons related to customer use of the Internet and e-commerce back to the parent. Wingspan Bank moved quickly to become one of the leaders in on-line banking transactions and customer relationships. In essence, Wingspan Bank delivered a new Web-based customer service and e-commerce banking system.

BankOne realized that to reinvent the current BankOne infrastructure and integrate the on-line effort to existing BankOne legacy banking systems would take too long. BankOne created two separate tracks—one for Wingspan.com Bank, which would have "state of the Net" on-line systems, and another for BankOne, which would progressively add new e-commerce and on-line customer services to (www.bankone.com) by linking to legacy systems that deliver on-line banking functions to existing customers.

"Revitalizing and Evolving" your e-service planning and development process includes both a marathon and a sprint. It requires dedication, long-term commitment, enterprisewide support, and a well-focused, long-range game plan. It also demands fast response, speed to market, and an action orientation. The technology is available today to transform your business into an e-healthcare business that actively embraces e-products, e-services, and e-solutions. The challenge is to support sustained organizational change and develop the required corporate

"e-mentality," facilities, and infrastructure to be successful and achieve stated company business objective. Evolution with a big E for electronic, multimedia Internet-based technology requires an attitude and an action perspective to win.

Your challenge as a leader is to catalyze e-action based on solid research, market opportunity, and customer needs. In the world of information overload, don't forget to trust your intuition and judgment, once you have become immersed in the market. The 100-meter sprint is half over and the e-marathon is just beginning!

The billion-dollar question is what percentage of specific markets for products and services will the virtual "e" competitors gain in the next several years? It may be 25% or more, but nobody knows for sure. Existing companies and emerging .com companies are writing the story every day. The only way to get in the game is with a series of well-funded e-commerce and e-care initiatives that can rapidly evolve over time. Learning by doing is the way to success in the e-world of today and tomorrow.

What are you waiting for? Stop reading and start accelerating the launch of the .com version of your health care business.

CHAPTER 18

Invent the e-Healthcare Future

Douglas E. Goldstein

"E" YOUR ORGANIZATION TODAY!

The new e-future is being imagined and created every cybersecond of every day. The e-healthcare revolution is rapidly evolving and transforming the very fabric of the health care system. Selling over-the-counter pharmaceuticals on line is easier than doing cyber home visits, but each is possible and there are hundreds of new ventures seeking to build cyberbrands and customer relationships. Health care executives and providers must understand that health care's e-future is not about just publishing and pushing information; *it is about offering e-services* within brand-new e-business and e-care paradigms and models!

Doing "e" means figuring out how to make health care better, faster, and more efficient through appropriate use of "e" technology. The last thing cybercitizens want is to be bombarded with more bytes of useless data. Consumers are drowning in a sea of health and medical Web sites with information that is sometimes more entertaining than scientific. Today's consumers want e-solutions, and they want them now. What e-customers and cyberpatients really need is decision support and cost-effective products and e-services—not more text-based tips about weight loss or stress management.

IT IS THE *NEW* E-CONOMY

Billions and billions of dollars are being pumped into complete re-engineering of the American and international economies using the Internet and associated technologies as a platform and tool. In 1999, President Clinton and the Federal Reserve Board recognized that a new economy is being built in which, says Alan Greenspan, "an impressive proliferation of new technologies is inducing major changes in the underlying structure of the American economy."[1(p.B7)] What is really being created is a new e-business cycle where technology makes workers more productive, improves corporate profits, and allows tremendous economic growth without inflation. Developing knowledge- and action-oriented e-commerce and e-care business plans can lead your organization to investing in this new economy, where new e-services sell products as well as advertise and support health care delivery.

The Internet is more than a comet burning briefly in the night sky. Why? Because the Net has altered the fundamental cost of moving data. What was once relatively expensive is now extremely inexpensive. Just compare the cost of sending educational sales materials by overnight delivery with the cost of sending the same information on line through an interactive multimedia message. Then compare the cost of sending an e-mail—fractions of cents—with the cost of sending a physical envelope—33 cents or more. Multiply this by the trillions of events and transactions that are moving from print space to cyberspace, and you will understand the magnitude of the Internet's impact.

Attention big corporations, small businesses, physicians, health systems, and all other elements of the health care industry. Take action now to

e-ducate
e-magine
e-mpower
e-volve
and
e-nergize

the "e" plans, services, and activities for your organization! The e-tsunami is here, and it is building great force. You can view it as a threat, or you can see it as an opportunity for renewal. The choices are clear—plod along with traditional care delivery, or be extremely proactive and embrace the new opportunities of e-communication, e-community, e-commerce, and e-care. Plodding will lead to rapid decline and extinction. Companies with leaders who think, do, and act to expand their Net initiatives will prosper and achieve the competitive advantage.

ACHIEVE INNOVATION IN YOUR E-CARE BUSINESS

Traditional business models are being reinvented across the entire spectrum of health and medical products and services through "e." Within the health and medical industry, there are tremendous savings in administrative costs and in on-line e-care services. Every sector of the economy and health care system will be part of this Net revolution.

The cyberworld is moving from low-bandwidth connections of 28.8K or 56K to high-speed bandwidth cable and digital subscriber line, from delivering text and graphics to offering real-time interactive audio and video. As people go from low-speed, hard-wired connections to high-speed wireless connections, they have anytime, anywhere, access to information, knowledge, products, and services anywhere on the planet—via "e" technology and the Net. On this high-speed e-highway are cyber medical visits. When home-based telemedicine is really possible, "bricks and mortar" health care will become "bits and bytes" e-healthcare.

SURF THE E-TSUNAMI

The e-future is not preordained. It is being invented by you and me. As Bill Gates once said, "there is no reliable map to uncharted waters." If you are idle and passive, the e-tsunami will swallow you. But if you build a cybercruiser with your e-team and develop e-care business models to surf the wave, the e-tsunami will energize your journey. In the e-healthcare game, it is not always clear which organizations will win and which will lose. Survival and prosperity will go to the organizations and e-teams that bring together knowledge, talent, capital, vision, and the power of "e" for unbelievable synergy and growth—without dwelling on the fact that it has not been done, tested, or proven yet.

Because of the large number of involved payers and employers and the fragmentation of providers, health care is a complex industry. But this complexity should not prevent you from taking action. Take the ideas, examples, and lessons discussed in this book, combine them with the cyberspace knowledge and lead your organization on the path to e-success.

In all your efforts, "Do It Better—On Line." Please take the time to tell me your success stories at DigitalDoug@aol.com. Share the e-strategies and e-services that have helped your e-customers and e-patients live better, healthier lives through the wise use of "e" technology.

REFERENCE

1. D. Ignatius, "Online in the New Economy," *Washington Post,* 11 July, 1999, B7.

Glossary

THE WORLD of "e" is continually evolving. The following glossary of terms is meant to provide an overview of the jargon common in the world of the Net. Visit www.netlingo.com or www.webopedia.com regularly to add new terms to your e-vocabulary.

Access
The ability to get into and use a system—in this case, an on-line system. Access to the Internet through commercial on-line services such as Mindspring or America Online requires an account, an access telephone number, a password, and special software designed for that service. Making a direct connection to the Internet through an Internet service provider requires a special connection and an Internet access account.

Address
A name that identifies a unique network component. On the Internet every file and every e-mail user has a unique address. When a file address is typed into a browser, the user is brought directly to that file.

Air Space
The communication space in which two or more people are in the same room, communicating, face-to-face without the use of any electronic intermediary such as a telephone, iPhone, Web browser, television, etc.

America Online (or AOL.com)
The most popular and fastest-growing major commercial on-line service. America Online features an attractive graphical interface, many content areas, e-mail discussion groups, file downloading, and Internet access. AOL offers content and services with their proprietary network for members only and is a leading ISP that allows access to the broader Internet such as the World Wide Web.

Bandwidth

The volume of data a transmission line can carry or transfer at one time. Telephone lines generally have the lowest bandwidth, while fiber optics have the highest bandwidth. In general, the wider a line's bandwidth, the more data it can move at once. As high-speed cable access offers increased bandwidth in consumers' homes, the speed of Net surfing increases, and on-line video communication becomes a reality. New technological advances such as digital subscriber lines (DSL), which deliver high-speed connections through standard phone lines, are rapidly bringing high-speed access to millions of consumers and businesses.

Banner Ad

An on-line advertisement on a Web page that, if clicked on, typically takes the user to the advertiser's site or delivers educational and product messages of the sponsor.

Baud

The speed at which information travels from one computer to another. Baud relates to the type of modem or communication device within a computer. Most new PCs now ship with a standard 56K, and cable modems are taking hold in many markets, making a baud of 256K or higher possible due to cable's ability to handle high bandwidth.

BBS (Bulletin Board System)

Public message areas that offer live chat, a file storage area, electronic mail, and other features. Imagine a corkboard at a grocery store where local residents post help wanted and for sale signs. A BBS works in the same way. BBSs were a popular form of Internet communication before the advent of the World Wide Web. Now many Web sites have created various message board services within their on-line services.

Bot

A term that comes from the word "robot," a bot is a computer program that runs automatically. Many bots are used by leading the search engine to index and categorize new and existing content within the ever-increasing number of Web sites.

bps

An abbreviation that stands for bits per second. Bps is the number of bits that transfer per second over a line. Baud and bps are the same up to 9600. However, at rates higher than 9600, the picture changes. Even though the transfer of information occurs at 9600, the compression of data increases the number of bits transferred per second.

Broadband

This is the term used to refer to the high speed Internet connections such as T1 telephone line, cable modem, DSL, and other very fast connections that facilitate moving real-time audio and video through Internet technology.

Browser

A software program used to navigate or move among the hypertext documents on the World Wide Web. While the original browsers were text only, today's browsers are multimedia graphical interfaces that are easy to use. Examples of browsers are Netscape and Internet Explorer.

BTW

This abbreviation for "by the way" is frequently found on the Internet and in e-mails. An example: "BTW, did you know they've discovered that one of the biggest problems of people with congestive heart failure is a protein produced by their own damaged heart?"

CGI (Common Gateway Interface)

A Web programming language that is an interface-creation scripting program that allows Web pages to develop in a customized fashion, based on information entered by users in check boxes or text input fields.

Chat

Real-time text-, audio-, or video-based conversation over the Internet between two or more people who type in questions and responses. Services such as America Online and TalkCity provide chat rooms for individuals interested in specific subjects with text-based chat. Keep in mind that chatting means writing, not talking. As a person types in a sentence, it appears almost simultaneously on the screens of others who occupy the chat room area of a Web site.

Chronic Health Seeker

A term coined by the author to refer to e-patients with chronic disease states who actively use the Internet to manage their conditions.

Circuit Technology

The communication methods used to avoid a telephone call by opening a dedicated voice (analog) circuit between two people making a call.

Clicks and Mortar
Refers to the integration of traditional business or customer service transaction processes of an existing bricks and mortar business that become partially Web enabled to better service customer interests.

Client
Simply put, a software application that runs on a personal computer or workstation that relies on a server to perform some operation. For example, a piece of software that allows a person to send e-mail is called an e-mail client.

Client/Server Architecture
A particular type of network in which each computer or application on the network is either a client or a server.

Compressed File (or "Zipped" File)
A file that is reduced in size so it takes up less disk space or bandwidth and transfers faster. Opening a compressed file is a process that often involves an extra step for the user. Before people use a compressed file, they must decompress it with a decompression utility (software that decompresses the file).

Cyberphysician
A physician who offers medical information on the Internet. For example, America's Doctor Online connects consumers with health and medical questions to its cyberphysicians in real time. With increases in bandwidth and data compression technology, actual medical triage, assessments, and diagnosis are being done on line.

Cyberspace
The entire Internet of all connected computers and user exchanging data. Coined by William Gibson in the novel *Neuromancer*, this term describes the territory or turf for on-line discussions, electronic mail, and information transfers as well as the culture of the Internet and electronic communications. Whenever people log on to a commercial on-line service or connect to the Internet, they are entering cyberspace.

Cybervisit
A visit between patient and provider that occurs over the Internet using two-way conferencing using advanced telemedicine or Internet technology. As bandwidth is increased to where high-speed access is readily available across the United States, cybervisits are likely to replace an increasing percentage of face-to-face visits in the areas of home care, disease management, and office visits.

Dedicated Connection

When people arrange for a dedicated connection between one computer and a host computer, they get a connection dedicated to that task. It has no other purpose. The advantage: direct connections are faster than dial-up terminal or dial-up direct connections and are therefore ideal for using high bandwidth video and audio applications. Cable modems are an example of "always on" connections into the home.

Dial-up Direct

Using a host computer to connect a computer to the Internet. Dial-up direct connections function in a way similar to dedicated connections, and they allow a person to surf the Web and send e-mail when they are connected.

Domain Name

The unique name of an Internet site. For example, www.cyberatlas.com is a domain name in the World Wide Web.

Download

To transfer a file from one computer to a second computer. When a file moves through the telephone lines from the second computer to the first, it is being downloaded to the first computer. A person can also transfer a file from the first computer to the second computer—a process called uploading. Downloads can be done through the public Internet.

Dynamic Hypertext Markup Language (DHTML)

A more advanced form of Web programming than HTML that handles interactive features such as audio and video better.

e-Business

It is the process of doing business electronically through the exchange of products and services through the Internet and its variations (e.g., Intranet, Extranet, virtual private networks, etc.).

e-Care Delivery or e-Care

e-care involves the delivery of health and medical services using proprietary or open platform telemedicine technology, on-line self-care management, and triage, as well as other Internet technology-based applications and services.

e-Commerce

Conducting business on line or through Internet-mediated transactions. The buying and selling of products on the Internet are aspects of e-commerce in health care. E-commerce refers to the sale of health and medical products.

e-Communications

Communicating in one form or another, on line. This could be through the use of e-mail or e-newsletters or through offering a Web service to customers. E-communications in health and medical services involve various levels including (1) information sharing; (2) education; and (3) decision support.

e-Communities

On-line communities such as support groups. Individuals go to e-communities to connect with people who have the same condition or situation. For example, in health care, at the Cancer Survivors Network (www.cancersurvivorsnetwork.org), people can connect with others who have survived cancer and share emotional experiences, discuss coping with the disease, etc.

e-Healthcare

The use of multimedia Internet-based technology for improved patient care and health care organization operations across dimensions of content, connectivity, e-commerce, and e-care.

e-Patient

A consumer with an acute or chronic health condition who uses the Internet and various Web sites and e-services to manage his or her condition.

e-Service

The conduct of service-based transactions through Internet-based connectivity and technology.

Electronic Mail or e-mail

Commonly referred to as e-mail, this revolutionary communication tool allows computers and e-mail programs to pass or transfer messages from one person to one or more people through public networks like the Internet. Whenever people use their computers to send and receive messages over a network such as the Internet, they are engaging in e-mail communication.

Emoticon

A set of symbols used to convey emotion in chat and electronic mail. A well-known example is the smiley face :).

Encryption

Through this process, information is coded and rendered useless to anyone without the keyword and software to decode it. Encryption is needed to protect sensitive information such as patient medical records or credit card data as it passes through several computers before arriving at its destination.

Extranet

An Intranet that is accessible in part to authorized outsiders within a defined affinity network. Whereas an Intranet resides behind a firewall and can be accessed by only members of the same company or organization, an Extranet provides connectivity using Internet technology and various levels of accessibility if the user has a username and password with a finite group of people. Extranets are extremely effective places to conduct e-commerce, since they allow manufacturers, vendors, and customers to do business on the Internet together, but through an invitation only to customers, suppliers, and others. In health care, an example of an Extranet would be where all the physicians within an IPA use Internet technology for payment, moving claims, and other business processes.

FAQs (Frequently Asked Questions)

FAQs are lists of questions on Web sites that help users obtain answers without calling directly and asking a person over a telephone line. For example, the FAQs on a physician's site could include "Which insurance plans do you accept?" "Can I pay with my Visa or MasterCard?" and "What do I need to take to my first appointment?" By answering these questions on a Web site without the aid of a person, the number of telephone calls to a human in the office can be reduced.

File

A single archive of information that stores a text document, a graphic image, a program that launches an application, or a sound or video clip.

Firewall

A software/hardware system that blocks unauthorized access to a private network or data. Firewalls are typically used to prevent unauthorized Internet users from accessing private networks or data connected to the Internet, such as Intranets, Extranets, or to protect entry from the public Internet to a private database or network.

Flame

An unrestrained series of insults, usually issued in the form of an e-mail message or a posting to a newsgroup or mailing list. Flaming is often brought about by people who use newsgroups or mailing lists to advertise products and services, engage in off-topic discussions, or take advantage of group members.

Forum

An electronic gathering place, similar to the newsgroups of Usenet or Web-based forums. Some forums exist to support professions, specific interests, and hobbies and offer people the opportunity to leave messages, make contributions, download files, and chat.

Freenet

Community-based networks that provide services such as Internet access to local users. People who cannot afford a regular Internet account or an account with a commercial on-line service such as America Online often take advantage of these freenets or community nets.

Freeware

Software that is distributed at no charge by the software owner, who then retains the copyright, but allows unlimited use without payment of fees.

FTP (File Transfer Protocol)

File transfer protocol allows a person to transfer files from one computer to another. Using a specific software program, a person logs in to a computer and requests that a file be transmitted. With FTP, a person can both upload and download a program from that host computer.

Health.net

The reference to the community of Internet health and medical companies owned by Hambrect and Quist focused on delivering products and services through content, commerce, community, and connectivity.

Health Net Retriever

A term coined by Cyberdialogue to refer to a consumer who looks for health information on line at least once a year.

Hit

Each time a Web server sends a file or data element to a Web browser that requests it, it is recorded in the server log file as a "hit." Hits are generated for every element of a requested page (including graphics, text, and interactive items). If a page containing two graphics is viewed by a user, three hits will be recorded—one for the page itself and one for each graphic. Webmasters use hits to measure their server's workload. Because page designs vary greatly, the number of hits is a poor guide for traffic measurement.

Home Page

The main page of a Web site or service. It typically includes a welcoming message and a brief description of the site's function and scope and is a launching pad to other pages within the service. Some people use "home page" and "Web site" as if they were synonyms, which is incorrect.

Host

A computer that is connected directly into a network such as the Internet. Whenever people dial into the Internet, they make a connection through their host computer.

HTML (Hypertext Markup Language)

A page layout programming language that can be interpreted by a Web browser. Before organizations put up pages of information on the Web, they convert them into HTML.

Hypertext

Text that appears as colored, underlined words on Web sites. Hypertext links to other related text on other Web sites or pages. For example, a Web site might mention leukemia in one place but explain it in greater detail in another place. A hypertext document would feature a link from the first mention of leukemia to the related explanatory text. When users click on the highlighted or underlined word, they are transported to a complete description of the disease or a list of resources or another Web site that has been linked to that text.

Internet

A vast public, international network of linked, decentralized computers linked by fiber optics and other networks that allows users to communicate with each other no matter what their location. The Internet is used to transmit electronic mail, find information, and engage in person-to-person or business-to-business exchanges of text, graphic, audio, video, and other data.

Internet Explorer

The popular Web browser developed and distributed by Microsoft.

Internet Protocol

Often abbreviated as IP, this is a series of rules concerning how information flows across computer networks within the Internet universe.

Internet Technology

A software application such as a Web browser that uses the Internet or other applications that take advantage of the global computer network.

Intranet

A network that is based on TCP/IP protocols and typically used by one corporation or company. An Intranet is accessible by only the organization's members, its employees, or others with a username and password. An Intranet's Web sites look just like any other Web sites, but the firewall surrounding the Intranet ensures that no one gets in without proper access.

iPhone

An Internet-enabled telephone with a graphical screen that can surf the Web and exchange data.

ISDN (Integrated Services Digital Network)

An ISDN is a digital, telephone-based connection methodology that allows for high-speed transfer of digital information at a speed of 128,000 bits per second or higher.

ISP (Internet Service Provider)

A company that sells access to the Internet for a monthly or annual fee to consumers or businesses. Most people use an ISP as their "ramp" to connect to the Internet.

Java

A popular high-level programming Web language developed by Sun Microsystems that allows for decentralized computing across Internet.

Link

An electronic connection between two Web sites. Users click on underlined text or a graphical image and are transported to the link.

Listserv

An Internet-based mailing list server that is automatic that distributes one e-mail to many subscribers across the Internet. When e-mail is addressed to a listserv mailing list, the e-mail is automatically broadcast to everyone on the list.

Login

The procedure for making a connection with a host computer. In most cases, it involves filling in a name and a password. In some cases, however, people may log in by typing in their real name, username or screen name, and password.

Modem

A device that enables a computer to send and receive data through telephone lines. There are two types of modems: internal modems, which are built into the computer, and external modems, which are connected to the computer with a cable.

Netiquette

Rules of etiquette that govern on-line communication through e-mail, mailing lists, and newsgroups. Some netiquette: Never write messages in all capital letters, always express appreciation to anyone who offers assistance, and never fail to answer messages within 24 to 48 hours.

Netscape Navigator

A popular Web browser, Netscape allows people to navigate, point, and click their way through the Web to enjoy its dazzling graphics, sounds, and video files. It is developed and distributed by Netscape Corporation, which is wholly owned by America Online, Inc.

Network

A group of two or more connected computer systems. There are several different kinds of networks. In a local area network, the computers are close together—within the same building, for instance. In a wide area network, the computers are farther apart and typically are linked via telephone line or some other telecommunications connection such as a T1 line.

Newsgroup

A topic-specific area where people have the opportunity to discuss common interests by posting messages for others to read. There are approximately tens of thousands of newsgroups worldwide organized by Internet area operating on the Internet.

On Line

Connected with another computer using telephone lines and a modem or other communications method (wireless, cable modem, etc.) and communications software. When people connect to the Internet, they are on line changing data.

Page

All Web sites are a collection of electronic "pages." Each Web page is a document formatted in HTML that contains text, images, or media objects such as Java applets. The "home page" is typically a visitor's first point of entry and features a site index. Pages can be static or dynamically generated. All frames and frame parent documents are counted as pages.

Page Views

Number of times a page within a Web site is requested by multiple users within a designated time period.

Phone Space

The communication space where two people are verbally interacting using the telephone and a direct analog circuit connection.

Portal (Web)

A high-volume Web site that serves as a gateway or starting point for many consumers or businesses.

Push

Sending data to a client (or user) without that client or user requesting it directly via e-mail, Web browsers, and other Internet technology. A popular use of push technology is the automatic delivery of customized news feeds based on stated customer preference.

Real-Time

The space that is created when time, distance, action, and response collapse simultaneously aided by technology to fulfill a customer need or transaction.

Server

A computer or device that operates on a network and manages network resources. For example, a file server is a computer and storage device that stores files. These files are then accessible to everyone on the network. Web server refers to a server focus on delivery of Web sites and Web services to consumer or business users requesting data from the site hosted by the server.

Shareware

Free software that is available for download from the Web. Most shareware is delivered free of charge, but the author usually requests a small fee if the person likes the program and uses it regularly. People can copy shareware for friends and colleagues using the honor system, but these friends and colleagues are also expected to pay a fee if they use the product.

Signature

Data (text, audio, or video) that is at the end of an e-mail message and is customized by the sender. Most signatures identify the author by name, title, organizational affiliation, credentials, address, telephone number, fax number, Web site, and even areas of expertise or interests.

SSL (Secure Sockets Layer)

A protocol developed by Netscape that allows private documents to be transmitted over the Internet safely and securely. SSL uses a private key to encrypt data while they are being transmitted.

Sticky Application

A term that describes a Web application or service that brings a user back time and again to a particular Web site. Sticky sites are those where visitors typically stay for an extended period of time. For instance, a banking site that offers a financial calculator is stickier than one that does not because visitors do not have to leave to find a resource they need.

T-1

A high-speed (1.54 megabits/second) network connection offered to businesses and consumers by telecommunications companies.

TCP/IP (Transmission Control Protocol/Internet Protocol)

A system for transferring data over the Internet. In most cases, a person must run a TCP/IP program to use a dedicated or dial-up connection.

Thin-Client Server

A client that is designed to be very small so that most of the processing it was built to perform happens on the server instead of the desktop. In many cases the server could be delivering applications over the public Internet.

Unique Users

The number of different individuals who visit a site within a specific time period. To identify unique users, Web sites rely on some form of user registration or identification system using advanced Web management software.

Upload

To transfer a file from one computer to a second computer. When a file moves through the telephone lines from one computer to the second, that file is being uploaded from the first computer. When a file moves from the second computer to the first computer, that file is being downloaded to the first computer.

URL (Uniform Resource Locator)

The global address of a document on the World Wide Web. Every Web site or page has an address that usually reads something like http://www.recon.com.

Usenet

Another use of the public Internet that is the home of more than 10,000 Internet newsgroups. People come to meet friends, discuss events, research trends, and find information on topics ranging from acquired immune deficiency syndrome (AIDS) and pharmacy to health care management and diabetes.

User

A person using a computer.

Virus

A damaging program that can "infect" a computer via e-mail, shared floppy disks, telephone lines, or the Internet. These programs reproduce and spread, just like a virus, and perform a variety of nasty functions. Some corrupt files, others delete them, and others send multiple e-mails to the people listed in a person's e-mail address book.

Visits

A sequence of requests made by one user at one Web site. If a visitor does not request any new information for a period of time, known as the "time-out" period, the next request by the visitor is counted as a new visit.

Webcasting

A broadcast of information or data using the Internet or World Wide Web and push technologies. For example, some hospitals and Web portals have begun webcasting live surgeries via the Web. Users visit the hospital's site, and the live surgery is broadcast to them live.

Web Service

An advanced use of Internet technology to deliver actual services as opposed to information content.

Wireless

The communications protocols and methods for transferring data through the air without use of dedicated phone lines or other fixed cable medium.

World Wide Web (or www or Web)

A system of Internet servers that supports documents that are formatted in HTML language. The WWW allows users to jump from one document to the next by clicking on "hot spots"—underlined text that is linked to pages in other Web sites.

Index

About the Editors

ABOUT THE AUTHOR AND EDITOR

Douglas E. Goldstein is a widely recognized expert in e-healthcare, e-commerce, and e-care. He leads organizations in achieving better customer e-service, lower costs, and improved performance through appropriate use of Internet and multimedia technology. As a "practical futurist," entrepreneurial executive, and management executive, Mr. Goldstein has helped the nation's leading health care organizations develop alliances and e-services necessary to survive and prosper in the Internet Age.

Prior to *e-Healthcare: Harness the Power of Internet e-Commerce and e-Care,* he was the lead author of five *Best of the Net Online Guide* Internet books, on consumer health, health care management, finance, and business on the Internet. Mr. Goldstein has written three widely respected health care management books: *Building and Managing Effective Physician Organizations* (Aspen Publishers, 1996), *Alliances: Strategies for Building Integrated Delivery Systems* (Aspen Publishers, 1995), and *Medical Staff Alliances: Building Successful Partnerships with Physicians.* He also writes "Medical Internet," a monthly column for *Managed Care Interface* magazine.

Mr. Goldstein has served as Founder and Chairman of Health Online, Inc., and as CEO/President where he was responsible for the company's strategy, operations, marketing, product development, and business expansion. He guided the development of HealthOnline.com, a syndicated on-line health and medical channel and community being used by health systems across the country. In 1999, the first on-line health and medical channel, *Medformation.com*, was launched with Allina Health System as a result of Mr. Goldstein's e-vision and e-business expertise.

He has also served as the President of Medical Alliances, Inc., a leading e-commerce business development firm, and Vice President, Market Development for Consumer Health Services (1-800-DOCTORS), which helped more than three million consumers per year select physicians.

He is the creator of "Health Adventure Online" (www.bayfront.org), a 1998 Smithsonian–ComputerWorld nominee; Teen Health Education Online (THEO), which was developed for the Pinellas County Schools and Bayfront Medical Center; MedSource.com, a leading interactive Web site dedicated to communicating knowledge to health care leaders; and "Greatest Hits" (www.greatesthits.com), the Web site for his first five Internet books. Mr. Goldstein has guided numerous other Web and e-service strategies and programs during engagements with leading health care organizations in many areas of e-healthcare, including virtual provider connectivity, patient education, and disease management.

Mr. Goldstein is a frequent keynote presenter on the future of e-health care and its impact on the trillion-dollar health care market place for organizations such as American Association of Health Plans, Medical Group Management Association, Pfizer U.S. Pharmaceuticals, and many others. He has delivered e-nergizing, e-ducational, e-mpowering, and e-ntertaining seminars and workshops for thousands of health care executives, physicians, and consumers. He has had numerous articles published in leading magazines and has been widely quoted by leading print, Web, radio, and television organizations. He graduated with honors from the University of Michigan with a Bachelor of Science degree, with dual majors in multimedia communications and business.

ABOUT THE QUALITY EDITOR

Cheryl L. Toth is a dynamic executive, speaker, and new media business development expert. Her consulting firm helps physicians and health care organizations use Web services and e-communication to strengthen physician–patient relationships and improve practice efficiencies. Ms. Toth's comprehensive knowledge of practice operations, managed care, technology, and e-services makes her a sought-after speaker and adviser.

Prior to organizing her own firm, Ms. Toth was a senior management consultant with KarenZupko & Associates, Inc., a national practice management consulting firm that works with hundreds of physician groups and provider organizations. During her tenure, Ms. Toth performed nearly 100 consultations and change management projects with physicians, MSOs, and integrated delivery systems. Improved efficiencies from these projects saved practices millions of dollars in recovered receivables and decreased operating costs.

Ms. Toth authors journal articles, newsletters, book chapters, and on-line content about physician practice management and e-business techniques. She has contributed to *Managed Care Interface*'s monthly column, "Medical Internet." Ms. Toth evaluates physician Web sites and provides practical improvements for transforming them into dynamic Web services that improve patient communications and reduce practice overhead. She develops interactive practice management and consumer tips, and has created three human resource management products on diskette. Recent e-projects include Web service and content development for several health care companies, including Bio-Portraits.com and Health Online, Inc.

Ms. Toth has presented management and marketing workshops to thousands of physicians and health care managers nationwide. Her lively e-health care revolution presentations have been given to physician societies such as the Texas Allergy Association and the American College of Gastroenterology. Ms. Toth is an adjunct faculty member of Scottsdale Community College and the University of Phoenix, where she teaches business communication and management courses. Ms. Toth holds a Bachelor of Science degree from Western Michigan University (1988) and an MBA from Loyola University Chicago (1992).